ASSAY OF DRUGS
AND OTHER TRACE COMPOUNDS
IN BIOLOGICAL FLUIDS

METHODOLOGICAL DEVELOPMENTS IN BIOCHEMISTRY   *Vol.5*

Series Editor: Eric Reid

Wolfson Bioanalytical Centre   *University of Surrey*

Other titles in the Series

SEPARATIONS WITH ZONAL ROTORS   *(1971; ranks as Vol. 1)*
   published by (and available from) the Centre at Guildford

METHODOLOGICAL DEVELOPMENTS IN BIOCHEMISTRY
   published by Longman Group Limited

Vol. 2 (1973): SEPARATION TECHNIQUES
Vol. 3 (1973): ADVANCES WITH ZONAL ROTORS
Vol. 4 (1974): SUBCELLULAR STUDIES

METHODOLOGICAL DEVELOPMENTS
IN BIOCHEMISTRY   VOL. 5

ASSAY OF DRUGS
AND
OTHER TRACE COMPOUNDS
IN
BIOLOGICAL FLUIDS

Edited by Eric Reid

Wolfson Bioanalytical Centre
University of Surrey

1976

NORTH-HOLLAND PUBLISHING COMPANY
AMSTERDAM · NEW YORK · OXFORD

ISBN North-Holland: 0 7204 0584 X

Publishers:
North-Holland Publishing Company – Amsterdam
North-Holland Publishing Company, Ltd. – Oxford

Sole distributors for the U.S.A. and Canada:
Elsevier/North-Holland, Inc.
52 Vanderbilt Avenue
New York, N.Y. 10017

Library of Congress Cataloging in Publication Data

Main entry under title:

Assay of drugs and other trace compounds in bio-
    logical fluids.

    (Methodological developments in biochemistry ;
v. 5)
    Bibliography: p.
    Includes index.
    1. Body fluids--Analysis. 2. Drugs--Analysis.
I. Reid, Eric, 1922-   II. Series.
QP519.7.M47 vol. 5 [RB40] 574.1'92'028s
ISBN 0-7204-0584-X [612'.01522'028]   76-22776

PRINTED IN THE NETHERLANDS

EDITOR'S PREFACE

Scattered amongst the 'analytical fraternity' there are experts familiar with the challenging problem of analyzing blood or urine samples for a drug or other small molecule present in trace amount. Seldom can the raw sample be put direct into the measuring instrument. Commonly it has to be freed from interfering material, or at least concentrated, by one or more sample-preparation steps, the choice and validation of which call for judgement and experience such as are manifest in pioneer papers published from B.B. Brodie's laboratory in the 1940's. All too often, however, authors produce methods 'out of a hat', or at least with no discussion of strategy as distinct from tactics. This remark is less applicable to toxicological papers concerned, for example, with drugs of abuse: but this literature is of limited help since the emphasis is largely on rapid identification rather than accurate quantitation, and the mode of extraction may have to sacrifice efficiency to versatility.

Altogether the design of an assay method for an organic trace substance of *known* identity depends largely on 'laboratory lore' and is ill served by literature or learned meetings. The 'Techniques Forum' held in September 1975 by this Centre (as a laboratory involved in assay work for industry) proved to be a most effective and stimulating exchange of experiences amongst practitioners, whose contributions have led to the present book.

For the sake of the novice, some editorial effort has been made to integrate the contents, and to provide reinforcing material. This falls largely in a specially written 'strategy' article (Art. G-1) which represents merely a personal viewpoint. (An idiosyncratic plea is now interpolated, for civilized recorder traces which read from left to right !) As is evident from the Contents list, the articles have been classified on a somewhat arbitrary basis into four Sections, viz.-
'E': The end-step: Advances in instrumental techniques.
'G': General analytical strategy.
'S': Sample preparation (approaches to working up the sample for the end-step).
'T': Tactical illustrations: 'Analytical Case Histories'.

The book will have served its purpose if, besides being of instructional value, it comes to be used in pharmaceutical and clinical laboratories as a desk book, of the nature of a guide rather than a handbook. The need for reliable micro-determinations on body-fluid samples is ever increasing, in connection with bioavailability and other approaches to establishing drug efficacy and safety, including therapeutic monitoring. Besides, notwithstanding the above remark about toxicological literature, a comment by a Forum participant (W.D.C. Wilson) is apt: "More and more the forensic toxicologist is involved in determining the drug levels in *therapeutic* amounts and interpreting these in the light of court evidence for the benefit of the court. Less and less is he concerned with *intoxication* and treatment". Much of the material in the book can be extrapolated beyond blood and urine, e.g. to culture fluids in the fermentation field and to water and effluents in the pollution-monitoring field.

Acknowledgements. - Thanks are due to all contributors, for sparing time to help others gain from their expertise, and to Mrs. R. Sarker for meticulous typing. For permission to use published material, acknowledgements are made in the text; especial thanks are due to the American Chemical Society, the Ciba Foundation, Massachusetts Medical Society, New York Academy of Sciences, and Wiley-Interscience, besides Journal Editors (e.g. *Acta Pharm. Suecica, Xenobiotica*).

Wolfson Bioanalytical Centre,
University of Surrey, Guildford GU2 5XH

Eric Reid

5 April 1976

CONTENTS

NOTE: Topics in individual contributions are not systematically cross-referenced. — The appropriate NOTES & COMMENTS and the Index should be consulted for other relevant material.

LIST OF AUTHORS

*Full addresses are given in the headings to the cited Articles (look up
CONTENTS to find page no.).   For the 'NC' Articles, listing of authors
below is confined to certain 'NOTES'.*

A.A.A. Aziz - Art. T-2
*Wolfson Bioanal. Centre, Univ. of
Surrey, Guildford, U.K.*

J.D. Baty - Art. T-NC
Univ. of Liverpool, U.K.

A.D. Blair - Arts. T-11 & T-15
*Harborview Medical Center,
Seattle, U.S.A.*

J.W. Bridges - Art. E-3
*Biochem. Dept., Univ. of Surrey,
Guildford, U.K.*

U.A. Th. Brinkman - Art. T-NC
*Academic Hosp. of the Free Univ.,
Amsterdam, The Netherlands*

S.S. Brown - Art. T-3
Clinical Research Centre, Harrow, U.K.

V.P. Butler - Art. G-2
Columbia Univ., New York, U.S.A.

R.A. Chalmers - Arts. S-3 & S-6
*M.R.C. Clinical Research Centre,
Harrow, U.K.*

J. Chamberlain - Art. S-4
*Hoechst Pharmaceutical Res. Labs.,
Milton Keynes, U.K.*

T.G. Christopher - Art. T-10
*Harborview Medical Center,
Seattle, U.S.A.*

J.M. Clifford - Art. T-6
*G.D. Searle & Co., High Wycombe,
U.K.*

D.A. Cowan - Art. T-5
Chelsea College, London, U.K.

T. Cowen - Art. T-7
*Squibb International Development
Lab., Moreton, Merseyside, U.K.*

S.H. Curry - Arts. S-2 & T-4
The London Hosp. Medical College, U.K.

R.E. Cutler - Arts. T-11 & T-12
*Harborview Medical Center,
Seattle, U.S.A.*

A. de Kok - Art. T-NC
*Academic Hosp. of the Free Univ.,
Amsterdam, The Netherlands*

D. Dell - Art. S-5
*Hoechst Pharmaceutical Res. Ltd.,
Milton Keynes, U.K.*

E.C. Dinovo - Art. T-NC
Univ. of California, Irvine, U.S.A.

N. Evans - Art. E-6
Univ. College, Cardiff, U.K.

D.B. Faber - Arts. E-4 & T-NC
*Academic Hosp. of the Free Univ.,
Amsterdam, The Netherlands*

J.B. Fairbrother - Arts. S-NC & T-8
*Squibb International Development Lab.,
Moreton, Merseyside, U.K.*

A.W. Forrey - Arts. T-11 & T-12
*Harborview Medical Center, Seattle,
U.S.A.*

T.C. Forster - Art. T-10
*Squibb International Development Lab.,
Moreton, Merseyside, U.K.*

L.A. Gottschalk - Art. T-NC
Univ. of California, Irvine, U.S.A.

A.D.R. Harrison - Art. E-NC$_1$
*Wolfson Bioanal. Centre, Univ. of
Surrey, Guildford, U.K.*

D.R. Hoar - Art. T-9
*Unilever Research Colworth/Welwyn
Lab., Sharnbrook, Bedford, U.K.*

A.H. Jackson - Art. E-6
Univ. College, Cardiff, U.K.

V.H.T. James - Art. T-1
*St. Mary's Hosp. Medical School,
London, U.K.*

C.R. Jones - Art. S-1
*Wellcome Research Labs., Beckenham,
Kent, U.K.*

L.J. King - Art. T-NC
*Biochem. Dept., Univ. of Surrey,
Guildford, U.K.*

J.P. Leppard - Art. T-2
*Wolfson Bioanal. Centre, Univ. of
Surrey, Guildford, U.K.*

S.A. Matlin - Art. E-6
Univ. College, Cardiff, U.K.

Barbara Maxwell - Art. T-11
*Harborview Medical Center, Seattle,
U.S.A.*

B.J. Millard - Art. E-1
*The School of Pharmacy, Univ. of
London, U.K.*

Michelle A. O'Neill - Art. T-12
Harborview Medical Center,
Seattle, U.S.A.

E. Reid - Arts. G-1 & T-2
Wolfson Bioanal. Centre,
Univ. of Surrey, Guildford, U.K.

P. Robinson - Art. T-NC
Univ. of Liverpool, U.K.

J.R. Salmon - Art. T-7
Squibb International Development
Lab., Moreton, Merseyside, U.K.

G. Schill - Art. G-3
Univ. of Uppsala, Sweden

D.J. Sissons - Art. T-9
Unilever Research Colworth/Welwyn
Lab., Sharnbrook, Bedford, U.K.

M.R. Smyth - Art. E-2
Chelsea College, London, U.K.

W. Franklin Smyth - Art. E-2
Chelsea College, London, U.K.

R. Whelpton - Art. S-2
The London Hosp. Medical College, U.K.

G.A. Wilson - Art. T-1
St. Mary's Hosp. Medical School,
London, U.K.

D.B. Campbell - Art. G-NC
Servier Labs., Greenford, U.K.

ABBREVIATIONS AND NOMENCLATURE

Apart from abbreviations used only in particular articles (and defined therein), there are some general abbreviations which are now set down together with some comments on nomenclature.

For different physical modes of chromatography the following terms have the merit of some consistency:-

ABBREVI-ATION	FULL TERM	DISFAVOURED ABBREVIATIONS/TERMS, and COMMENTS
(PC)	Paper chromatography	General policy has been to use the full term.
TLC	Thin-layer chromatography	For 'PMD' see Art.
GC	Gas chromatography	*NOT* GLC (why specify the stationary phase?) or VPC. *For derivatizing agents, e.g. 'BSA', see p.11.*
HPLC	High-pressure liquid chromatography *or (novel suggestion!)* Highly particulate liquid chromatography *— inelegant, but not open to criticisms as on right*	HPLC is widely used; but 'High presssure' is sometimes a misnomer, and 'High performance' pre-judges the results! — as does 'High efficiency' (HELC) or 'High resolution' (HRLC), such terms and also 'High speed' (HSLC) being popular in sales literature. The bald term 'Liquid chromatography' (LC) inexcusably disregards classical column chromatography. *[A criticism of 'LC'* [1] *needs to be read in conjunction with the correction of a typographic mis-setting at the printing stage; criticism of 'HSLC' etc.* [1] *escaped this garbling.]* Editors are at sixes and sevens, and confusion reigns.

Ref. 1: Leppard, J.P. & Reid, E., *Annu. Repts. Chem. Soc. 71B* (1974) 44-56.

For chromatographic media such as Sephadex or porous glass beads, the Editor favours the term 'steric exclusion': *not* 'gel filtration' (a filter does *not* retain small molecules!) or 'gel permeation' or 'molecular sieving'. For chosen types of HPLC media the Editor deplores the bald use, even in reputable journals, of trade names unaccompanied by any indication of type.

The following abbreviations are convenient and widely accepted:
MS = mass spectrometry, and (in GC) FI(D) = flame ionization (detector)
EC(D) = electron capture (detector).

In the spectrophotometric context the following terms are used:
E = extinction (absorbance, optical density), UV = ultra-violet.

For temperatures, ° signifies °C.   RIA = radioimmunoassay.

In the context of preparing a chemical derivative for GC, the usefulness of the term 'derivatize' is felt to outweigh its inelegance. Where deuterium is introduced into a molecule, U.K. usage seems to lean towards 'deuteriated', and American usage towards 'deuterated' *(comment by B.J. Millard)*. The Editor deplores 'lyophilize' (= freeze-dry) but, in good company, encourages the term 'spike' for supplementing an assay tube with a standard or other trace additive. Where an 'internal standard' is thus added, readers should beware of assuming that this is the authentic test substance; usually the term signifies a different compound (p. 61). 'Accuracy' does not mean reproducibility (precision) but nearness to the true value.

E-1

MASS-SPECTROMETRIC QUANTITATION IN GAS CHROMATOGRAPHY, AND OTHER GAS CHROMATOGRAPHY ADVANCES

Brian J. Millard[*]

The School of Pharmacy, University of London,
Brunswick Square, London, WC1N 1AX, U.K.

The advantages and disadvantages of open tubular columns over packed columns are discussed. The superior separation achieved by open tubular columns is offset by the low loading which can be tolerated relative to packed columns. Support-coated open tubular (SCOT) columns, while sometimes less effective at higher temperatures than the open tubular type, may give a better performance for the same length due to a thinner and more evenly distributed stationary phase. The principal advantage of SCOT columns is in the larger permissible sample load.

Specific detectors other than mass spectrometers are discussed with particular reference to sensitivity. These include electron capture (EC), flame photometric, coulometric and thermionic detectors.

The mass spectrum of a compound is unique to that compound; hence the mass spectrometer can be considered to be the ultimate in specific detectors. For quantitative work, the scan mode is inappropriate: the mass spectrometer monitors a few ions, from 1 to 4, which are chosen so as to be diagnostic for the compound being determined. When single ion monitoring is employed, the instrument is about 1000 times more sensitive than when it is in the scanning mode.

Internal standards in GC-MS quantification are of two types, either the compound itself labelled with a stable isotope, this version eluting about the same time but giving ions higher in mass than the unlabelled compound by virtue of these isotopes, or a homologue of the compound which gives some of the same ions but at a different retention time. The first method has the virtue that if the labelled compound is used in large excess, a carrier effect operates both for extractions and for passage through the GC column, thus minimizing losses. The second method uses the mass spectrometer in its most sensitive mode of single ion monitoring. It is shown that the two methods can be combined to give the advantages of both.

Due to its unique sensitivity and selectivity, mass spectrometry is one of the most powerful tools available for the structural determination of organic compounds. A major requirement of the technique is that compounds should be relatively pure, so that it is necessary to employ separation techniques when studies of complex mixtures such as biological fluids are undertaken. The advent of combined GC-MS about ten years ago was a highly significant event for two reasons, firstly because complex mixtures could be injected directly into the system, avoiding manipulative losses, and secondly, the combined instrument enabled the quantitative power of GC to be enhanced by several orders of magnitude. This paper discusses the essential features of GC-MS as a quantitative analytical technique and covers the more recent advances in this technique and in GC itself.

DISCUSSION

The major components of any GC system are the column and the detector. Both of these have undergone extensive development and improvement.

[*]*Present address: Dept. of Chemical Pathology, Inst. of Neurology, Queen Square, London, WC1N 3BG.*

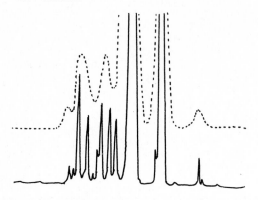

Fig. 1. Comparison of packed
column and open tubular column.
Separation of hop sesquiter-
pene hydrocarbons on a 3 m,
6.25 mm o.d. packed column
(dotted line) and a 45 m, 0.25 mm
i.d. capillary column *(solid
line)*. *From ref. 1, courtesy
of the author and the publisher.*

Table 1. Operating characteristics of different columns in GC-MS.

Column size, mm	Helium flow, cm³/min	% Helium to MS	Minimum amount of sample needed, g	Maximum sample load, g
0.25	1	100	10^{-9}	5×10^{-6}
0.5	5	20	5×10^{-9}	5×10^{-5}
0.5 SCOT	5	20	5×10^{-9}	2×10^{-4}
0.75	10	10	10^{-8}	2×10^{-4}
3.2 packed	30	3	3×10^{-7}	10^{-2}

Columns

Two types of column are in use at the present time, packed columns and open tubular
columns. The latter are further subdivided into two types, wall-coated (WCOT) —
generally called capillary columns — in which the stationary phase is coated on
the wall of the column after prior cleaning, and support-coated (SCOT) columns in
which the coating also contains a porous layer of very fine support material. This
allows a greater amount of stationary phase per unit length. Whilst packed columns
usually have an internal diameter of ¼ or ⅛ in., capillary columns are of 0.25,
0.5 or 0.75 mm internal diameter and give much better separation than packed
columns, as can be seen in Fig. 1. This compares the separation of some sesquiter-
pene hydrocarbons on a 3 m ¼ in. packed column with a 45 m 0.25 mm capillary
column [1].

     SCOT columns are somewhat less effective than capillary columns, especially
at higher temperatures, and the principal advantage is in the higher loading that
can be tolerated. This means that frequently a large gain in sensitivity can be
made without too large a sacrifice of separation efficiency.

     The operating characteristics of these various columns when used in a com-
bined GC-MS system are shown in Table 1 [2]. In general it can be seen that if
chromatographic efficiency is of secondary importance and the sample contains a
large amount of solvent, an ⅛ in. packed column is the answer. If the total sample
sample is only a few micrograms, a 0.25 mm capillary column will be an advantage.
Many laboratories find a 0.5 mm SCOT column to be the best general-purpose column.

     Considerable improvements have been made in stationary phases in the last
few years, and this is of importance for workers analyzing drugs or metabolites,

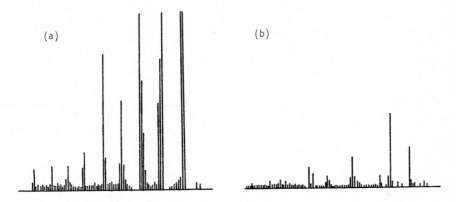

Fig. 2. Bleed from a Tergitol NP-35 column (a) before and (b) after fitting a short bleed-absorbing Carbowax 20M-TPA column. *From ref. [3], courtesy of the authors and the American Chemical Society.*

since temperatures of 250-300° are frequently employed. At these temperatures, column bleed becomes important. In ordinary GC work a dual column system can be used so that the bleed signal from the control column tends to cancel out that from the analytical column. However in GC-MS this cannot be done, and high stability columns become essential. The temperature limits of some commonly used columns are given in Table 2.

When column bleed is high and a GC-MS analysis is to be undertaken, one solution is to add an extra short length of a bleed-absorbing column, which contains a different stationary phase. Fig. 2 shows how a high bleed, as evidenced by a blank mass spectrum, can be reduced by the use of such a bleed-absorbing column [3].

GC detectors, including MS

The more general availability of GC-MS systems which represent almost the last word in specificity has tended to take the steam out of dramatic advances in specific detectors for GC. The main types of specific detector need not be described here, but they are listed with references in Table 3. Some comments on them may be made. Thus,

Table 2. Temperature limits of common stationary phases.

Stationary phase	Maximum temp., °C	Polarity
Apiezon L	300	non-polar
Carbowax 20	250	polar
Dexsil 300	500	intermediate
SE 30	320	non-polar
OV-1	320	non-polar
Versamide 900	250	polar

Table 3. Main types of GC detector

Detector	Selectivity	Sensitivity, g/sec
Thermal conductivity	Responds to all compounds	6×10^{-10}
Flame ionization (FI)	Responds to all organic compounds	9×10^{-13}
Electron capture (EC)	Halogens, nitro compounds, conjugated carbonyls	2×10^{-14}
Mass spectrometer (MS)	Virtually 100% compound-specific	1×10^{-15}

while the EC detector is the most sensitive of these, it is the least selective, and has some measure of response to a wide range of compounds. The flame photometric detector is an excellent detector of admirable sensitivity. The characteristic emissions at 526 nm for phosphorus or 394 nm for sulphur compounds are selected by a filter and fall on a photomultiplier. Thermionic detectors are varied. The detector has a hydrogen flame which burns near an alkali metal salt, such as rubidium sulphate or caesium bromide. Both of these detectors are very good for phosphorus and almost as good for nitrogen.

The mass spectrometer is the ultimate in specific detectors, since it can be tuned to respond to only the one component that is of interest in a GC effluent. However, this would mean monitoring almost all the fragment ions produced by a compound. A substantial reduction of the number of ions monitored can be achieved without too much loss of specificity. When the added selectivity of the GC apparatus is taken into account, there is probably only about one chance in 10^6 that four ions selected as being diagnostic of a particular compound have been formed by some other compound with exactly the same retention time. If only one ion is chosen, provided it is relatively high in mass, the chance of some other compound having this ion in its mass spectrum and having the same retention time is still only about 1 in 10^4. Since the mass spectrometer is in its most sensitive mode when monitoring a single ion, it is therefore perfectly feasible to operate the instrument at maximum sensitivity and still retain high selectivity.

Although the low flow rates of capillary columns allow a direct connection between the GC and the MS, this is not possible with packed columns. It is then essential to use a molecular separator to remove the carrier gas, since the MS source is operating at high vacuum. There are many separators on the market, such as the jet type [4], the porous glass type [5] and the membrane type [6]. The membrane separator, which depends on the passage of organic compounds through a silicone rubber membrane by dissolution, has the advantage of high efficiency (the proportion of compound allowed through) but the disadvantage of a low temperature limit of about 230°. The porous glass type presents a large surface area to compounds and thus causes problems of adsorption with polar compounds. Jet separators were originally made of stainless steel, which can cause catalytic decomposition of thermally sensitive compounds, but later versions are made of glass and seem to be superior to other types. Their efficiency varies according to such parameters as the relative molecular mass and polarity of the particular compound.

There are many variables in a GC-MS system, at the injection port, gas flow, efficiency of the molecular separator, electron-beam voltage, source temperature, accelerating voltage, electron-multiplier voltage, etc., so that the use of an internal standard is obligatory for quantitative work.

Internal standards

Internal standards are usually of two types. Firstly, a homologous compound producing a fragment ion of the same composition and hence m/e value as the compound being measured [7-9]. This must have a different retention time so that the particular m/e value can be monitored and the ratio of the responses given by the two compounds determined. Secondly, an analogue of the compound labelled with a stable isotope can be used which will produce a fragment or molecular ion higher in mass than that formed by the compound under measurement by virtue of the heavy isotope. These two compounds will have usually the same retention time and will produce signals at two different m/e values which have to be compared [10-12].

Most workers favour the use of the labelled analogue, since when used in an excess, say 100 to 1, it acts not only as a carrier through the GC-MS system, but also for extractions. This is of particular value when dealing with small quantities of substances, since absorption of these on the column and separator and in the MS source, together with losses in extraction, result in a low or even zero MS response. However, the use of a labelled analogue means that at least

two ions have to be monitored. The act of switching between peaks may introduce
instability so that drift occurs from the top of the peaks. This will be reflected in a high standard deviation for the peak ratios being determined. The variance in the measurement of a peak intensity is inversely proportional to the
square root of the number of ions received in that peak, which itself will depend
on the length of time for which the peak is measured. The variance of each channel
in an n-channelled multiple ion monitor will therefore be at least $\sqrt{n}$ times the
variance of a single channel ion monitor. The sensitivity of the technique will
also be proportional to the number of ions received in the peak. When all these
facts are taken into consideration, the use of a homologue rather than a labelled
analogue is indicated, since then single ion monitoring can be employed. This
will not be true when small quantities of substances are being determined for the
reasons of absorption mentioned earlier. This can be illustrated by reference to
measurements we have made on allobarbitone, as the dimethyl derivative formula (1).
This produces an intense fragment ion at m/e 195 as shown, so the compound
dimethylquinalbarbitone (2), which produces the same ion, is an ideal homologous
internal standard. An alternative is to use a deuteriated dimethylallobarbitone
(3) which produces by the same fragmentation an ion of m/e 199.

Preliminary experiments using mixtures of (1) and (2) showed that the responses at m/e 195 for both these components tailed off rapidly in a non-linear
fashion for decreasing amounts injected, so that the lower limit for detection
through the GC-MS system was approximately 0.5 ng. Since it was necessary to
measure plasma levels lower than this, the method was abandoned without any determination of the coefficients of variation. The use of (3) as both an internal
standard and carrier was then examined in a series of experiments in which varying amounts of (1) with 100 times the amount of (3) were injected into the GC-MS.
This easily enabled the range from 1 ng down to 40 pg of (1) per injection to be
covered. The CV values for these injections are given in Table 4. The value is
19.8% for the 40 pg injections. It was then decided that the great virtue of (3)
was in its function as a carrier rather than as an internal standard, and a series
of injections were carried out in which mixtures of (1), (2) and about 100 times
the amount of (3) were injected. The mass spectrometer was then set up in its
single ion monitoring mode and m/e 195 was monitored. This resulted in a dramatic
improvement of the CV values compared with the previous experiment, as shown in
Table 4, where now it can be seen that the CV for the 40 pg injection has been
almost halved to 11.5% [13].

It was decided to try the same type of experiment with prostaglandins, since we were at the time interested in the measurement of prostaglandin F2α in cerebrospinal fluid. After methylation and formation of the tris-trimethyl silyl derivative, this compound fragments to form an intense ion at *m/e* 423. A cyclohexyl analogue was available which also gave the same ion, while a tetradeuteriated analogue of prostaglandin F2α gave an ion of *m/e* 427. The first pair of compounds could be analyzed by conventional multiple ion monitoring and gave the results shown in Table 5, where down to 10 pg of F2 could be measured with a CV of 30%. The much lower level detectable here compared with the barbiturates was probably due to a lower polarity and the fact that the instrument had been used exclusively for the determination of F2 for several weeks, so that all parts were saturated. When the new method was used with a mixture of all three compounds with the deuteriated analogue functioning solely as a carrier, the lower limit was 0.1 pg with a CV of 50% (Table 5).

Table 4. Coefficients of variation for the determination of dimethyl allobarbitone (*formula* 1) by co-injection of dimethylquinalbarbitone (2) and deuteriomethylallobarbitone (3).

	Amount of (1) injected, ng			
	0.04	0.1	0.4	1.0
Multiple ion monitoring (3) as internal standard	19.8	15.3	1.9	1.3
Multiple ion monitoring (2) as internal standard	23.1	6.5	4.0	0.9
Single ion monitoring of *m/e* 195	11.5	2.0	0.8	0.6

Table 5. Comparison of multiple (MIM) and single (SIM) ion monitoring for prostaglandin F2 measurement.

	Amount of F2, pg				
	1000	100	10	1	0.1
CV of MIM, %	3.5	4.5	30	-	-
CV of SIM, %	3.0	3.5	8.5	25	50

It is a widely held view which does not appear to have been experimentally verified that labelled analogues are extractable by solvents to the same extent as the unlabelled compounds. If homologues are used, as in the above work, the criticism could be levelled that the homologues do not extract to a similar extent. This was checked by using plasma to which a certain ratio of (1), (2) and (3) had been added. The plasma was then extracted with ethyl acetate and the ratios of these compounds in the extracts determined. This indeed showed that the ratios had been changed (Table 6) because although about 25% of (1) was recovered, about 30-35% of

Table 6. Extraction of dimethylallobarbitone (1) and dimethylquinalbarbitone (2) from plasma by ethyl acetate.

ORIGINAL MIXTURE		ETHYL ACETATE EXTRACT	
Amount of (1) per ml of plasma, ng	Ratio of (1) to (2)	Amount of (1) extracted, ng	Ratio of (1) to (2)
1	3.7	0.25	1.3
2.5	1.93	0.6	1.2
5	0.89	1.25	0.53
10	0.87	2.5	0.51
20	0.86	5	0.50

(2) was recovered, thus decreasing the ratio of (1) to (2). This fact does not invalidate the method as might appear at first sight, since all that is necessary in using this method for the determination of allobarbitone in plasma is that the usual series of standard solutions made to prepare a calibration curve should adequately cover the range of levels to be expected.

The conclusion from this work is that the best GC-MS method for the quantification of small amounts of compounds in urine or plasma is to add a large excess of a stable isotope labelled compound solely to act as a carrier while a homologue is added as internal standard. This homologue should be chosen so as to produce the same ion as the compound to be measured, and there should be fairly intense ions in the respective mass spectra in order to maintain sensitivity.

References

1. McFadden, W.H., *Techniques of Combined Gas Chromatography/Mass Spectrometry.* Interscience, New York (1973) p. 85.

2. *As for* Ref. 1, **p. 86.**

3. Levy, R.L., Gosser, H.D., Herman, T.S. & Hougen, F.W., *Anal. Chem. 41* (1969) 1480-83.

4. Ryhage, R., *Anal. Chem. 36* (1964) 759-764.

5. Watson, J.T. & Biemann, K., *Anal. Chem. 36* (1964) 1135-1136.

6. Llewellyn, P.M. & Littlejohn, D.P., *Conference on Analytical and Applied Spectroscopy,* Pittsburgh (1966).

7. Agurell, S., Boreus, L.O., Gordon, E., Lindgren, J.-E., Ehrnebo, M. & Lonroth, U., *J. Pharm. Pharmacol. 26* (1974) 1-8.

8. Gilbert, J.N.T. & Powell, J.W., *Biomed. Mass Spectrom. 1* (1974) 142-144.

9. Narasimhachari, N., *Biochem. Biophys. Res. Comm. 56* (1974) 36-46.

10. Horning, M.G., Nowlin, J., Lertratanangkoon, K., Stillwell, R.N., Stillwell, W.G. & Hill, R.M., *Clin. Chem. 19* (1973) 845-852.

11. Clarke, P.A. & Foltz, R.L., *Clin. Chem. 20* (1974) 465-469.

12. Garland, W.A., Trager, W.F. & Nelson, S.D., *Biomed. Mass Spectrom. 1* (1974) 124-129.

13. Lee, M.G. & Millard, B.J., *Biomed. Mass Spectrom. 2* (1975) 78-81.

E-NC₁ NOTES AND COMMENTS RELATING TO INSTRUMENTAL TECHNIQUES

Editor's explanation.— *Discussion remarks made at the Techniques Forum on which this Volume is based, together with supplementary material, are gathered together here and, hereafter, at the ends of Sections. The resulting 'Articles' inevitably lack the coherence of the foregoing individual contributions. Yet they may, in conjunction with the Editor's contribution (Art. G-1), help knit the strands of the Volume together.*

GAS CHROMATOGRAPHY, and GC-MS

Contribution by B.J. Millard (Article 1) - *Questions and replies*

In multiple ion monitoring, are all ions produced simultaneously or does the mass spectrometer switch from one ion to another ? *(question from* J. Chamberlain*)*. — Although all of the ions in the mass spectrum are produced simultaneously in the source of the instrument, they cannot all be focussed at the same time. The spectrometer is switched between those ions (usually 2 to 4) of interest, the cycle taking a fraction of a second. The recording appears to be simultaneous because sample and hold amplifiers are used.

Question by D.A. Cowan.— Do you consider that a radical re-design of the mass spectrometer is required to reduce the variation in the assay results ? Was the variation you obtained due mainly to the poor electron multiplier ? - *Answer:* Yes, I think the poor results obtained in some cases were due to an electron multiplier that was considerably down on gain. The better results shown in Table 4 were obtained with a new electron multiplier. I think that this tends to show that, rather than a radical re-design of the mass spectrometer, all that is required is that all parts of the system should be operating up to specification.

Can the vacuum of the MS be used as the driving force of the GC ? (J. Chamberlain). — Definitely not ! The resolution of the column would be degraded if it operated under vacuum. The question also implies that the carrier gas would then be the small amount of air present at less than atmospheric pressure. The objections to air as carrier are of course well known.

Have you any experience in using ^{13}C-labelled internal standards ? Rather cheap [^{13}C]benzene, about 90% enriched, is now available (H. de Bree). — These are not usually as cheap as deuterium-labelled compounds, which are usually fairly easily synthesized from such reagents as lithium aluminium deuteride, or exchange reactions. A much greater variety of starting materials is available.

Remark by B. Scales. — In our hands, problems with the use of deuterated prostaglandins as carrier occur because of the large proportion of carrier used to get good GC. The significant percentage of unlabelled material present allows only poor limits of detection. Has Dr. Millard had this sort of experience using deuterium-labelled compounds ? — *Answer:* This is a problem where there are only a few deuterium atoms present in the standard. If standards with, say, four or more atoms are used, the proportion of unlabelled compound present in the standard should be vanishingly small if the original source of deuterium was over 99% isotopically pure. We normally use a carrier - compound ratio of about 100 : 1 rather than 1000 : 1 as do some workers.

Comment (relating to the above remark by B. Scales*) by* W. Snedden. — We find that, in prostaglandin assay, it is possible to omit the deuterated carrier provided that the GC column is pre-saturated with about a 100-fold excess of the material to be measured. Using this technique, we have been able to measure 5×10^{-14} g of PGF2 methyl ester tri-TMS ether with a standard error of about 11%. *Answer by* W. Snedden *(to a question by* L.E. Martin*)*.— We have measured sub-picogram levels of PGF2 in about 1 ml specimens of plasma. We were interested in following the PGF2 level in female plasma throughout the progress of the pregnancy.

Further comment by W. Snedden. — Concerning Dr. Millard's point (cf. Art. 1) about the danger of wash-off of substance after saturating the column, wash-off does indeed take place. We investigated this by saturating the column with deuteriated PGF2 derivative and then injecting a series of non-deuteriated PG samples and observing the change in isotope abundance. We found that wash-off decreased steadily and the column stabilized after about 20 min. Re-saturation is not required for about a further hour.

Cost aspects of GC-MS systems

Remarks by B.J. Millard.— We should keep the cost of GC-MS in perspective, the technique being hardly as expensive as is sometimes thought. Prices for complete GC-MS instruments start at about £30,000, and go up to about £120,000 with computer systems included. However, with a high throughput of analyses, the cost per analysis can work out to about £10-£20. If the technique is used only for those analyses whuch cannot be carried out readily by other techniques, due to (say) a high sensitivity or specificity requirement, one could say that almost any cost may be acceptable. A cost of £10 per analysis in these circumstances would be regarded as very reasonable.

Supporting remarks by R.A. Chalmers.— Low costs hinge on full use of the techniques and instrumentation available. In my own laboratory, the main 'workhorse' GC is fully automated with automatic injection, integration and data fractionation, and operates 6 days per week, 24 h per day during full utilization. Large numbers of samples can be processed, and per-sample costs are greatly reduced.

Nitrogen detectors for GC

Amongst those who mentioned problems with nitrogen detectors was P.F. Carey: With a Hewlett Packard nitrogen detector, problems of detector stability have been encountered which would appear to apply to other detectors which rely on maintaining the optimal ionization atmosphere by flow rate of hydrogen, air and carrier gases alone. Time taken in setting up this particular detector is also excessive. *Remark by* D.B. Faber: Nitrogen detectors are of some use, but at present are better for qualitative than for quantitative analyses, the latter being difficult unless there is a constant response factor. *Confirmatory remark by* E. Reid: Run-to-run variation is indeed a problem, in our experience.

Favourable comments by A.J. Clatworthy.— The routine use of nitrogen detectors in forensic toxicology is a screening procedure to be praised and not decried. Our laboratory (Metropolitan Police Forensic Science Laboratory) has had two Varian nitrogen detectors (rubidium sulphate) since October 1973. This has allowed the routine screening of samples of blood, both post-mortem and clinical, for a wide range of nitrogen-containing drugs such as barbiturates, methaqualone, glutethimide and the benzodiazepines, at therapeutic levels. For many compounds such as caffeine (a trimethylxanthine) a massive increase in sensitivity is found, and likewise with barbiturates after methylation with diazomethane. The main advantage is the minimal response, at high sensitivity, or background co-extractions from biological samples which create a problem when FID is used. Once set up, the instrument response is reproducible and does not need checking daily. The instrument is also relatively easy to use, so that tht GC can be used routinely by technicians and 'scientists' alike. *Added by* W.D.C. Wilson: The sensitivity of the nitrogen detector is better than that of the normal FID; but the greatest advantage in forensic toxicology is the specificity.

Further remarks by A.J. Clatworthy.— The main problem lies in theoretical ignorance: why and how does a nitrogen detector work ? Very little has been published on the subject. The formation of a 'cyanide' radical is most likely, as is shown by the increase in the absolute response of AFID over FID when barbiturates are methylated. Not all nitrogen-containing compounds will give a response to the nitrogen detector, as exemplified by nitroglycerin; but recent work has shown that whilst most nitrogen-containing compounds can be detected, the best increase in sensitivity of AFID over FID occurs on substituted nitrogen atoms.

SOME REPORTED APPROACHES TO DERIVATIZATION FOR GC-ECD

A.D.R. Harrison
Wolfson Bioanalytical Centre
Univ. of Surrey, Guildford GU2 5XH, U.K.

The GC-ECD technique hinges on having volatilizable molecules containing an electron-capturing group, usually halogen although the nitro, hydroxy and carbonyl
groups also have some electron-capturing capacity. Derivatization is usually
necessary, since only exceptionally is the compound to be estimated already a volatilizable halogenated compound (as in the case of blood halothane estimations); such
compounds are in fact valuable in checking GC-ECD performance without reliance on
efficient derivatization. An example of derivatization for the purpose of rendering volatile a molecule that already contains a halogen atom is a reported procedure for estimating frusemide TMS*-derivatized by extractive alkylation [1].

A novice seeking to acquire judgement and skill in preparing suitable derivatives will fare better by talking to an expert than by scrutinizing the literature, although some useful publications do exist [e.g. 2-4] besides a plethora of
sales literature of varying objectivity. The reward may be a single, reproducible
GC peak which is a sensitive and selective measure of the trace compound in the
original biological fluid. This ideal outcome is likely to hinge on design of a
sample preparation procedure to furnish a cleaned-up concentrate for derivatization, as well as on optimized derivatization conditions which, typically, may entail use of an acid anhydride under strictly anhydrous conditions.

Amongst published GC-ECD assay procedures which entail a derivatization step,
those which document and discuss the choice of conditions will repay study. Such
papers have been encountered in our assay studies on metadrenalines and on drugs
such as β-blockers, and are the basis of the following Notes, which do not purport
to be systematic. Innovations in derivatizing agents have largely entailed the
introduction of polyhalogenated compounds, usually polyfluorinated (in which connection a classical book [5] is recommended). The -CF_3 group is strongly electron-
withdrawing, and by replacing active hydrogens it confers stability on the molecule
and reduces its polarity, such that a GC stationary phase can advantageously be of
lowered polarity. By comparison, the -CH_3 group is electron-releasing and, in
consequence, signal-reducing. For acylation the targets are amino and hydroxyl groups.

Amongst possible fluoroacyl groups, introduced by use of the appropriate
acid anhydride, TFA as used for β-blockers [6-8] or for metadrenalines [2, 9] has retained its popularity. The reagent (b.p. 37°) should be colourless [7]. Overnight storage of the derivatives, cold and dry, seems to be permissible. For catecholamine
metabolites at least (which, in our experience, tend to give multiple TFA peaks),
PFP and HFB derivatives may surpass TFA in stability and in ECD response [10]. PFP
has been regarded as preferable to HFB [11], since excess reagent is more easily
evaporated off and since there is earlier peaking (with benefit to the EC response)
and better resolution. For GC of PFP-catecholamines, breakdown was minimized by
silylating the pipework with Dexsil or by replacing it with glass-lined metal capillary tubing [12]. An erratic GC baseline could arise from a trace of moisture in
the derivative solution, such that repeated samplings by syringe from the 'Reacti-
vials' via the septum in the cap called for re-sealing of the hole with a pin.

For basic compounds possessing hydroxyl groups, the latter may usefully be
reacted initially with TMS-imidazole (TSIM; ether formed) followed by acylation of
amino groups with HFB-imidazole [13]. For sulphonamides, PFB acylation was useful

---

*
HFB = heptafluorobutyrl	TMS = trimethylsilyl	TSIM= *N*-trimethylsilyl-
PFB = pentafluorobenzyl	BSA = *N,O*-bis(trimethyl-	imidazole *(reagent)*
PFP = pentafluoropropionyl	silyl)acetamide *(reagent,*	
TFA = trifluoroacetyl	≢ *bovine serum albumin !)*	

but the TFA and HFB derivatives had better volatility [14]. However, for amphetamine the ECD response was vastly better for PFB than for TFA [15].

Acidic groups can be alkylated by PFB bromide, more rapidly if by 'extractive alkylation', or they can be silylated by BSA along with other groups possesing an active hydrogen [4]. Oxo groups can be converted into pentafluorophenylhydrazones for GC-ECD [16]. A possible approach for prostaglandins, which may give heat-labile HFB derivatives, is formation of a PFB ester and then of a TMS ether [17]. For substituted biguanides such as phenformin, an interesting approach has been described entailing ring-closure to 2,6-disubstituted 4-monochlorodifluoromethyl-1,3,5-*s*-triazines suitable for GC-ECD; the chlorine atom served to help MS identification [18]. With PFB-TMS-catecholamines, the benzyl group helps MS assay [19].

Ideally the identity of derivatives prepared in exploratory work should be be confirmed by MS, as was done in a study of β-blockers [8] which serves to illustrate certain points. All glassware was coated with dimethyldichlorosilane. Trimethylamine was added to aid TFA derivatization (which was superior in selectivity to HFB derivatization), and the benzene reaction mixture was finally extracted with pH 6 phosphate buffer without detriment (up to 24 h) to the benzene solution of the derivative. The EC detector was run at 270° to minimize contamination. It was vital that TFA or HFB anhydride be protected from moisture, since free acid impedes derivatization. Derivatization could be done on the hydrochloride of the drug as well as the base; but some salts need a higher reaction temperature, as in the case of normetadrenaline hydrochloride derivatized with TFA anhydride (advantageously with trimethylamine present) [9]. We reiterate that anhydrides must be in 'top' condition.

It can never be taken on trust that all derivatizing groups in a molecule will survive storage. Even in the dry state, TFA or HFB derivatives of β-blockers may not survive several days. For derivatized compounds in moisture-free solution there may be decomposition within hours at the one extreme (which handicaps overnight GC runs with an automatic injector); yet for some [e.g. 19] even several weeks is allowable with a suitable solvent. Traces of water in ethereal extracts had an interesting effect on the on-column acylation (e.g. propionyl or HFB) of primary or secondary amines: unlike the *N*-acyl derivatives, any *o*-acyl derivatives failed to survive [20]. Storage with the derivatizing agent present may be worth trying [4].

The foregoing assorted observations exemplify approaches and possible problems in the skilful art of derivatization, prior to which an appropriate sample preparation procedure has to be chosen [9]. A recent terse survey of drug derivatization [4] is particularly worth consulting; it is not confined to halogen substitution as practised for GC-ECD.

1. Lindström, B. & Molander, M., *J. Chromatog. 101* (1974) 219-221.

2. Kroman, H.S. & Bender, S.R. (eds.) *Theory & Applications of Gas-Liquid Chromatography in Industry and Medicine,* Grune & Stratton, New York (1968).

3. Riedmann, M., *Xenobiotica 3* (1973) 411-434.

4. Nicholson, J., *Proc. Analyt. Div. Chem. Soc. 13* (1976) 16-18.

5. Sheppard, W.A. & Sharts, C.M., *Organic Fluorine Chemistry,* Benjamin, New York (1969).

6. Scales, B. & Cosgrove, M.B., *J. Pharmac. Exp. Ther. 175* (1970) 338-347.

7. Desager, J.P. & Harvengt, C., *J. Pharm. Pharmac. 27* (1975) 52-54 *(& pers. commun.)*.

8. Walle, T., *J. Pharm. Sci. 63* (1974) 1885-1891.

9. Wilk, S., Gitlow, S.E. & Bertani, L.M., in *The Thyroid and Biogenic Amines* (Rall, J.E. & Kopin, I.J., eds.), North-Holland, Amsterdam (1972) pp. 452-473 *(& pers. commun. from Dr. Bertani)*.

10. Änggård, E. & Sedvall, G., *Anal. Chem. 41* (1969) 1250-1256.

11. Karoum, F., Cattabeni, E.C., Ruthven, C.R.J. & Sandler, M., *Anal. Biochem. 47* (1972) 550-561.

12. Wong, K.P., Ruthven, C.R.J. & Sandler, M., *Clin. Chim. Acta* 47 (1973) 215-222.

13. Horning, M.G., Moss, A.M. & Horning, E.C., *Anal. Lett.* 1 (1968) 311-321.

14. Gyllenhaal, O. & Ehrsson, H., *J. Chromatog.* 107 (1975) 327-333.

15. Wilkinson, G.R., *Anal. Lett.* 3 (1970) 289-298.

16. Horning, M.G., Ikekauwa, N., Chambaz., E.M., Jaakonmaki, P.I. & Brooks, C.J.W.,
    J. Gas Chromatog. 5 (1967) 283-289.

17. Wickramasinghe, A.J.F. & Shaw, R.S., *Biochem. J.* 141 (1974) 179-187.

18. Matin, S.B., Karam, J.H. & Forsham, P.H., *Anal. Chem.* 47 (1975) 545-548.

19. Lhuguenot, J.-C. & Maume, B.F., *J. Chromatog. Sci.* 12 (1974) 411-418.

20. Beckett, A.H., Tucker, G.T. & Moffat, A.C., *J. Pharm. Pharmac.* 19 (1967) 273-294.

GC operational points

Remark by D. Hoar.— Carbon disulphide used as a GC solvent tends, in our experience, to strip stationary phases within a few weeks.

Points presented by D.B. Campbell *(Servier Labs., Greenford, U.K.):*
Assay of amphetamine and related amines in plasma by GC has in the past proved difficult owing to the low concentrations (5-100 ng/ml) found after therapeutic doses. The insensitivity of the FID mode has to

Economics of gas usage in GC-FID.[*]

CYLINDER DETAILS			USAGE & RUNNING COST			
Gas	Capacity, lit.	Cost, p	Inlet press., psi	Flow rate, ml/min	Life, h	Cost, p/h
Nitrogen	6240	165	20	60	1733	0.095
Hydrogen with oxygen	7800	268	15	45	2889	0.093
Hydrogen with comp. air	"	"	20	60	2167	0.124
Oxygen	6800	160	10	300	378	0.423
Compressed air	4640	73	20	600	129	0.566

[*]*R. Flanagan, personal communication to D.B. Campbell*

some extent been overcome by the use of ECD, although to detect halogen derivatives of the amines by this technique is not without problems, especially when many samples have to be analyzed. In developing a more sensitive FID procedure for amphetamines [1], it was shown that the use of oxygen in place of compressed air doubled the detector sensitivity, enabling an ultimate sensitivity of 1 ng/ml to be attained. Similar increases in sensitivity have been found for many other compounds. Although gas costs were not at the time examined, it has recently been shown (*see* Table, *above*) that the use of oxygen is less expensive than compressed air and needs less hydrogen. It is suggested that oxygen be used on a more regular basis with FID operation than has hitherto been the practice.

1. Campbell, D.B., *J. Pharm. Pharmac.* 21 (1969) 129-131.

Remark by B. Scales.— In comparison with FID, nitrogen or EC detectors may improve sensitivity, but may have the disadvantages of excessive background peaks or of severe quenching due to water and solvent.

Points contributed by the Editor
[N.B.- *Further points are made in Art. G-1; see also* GC *entries in the Index.]*

1. Bach, P.H., *Lab. Pract.* 24 (1975) 817.

   Silylation device for glass columns as used for compounds that decompose thermally in metal columns.

2. Ryan, P.L., *Clin. Chem.* 21 (1975) 1041.
   [*Inapplicable if nitrogen used even for pulsed ECD* - ED.]

   Adaption of dual-column GC apparatus so that when a column + ECD is merely undergoing 'conditioning' or being used in the non-pulsed mode, it can be swept with nitrogen instead of argon/methane (dearer).

3. Solow, E.B., Metaxas, J.M. & Summers, T.C., *J. Chromatog. Sci.* 12 (1974) 256-260.

Example of GC-FID with on-column methylation — for determining antiepileptics in multiple drug therapy. (Accompanying articles deal with other drug assays.)

4. Greeley, R.H., *Clin. Chem.* 20 (1974) 192-194.
   [Ref. 16 on p. 13, top, also concerns FID derivatization.]

To make (e.g.) butyl derivatives of barbiturates for GC, reaction with 1-iodobutane is performed in *N,N*-dimethylacetamide containing phenyltrimethylammonium hydroxide, which furnishes a soluble salt.

5. Berry, D.J., *Scan [Pye Unicam]*, 5 (1974) 14-19. - Cf. Berry, D.J., & Grove, J., *J. Chromatog.* 80 (1973) 205-219.

Useful survey of drug assay (FID). A few columns suffice for toxicological needs: *general use*, SE30; *hypnotics*, C.D.M.S.; *amphetamines*, Apiezon L + KOH; *anticonvulsants*, SP1000; *alcohol*, Chromosorb 101. For primary screening identification, TLC and other tests are used initially, and GC subsequently [cf. 'primary' use of GC in the following Note - *Ed.*]

Forensic drug screening with the aid of GC

Answer to R.A. Chalmers, *by* A.J. Clatworthy *(Metropolitan Police Forensic Science Laboratory).—* When small blood samples have to be analyzed for drugs in the forensic laboratory, use is made mainly of GC and the alkaline flame-ionization detector (AFID, nitrogen detector). Thereby we can routinely detect and identify some 30 common acidic and neutral drugs in a 1 ml blood sample at levels below 1 µg/ml. The suspect drug is often derivatized using diazomethane in ether, particularly if it is believed to be a barbiturate (the dimethylbarbiturate derivative is formed), and then confirmed by GC-MS. If other drugs are suspected, derivatives are not usually made and the compound is confirmed by GC-MS. In the event of metabolites being found, e.g. 2'-OH-methaqualone, longer retention times and tailing peaks are found, and the metabolite will nearly always be derivatized, perhaps as TMS.

We therefore use not less than two parameters in every case of detection and identification of small amounts of drugs in blood, usually GC-AFID and GC-MS. In cases where large biological samples are available, other techniques such as UV spectrophotometry and TLC may be used as well.

E-2 POLAROGRAPHY AS APPLIED TO THE ANALYSIS OF CERTAIN DRUGS AND THEIR METABOLITES IN BODY FLUIDS

M.R. Smyth and W. Franklin Smyth
*Chemistry Dept., Chelsea College,
Manresa Road, London, SW3 6LX, U.K.*

This review deals with the methodological aspects of the application of polarographic methods to the analysis of drug species in body fluids and stresses the need to employ relevant separation techniques prior to the determination step.

With the advent of commercially available, sensitive polarographic equipment, there has been a noticeable increase in the number of applications of the technique to the determination of electroactive drug substances in body fluids. It is the purpose of this article, therefore, to present a methodological approach to this subject, quoting relevant examples from the literature and stressing the constituent processes which go to make up the analytical method as a whole.

SAMPLING AND INITIAL TREATMENT OF SAMPLE

As with other methods of analysis, care must be taken to obtain a representative sample, especially for the 'blank' since errors in its measurement, while less important at early post-dose times, may have a pronounced effect on the determination of small concentrations of drug species at later sampling times.

The body fluids which have been most analyzed using polarography are blood and urine although cerebrospinal fluid, sweat and saliva samples are also amenable to the technique. In the case of blood, 2-3 ml samples are usually taken from the appropriate vein and centrifuged to separate off the red cells from the serum. It is imperative at this stage to prevent any haemolysis of the red blood cells since traces of haemoglobin or its degradation products in the serum (or plasma) can cause interference in the subsequent polarographic analysis. It is, then, advisable to analyze this sample immediately or freeze it in order to prevent further metabolic, physico-chemical or chemical changes occurring in the sample.

There are special problems concerned with sampling urine since this body fluid has been found to have a much greater and more variable electroactive composition than plasma. This variation is dependent to a certain extent on the physiological state of the organism at the time of sampling. As with plasma, it is advisable to analyze the sample immediately or to freeze it.

SEPARATION

Although there are several reported cases of polarography being carried out directly on body fluids (particularly serum or plasma) [1, 2], these methods suffer both from 'direct' interferences (i.e. reduction, oxidation, catalytic or adsorption currents caused by naturally occurring electroactive substances) and from 'indirect' interferences (e.g. with proteins present the i_p *versus* concentration curve at low drug concentrations may be non-linear) which greatly affect the sensitivity of this method of analysis. It is more common, therefore, to separate the drug species of interest prior to the determination step.

(1) Ultracentrifugation/filtration methods

These methods are generally employed to remove the interference caused by the presence in the sample of molecules of relatively high molecular mass. For example, in the determination of penicillins and cephalosporins in serum [3], protein was

removed by filtering through a UM-2 filter at a pressure of 50 psi and the fil-
trate was subjected to polarographic analysis. These methods suffer, however,
from less than quantitative recovery and from being unable to remove other
electroactive interferences from the sample. They could find greater application
where, as in the pharmacokinetic area, drug binding *in vivo* has to be studied.

(2) TLC

This chromatographic procedure has been widely employed to separate structurally
related drug substances when polarographic methods have been unable to resolve the
parent compound from its metabolites. Following a suitable solvent extraction
from the body fluid and solvent evaporation, the concentrate is spotted onto a
TLC plate and separation achieved in the appropriate solvent system. The areas
with spots are then scraped off, eluted with a small volume of methanol or
dimethylformamide (the latter solvent is recommended to prevent re-adsorption of
the compound onto the silica) and taken up in supporting electrolyte prior to the
determination step.

The main source of interference from this procedure comes from metal ions,
e.g. Zn^{2+}, which are constituents of the support material and can be removed by
complexation with EDTA. This method of separation has found most application in
the determination of urinary metabolites, e.g. of flurazepam [4] and 2-hydroxy-
nicotinic acid [5].

(3) Ion-exchange and XAD-2 chromatography

Resin-column chromatography has been used both to remove electroactive urinary
interferences, e.g. in the determination of chlorpromazine [6] and morphine [7]
in urine, and to separate free and conjugated compounds in this fluid, e.g. in
the separation of oxazepam and its glucuronide conjugate by use of XAD-2 [8].

(4) Gel filtration

This method of separation has been little applied in polarographic methodology
due to being time-consuming and resulting in a dilution of the original sample.
It has been applied, however, to the determination of meprobamate in serum [9]
following separation with Sephadex G-25.

(5) HPLC

With the development of electrochemical detectors for liquid chromatography, the
authors anticipate that this will become a powerful tool in the analysis of body
fluids, both to remove interferences prior to electroanalysis and to resolve mixtures of structurally related drug substances. With the extension of the potential range to include many more oxidation processes, there is a considerable increase in the number of molecules amenable to polarographic analysis. Derivatization procedures can also be carried out on-line, e.g. the conversion of citral
into its semicarbazone derivative [10].

(6) Solvent extraction

Optimization of solvent extraction methods has been carried out following systematic studies of the acid-base equilibria and distribution characteristics of
structurally related drug species, e.g. the 1,4-benzodiazepines [11-12] and phenothiazines [13-14].

The effect of solvent on the extraction of naturally occurring electroactive constituents from blank serum (buffered at pH 7.4 with phosphate buffer)
is illustrated in Fig. 1. This shows that benzene co-extracts less electroactive interference than more polar solvents, e.g. diethyl ether or chloroform.

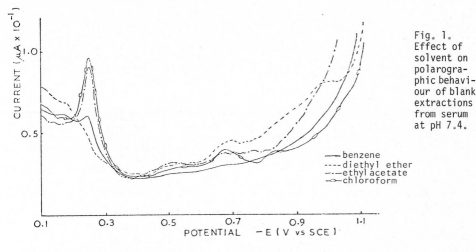

Fig. 1.
Effect of
solvent on
polarogra-
phic behavi-
our of blank
extractions
from serum
at pH 7.4.

—— benzene
---- diethyl ether
—·—ethyl acetate
—○—chloroform

The peak obtained at -0.25 V *versus* SCE (B.R. buffer* pH 3.0) following extraction with chloroform, ethyl acetate and to a lesser extent benzene has also been shown to occur following extractions from urine [15], and can be a major source of inter-ference in the analysis of trace amounts of compounds which reduce at relatively positive potentials (e.g. $-NO_2$ compounds) unless some form of chromatographic separation is also employed.

Another factor which governs the level of interference obtained from sol-vent extraction procedures is the pH at which the extraction is carried out. It is generally advisable to maintain the body fluid at physiological pH, but since this is not always possible certain 'clean-up' procedures can be employed to obtain a better background, for example back-extraction, addition of anhydrous salts (e.g. Na_2SO_4) to the organic solvent or, as suggested previously, some form of chromato-graphy (e.g. TLC).

POLAROGRAPHIC ANALYSIS

It is the aim of this Section to deal with the factors affecting the sensitivity and selectivity of polarographic methods of analysis.† In polarography the cur-rent flowing at a dropping mercury electrode (dme) is measured as a function of the applied potential. The total observed current in an electrochemical process results from two main components,
(i) the faradaic current (i_F) which arises as a result of the transfer of elec-trons at the dme,
(ii) the capacitive current (i_C) which is the current required to charge the electrode,
and it is the ratio of these currents (i_F/i_C) that determines the sensitivity of the technique one employs. Advances in instrumentation have therefore had to find means of increasing i_F or of discriminating against i_C.

(1) Instrumentation

Most of the theory concerning polarography has been carried out using conventio-nal D.C. polarography and is well documented elsewhere [16-17]. When polarogra-phy is adopted as a method of choice, it is advisable to carry out a systematic study of the polarographic behaviour [i.e. determination of the nature of the current, variation of the limiting current (i_{lim}) and half-wave potential ($E_{\frac{1}{2}}$)

---

* B.R. *denotes Britton-Robinson buffer.* † *For recapitulation of methods see p. 51 -ED.*

with pH, effect of organic solvent on i_{lim} and $E_{\frac{1}{2}}$, determination of electrode mechanism] of the drug and its metabolites using this technique prior to the application of more sensitive instrumentation for trace analysis. D.C. polarography has, however, found application in those cases where the concentration of a drug or its metabolites has been greater than 1-2 µg/ml, a notable example being the determination of 2-ethylthioisonicotinamide in urine [18].

The increase in sensitivity offered by cathode ray polarography (the limit of detection lies between 30 and 50 ng/ml) is brought about by the application of a rapid voltage sweep towards the end of the lifetime of a single drop, which results in an increase in i_F and a decrease in i_c. In addition, the peak wave form is easier to measure than the conventional D.C. wave and there is increased resolution between adjacent peaks (especially if a derivative circuit is employed). It suffers, however, from the need to employ a relatively large charging current, which can be compensated for by the use of twin-cell operation. This latter technique is known as 'differential polarography', and with the choice of suitably matched capillaries can offer a limit of detection between 2 and 10 ng/ml. This method has been applied to the determination of metronidazole directly in body fluids [19], whereas cathode ray polarography has found application in the determination of diazepam [20] and chlorpromazine [13].

A.C. polarography consists of superimposing a small alternating voltage (10-20 mV) on a linearly increasing D.C. potential ramp. The technique has been found to be more sensitive for reversible than for irreversible processes, although the sensitivity towards molecules undergoing irreversible processes can be increased if the species is adsorbed onto the electrode surface. The technique, with a limit of detection of the order of 1 µg/ml for organic molecules, offers an increased resolution over both D.C. and cathode ray polarography, as is best illustrated by the determination of ethionamide and its metabolites in urine (Fig. 2) [21].

Oscillopolarography, widely applied in Eastern Europe, suffers from a lack both of sensitivity (limit of detection 2-5 µg/ml) and of precision (rarely better than ±5%). Its main use lies in the elucidation of electrode processes and in the assessment of reversibility. In addition, calibration curves are generally non-linear, as has been demonstrated in the determination of meprobamate in serum [9].

In differential pulse polarography (DPP) a linearly increasing D.C. ramp is applied to the electrodes and a fixed-height pulse is superimposed near the end of the life of each drop. The current flow is sampled just before and at the end of each pulse, giving rise to a peaked representation of the data. The technique, although offering increased sensitivity (limit of detection of the order of 10 ng/ml), suffers from being time-consuming since one generally needs to employ a slow scan rate (1-2 mV/s) [22]. This technique has found most application in the determination of 1,4-benzodiazepines in body fluids [23], and with the development of subtractive techniques should provide a sensitivity of the order of 1 ng/ml under optimum conditions.

(2) Molecules amenable to polarographic analysis

The drug substances which have been studied by polarography have been reviewed elsewhere [24], and it is the intention here only to cite the various functional groups which are amenable to the technique. These are given in Table 1, and it should be borne in mind that the main factors affecting the sensitivity of polarographic methods for drugs containing these groups are (i) the number of electrons involved in the electrochemical process, (ii) the nature of the electrode process, and (iii) the degree of separation between the potential of the reduction or oxidation process and the decay potential of the supporting electrolyte.

In the absence of one of these functional groups, there are a variety of

Table 1. Functional groups amenable to sensitive polarographic analysis. *Where only one E_p value appears without a range of values, it refers to the particular example in the penultimate column.*

Functional group	Normal range of $E_{\frac{1}{2}}$ values (V *vs.* SCE)	Supporting electrolyte & pH	Reduction/oxidation mechanism	Comments & examples		Ref.
—CO.NH—	0 ±0.1	borax buffer pH 9.2	formation of Hg salt	Oxidation potential of anion in supporting electrolyte must be sufficiently +ve. N-containing heterocycles, e.g. barbiturates.		25
-SH	-0.3 ±0.05	B.R. buffer pH 9.45	formation of Hg salt	E.g. thiobarbiturates thioamides		←26 ←27
Hydro-quinones	0.0 (E_p value) 0.2	acetate buffer pH 4.7	oxid^n. to quinones (partially reversible)	E.g. Vitamin K_3 ascorbic acid		←28 ←29
—NO$_2$ (aromatic)	-0.15 ±0.05 -0.75 ±0.05	B.R. buffer pH 2.0	$-NO_2 \xrightarrow{4e} NH.OH$ $-NH.OH_2^+ \xrightarrow{2e} -NH_2$	1st wave recommended for analyses (in buffers pH 10-12). In some cases the $NH.OH_2^+$ reduction does not occur & in some cases it occurs simultaneously with the NO_2 reduction to give the amine.	E.g.- nitraze- pam chloram- phenicol nitrofu- rantoin	11 30 31
$>$N-NO	-0.75 ±0.1 -1.45 ±0.1	B.R. buffer pH 2.0 B.R. buffer pH 10.0	$>N-NO \xrightarrow[H^+]{4e} >N-NH_2$ $>N-NO \xrightarrow{2e} >NH + N_2O$	Conjugated cpds. give rise to better defined waves. E.g. N-nitrosamines.		32
$>$C-NO	-0.39 (E_p value)	B.R. buffer pH 10.0	complicated mechanism	Well-defined DPP peaks. E.g. *p*-nitrosophenol.		32
$>$C=N-	-0.75 ±0.05	B.R. buffer pH 2.0	$>C=N- \xrightarrow{2e} >CH.NH-$	E.g. 1,4-benzodiazepines.		11
$>$C=N-N$<$	-0.5 ±0.05	B.R. buffer pH 3.0	$>C=N-N< \xrightarrow{4e} >CH.NH_2 +HN<$	Competing hydrolytic reaction. E.g. nitrofurantoin.		31
-N=N-	-0.2 ±0.1	B.R. buffer pH 3.0	$-N=N- \xrightarrow{2e} -NH.HN-$	4e reduct^n. can occur when adjacent phenyl rings contain electron-donating substituents. E.g. *p*-OH azo dye derivatives.		33
$>$N→O (aliphatic)	-0.8	0.05 M HCl	$->N→O \xrightarrow{2e} >NH$	E.g. chlorpromazine N-oxide.		13
$>$N→O	-0.095, -1.19	0.01 M H_2SO_4	$>N→O \xrightarrow{2e} >N +H_2O$	E.g. trimethoprim N-1-oxide. ←Heterocyclic ring also reduced		34
S→O (aromatic)	-0.8	0.05 M HCl	$>S→OH^+ \xrightarrow{2e} >S + H_2O$	E.g. chlorpromazine S-oxide.		13
$>$C=O	large range	various electrolytes	$>C=O \xrightarrow{2e} >CH.OH$	Occurs at -ve potentials. Analytically usable waves exist when the $>$C=O is conjugated with $>$C=C$<$ as in αβ-unsatd. ketones or when $>$C=O is adjacent to an aromatic nucleus. E.g. haloperidol.		35
$>$C=C$<$	large range	various electrolytes	$>C=C< \xrightarrow{2e} >CH.HC<$	Occur at -ve potentials. Analytically usable waves occur when electron-withdrawing substituents are attached to the double bond. E.g. cephalosporins.		3

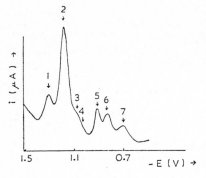

Fig. 2. A.C. polarographic differentiation
of urinary metabolites of ethionamide
(Bieder & Brunel [21]).
1 = 2-Et isonicotinic acid
2 = E.C.P.
3 = M.E.T.O.D. + M.E.S.T.O.D.
4 = *not identified*
5 = Ethionamide + *compound 7*
6 = *N*-Me ethionamide·
7 = Ethionamide sulphoxide.

derivatization procedures which can be employed to make a drug substance amenable
to polarographic analysis.

(i) Nitration

This is the most widely used derivatization procedure since it can be carried out
with relative ease and rapidity and gives rise to well defined reduction waves
which can be used for polarographic analysis with high sensitivity. It has been
carried out mainly on aromatic nuclei and, where possible, it is advised to employ
the mildest conditions which give quantitative recovery of the mono-nitrated derivative, e.g. nitration of paracetamol in $NaNO_2/HCl$ results in a 90% yield of the
2-nitro derivative [36]. The nitration of micro quantities of material leads,
however, to larger errors than a method not requiring a derivatization procedure
(generally between 5-10% for the nitration of 1 µg of material) [37]. The main
source of interference in this procedure comes from impurities in the nitrating
mixture (especially in fuming HNO_3 or HNO_3/H_2SO_4 mixtures) and from the nitration
of naturally occurring substances which remain following the preliminary separation. It is advisable, therefore, to employ a further solvent extraction step
rather than analyze the derivative directly in the nitration mixture.

(ii) Nitrosation

Nitrosation can also be carried out using $NaNO_2/HCl$. As with the nitration procedure, product(s) of the reaction should be identified by MS. Nitrosation occurs
with highly activated aromatic compounds and with molecules possessing centres
of high electron density, e.g. phenols and secondary amines. This method of derivatization has been applied to the determination of morphine in blood following
extraction with $CHCl_3$/isopropanol and separation by paper chromatography [38].
As with the nitration procedure, care should be taken to separate naturally occurring substances which are also amenable to nitrosation procedures, e.g. creatine
and creatinine [39].

(iii) Condensation

The most common condensation reactions that result in polarographically active
products are those involving the reaction of keto-compounds, e.g. steroids, with
either 2,4-dinitrophenylhydrazine or primary amines to give hydrazone or semicarbazone derivatives respectively. These procedures suffer, however, from the
susceptibility of the products to hydrolysis at the trace level, and should be
carried out only under strictly controlled conditions.

(iv) Other derivatization procedures

Other procedures have been developed to deal with particular cases. Thus, in the
determination of disulfiram in blood [40] the procedure involved heating the

compound with 50% H_2SO_4 to produce CS_2 which was then converted to copper diethyl-thiocarbamate (using Cu^{2+} and diethylamine) with 85-105% recovery. Another example is that of the conversion of sulphonamides (which are themselves polarographically active in non-aqueous media) to their azo-derivatives following diazotization and coupling with 1-napthol [41].

In the development of any derivatization procedure, however, it should be remembered that the specificity of the method will be lowered if one forms a derivative which is itself a product of metabolism. For this reason one should avoid procedures such as *N*-oxidation unless one has separated the metabolic product prior to derivatization.

PERFORMANCE OF THE DETERMINATION

After a consideration of (a) the degree to which polarographic methods of analysis can offer adequate resolution of the parent drug and its metabolites (this aspect is adequately dealt with elsewhere [42]), (b) the separation (and possibly derivatization) procedures necessary to improve the selectivity and sensitivity of the method and (c) the polarographic wave most suitable for analytical purposes, it is necessary to be acquainted with the parameters which affect the actual determination step so that one can optimize conditions for the measurement of the response.

(i) Choice of supporting electrolyte

This will depend to a great extent on the pH dependence of the electrochemical process one is monitoring, as ascertained initially by conventional D.C. polarography at the 10^{-4} M level. In general, it is advisable to employ a simple buffered system, e.g. acetate buffer, although many determinations have been carried out in mixed buffer systems, e.g. Britton-Robinson (B.R.) buffers, which have a buffering capacity over a wider pH range. The composition of the electrolyte is important in those cases where the electrochemical process is affected by certain ions in the buffer. For example, the reduction of chlortetracycline is affected by the presence of borate ions in the supporting electrolyte [43]. This of course can be important for identification purposes, as can be the incorporation of small concentrations of metal ions known to complex with a certain species; Thus, complexation of metronidazole with Cu^{2+} causes a reduction in the wave height due to free Cu^{2+} in the solution [44].

Following the separation/derivatization stages it is advisable to take the residue up in a small volume of methanol (or ethanol) to prevent loss of the substance on the glass. This can then be diluted with supporting electrolyte although it is advised to limit the concentration of alcohol in the final solution to 5-30% since this can result in a decrease in the limiting current. The other effect of incorporating alcohol in the final solution is that it discriminates against interfering adsorption currents [33] which can be identified by use of the D.C. technique. D.C. polarography can also be used to characterize maxima which can cause ill-defined waves for analytical purposes and which can be removed using a suitable suppressor chosen for maximum effectiveness (e.g. Triton X-100).

In cases where the electrochemical process occurs near the supporting electrolyte's decay potential, advantage may be taken of tetra-alkyl ammonium salts as the supporting electrolyte since these can extend the 'working potential' range by about 500 mV.

In the development of any polarographic assay, the 'ultimate' sensitivity of the method is determined by the behaviour of the 'blank', and care must be taken to ensure the purity of the supporting electrolyte, e.g. use of de-ionized water, Analar-grade chemicals, etc. Interference from metal ions can be minimized by including 10^{-3} M EDTA in the analyte, which has the effect of shifting their potential of reduction to more negative values. Decreased background can also be achieved by the incorporation of tetra-alkyl ammonium salts into the supporting electrolyte, as has been demonstrated for the behaviour of 0.1 M H_2SO_4 in the DPP mode [45]. It is also stated [45] that the concentration of the electrolyte should be maintained above 0.04 M, since below this value an increase is obtained in the background current, as one would expect from double-layer effects.

(ii) Choice of cell design and auxiliary electrode systems.

Brooks has reported [46] an increased sensitivity for the determination of the benzodiazepine class of drugs using a micro-cell of volume 0.5 ml with a 3-electrode system having a platinum anode and an SCE reference electrode. The main disadvantage of the SCE is that Cl^- ions can escape into the bulk of the solution and can then interfere with waves due to electrochemical processes occurring at relatively positive potentials, e.g. oxidation of barbiturates.

The sensitivity can also be improved by using a capillary which delivers a relatively large amount of mercury in unit time (e.g. 2.5-3.0 mg/sec in KCl under a pressure of 55 cm of mercury). This also leads to an increase in the background current, and there is usually a point above which the small increases in sensitivity or selectivity offered by changes in parameters such as scan rate, drop time, etc., are counteracted by considerations of the time and cost of analysis.

(iii) Calculation

The calculation of concentrations from polarographic data is made from measurement of the limiting current (as in the case of D.C. or pulse polarography) or from measurement of peak height (as in the case of cathode-ray polarography or DPP), and then reference of these current measurements to the linear portions of calibration plots of current *versus* concentration of electroactive species in the bulk of the solution. Most difficulty is encountered in cathode-ray polarography when the current does not return to the base level, thus making quantitation in the lower nanogram range very difficult. The other main source of difficulty arises from the 'blank' current (i_b), and unless this follows the line drawn for the measurement of peak height (i_p) it is analytically sounder to subtract this 'blank' current from the sum of $i_b + i_p$ in order to obtain the most satisfactory results. This is the principle behind 'subtractive' polarography, and furnishes reproducible results if one has been able to obtain a representative 'blank' sample. Other methods can be employed to improve the precision of the method, e.g. the standard addition method or the use of an 'internal standard', but these are generally not required since in the polarographic analysis of drugs and their metabolites in body fluids an error of ±5-10% can usually be tolerated.

FUTURE APPLICATIONS OF POLAROGRAPHY IN DRUG ANALYSIS

For polarography to become a powerful tool in the study of metabolism, it must not only be a sensitive method of analysis but should also (a) provide information on the structure of unknown metabolites, and (b) be amenable to some form of automation.

Concerning (a), there have been several approaches which warrant consideration. Firstly, linear relationships exist between $E_{\frac{1}{2}}$ and the Hammett (or polar) functions of substituent groups contained in electro-active benzenoid compounds. These studies have been particularly carried out by Zuman [47] and applied to the 1,4-benzodiazepines by de Silva *et al.* [48]. Secondly, there is the approach with which we ourselves are engaged, concerned with the establishment of linear relationships between $E_{\frac{1}{2}}$ and the energy of the lowest vacant molecular orbital (m_{m+1}) [49]. This approach has previously been applied to a series of heterocycles in organic media [50], whereas our studies have been directed towards the relationship of this function to the $E_{\frac{1}{2}}$ values of substituted nitrobenzenes in aqueous solutions [51]. Both approaches can be used to evaluate the structure of an unknown metabolite, but demand a detailed knowledge of the polarographic behaviour of a series of structurally related compounds since the relationships will be valid only if the same electrode process is in operation for each of the compounds.

Some useful information can also be obtained from a systematic study of the dependence of the unknown metabolite peak on pH, height of the mercury column, composition of the supporting electrolyte, etc., but definitive evidence concerning an unknown peak should await MS investigation.

Concerning the automation aspect, (b), there is now instrumentation available which incorporates a pressurized mercury electrode in an automatic system; this instrumentation also contains a micro-processor which is capable of subtracting the 'blank'. Moreover, significant advances will take place with the linking of reliable electrochemical detectors to HPLC.

Acknowledgements

One of us (M.R.S.) thanks G.D. Searle Ltd., High Wycombe, for the provision of a research grant and Dr. J.A.W. Dalziel for helpful discussions.

References

1. Kane, P.O., in *Advances in Polarography*, Vol. 3 (Longmuir, I.S., ed.), Pergamon Press, Oxford (1959) pp. 1076- 1086.

2. Halvorsen, S. & Jacobsen, E., *Anal. Chim. Acta 59* (1972) 127-136.

3. Benner, E.J., *Antimicrob. Agents Chemother. 10* (1970) 201-204.

4. De Silva, J.A.F., Puglisi, C.V., Brooks, M.A. & Hackman, M.R., *J. Chromatog. 99* (1974) 461-483.

5. De Silva, J.A.F., Strojny, N. & Munno, N., *Anal. Chim. Acta 66* (1973) 23-38.

6. Porter, G.S. & Beresford, J., *J. Pharm. Pharmacol. 18* (1966) 223-227.

7. Orlov, Y.E., Ignatov, Y.L. & Shostenico, Y.V., *Med. Prom. SSSR 18* (1964) 44.

8. Marcucci, F., Bianchi, R., Airoldi, L., Salmona, M., Fanelli, R., Chiabrando, C., Frigerio, A., Mussini, E. & Garattini, E., *J. Chromatog. 107* (1975) 285-293.

9. Hynie, I. & Prokes, J., *Chem. Zvesti. 18* (1964) 425-428.

10. Little, C.L., *Ph.D. thesis,* University of London (1974).

11. Clifford, J.M. & Smyth, W. Franklin, *Analyst 99* (1974) 241-272.

12. Clifford, J.M., Smyth, M.R. & Smyth, W. Franklin, *Z. Anal. Chem. 272* (1974) 198-201.

13. Beckett, A.H., Essien, E.E. & Smyth, W. Franklin, *J. Pharm. Pharmacol. 26* (1974) 399-407.

14. Whelpton, R. & Curry, S.H., *present Volume,* pp.

15. Smyth, M.R., *Ph.D. thesis,* University of London (1976), *to be submitted.*

16. Meites, L., in *Polarographic Techniques,* 2nd edn., Interscience, New York (1965).

17. Milner, G.W.C., *The Principles and Applications of Polarography,* 3rd edn., Longman, London (1962).

18. Okuda, Y., *Rev. Polarog. (Kyoto) 11* (1963) 197-203.

19. Kane, P.O., *J. Polarog. Soc. 7* (1961) 58-62.

20. Berry, D.J., *Clin. Chim. Acta 32* (1971) 235-241.

21. Bieder, A. & Brunel, P., *Ann. Pharm. Franc. 29* (1971) 461-476.

22. Christie, J.H., Osteryoung, J. & Osteryoung, R.A., *Anal. Chem. 45* (1973) 210-215.

23. De Silva, J.A.F. & Brooks, M.A., *Talanta 22* (1975) 849-860.

24. Smyth, W. Franklin, Hill, D.E. & Rendell, T.C., in *Polarography Fifty Years On* (Fleet, B., ed.), Macmillan, London (1976)

25. Smyth, W. Franklin, Jenkins, T.C., Siekiera, J. & Baydar, A., *Anal. Chim. Acta 80* (1975) 233-244.

26. Smyth, W.F., Svehla, G. & Zuman, P., *Anal. Chim. Acta 51* (1970) 463-482.

27. Davidson, I.E., in *Polarography in the Life Sciences,* a Symposium held at Chelsea College (1975). *[Proc. Analyt. Div. Chem. Soc. (1976) in press]*

28. Lindquist, J. & Farroha, S.M., *Analyst 100* (1975) 377-385.

29. Owen, R.S. & Smyth, W. Franklin, *J. Food Technol. 10* (1975) 263-272.

30. Fossdal, K. & Jacobsen, E., *Anal. Chim. Acta 56* (1971) 105-115.

31. Burmicz, J.S., Palmer, R.F. & Smyth, W. Franklin, *to be published.*

32. Smyth, W. Franklin, Watkiss, P., Burmicz, J.S. & Hanley, H.O., *Anal. Chim. Acta 78* (1975) 81-92.

33. Florence, T.M., *J. Electroanal. Chem. 52* (1974) 115-132.

34. Brooks, M.A., De Silva, J.A.F. & D'Arconte, L.M., *Anal. Chem. 45* (1973) 263-266.

35. Volke, J., Wasilewska, L. & Ryvolova-Kejherova, A., *Pharmazie 26* (1971) 399.

36. Cooper, R.G., *Lecture at private meeting at Shrivenham,* Royal Military College of Science (1975, July).

37. Hart, J.P., *Lecture at Euroanalysis II,* Budapest (1975, Aug.).

38. Mithers, K., *Acta Pharm. Toxicol. KBH 18* (1961) 199.

39. Velisek, J., Davidek, J. & Klein, S., *Z. Lebensm. Unters-Forsch. 155* (1974) 203-208.

40. Brown, M.W., Porter, G.S. & Williams, A.E., *J. Pharm. Pharmacol. 26 Suppl.* (1974) 95p-96p.

41. Fogg, A.G. & Ahmed, Y.Z., *Anal. Chim. Acta 70* (1974) 241-244.

42. Smyth, W. Franklin & Smyth, M.R., in *Polarography in the Life Sciences,* a Symposium held at Chelsea College (1975). *(As for ref. 27)*

43. Caplis, M.E., in *Electroreduction of the Tetracycline Antibiotics, Ph.D. thesis,* Purdue University, Lafayette (1970).

44. Chien, W.E., Lambert, H.J. & Sanvordeker, D.R., *J. Pharm. Sci. 64* (1975) 957-960.

45. Hasebe, K. & Osteryoung, J., *Anal. Chem. 47* (1975) 2412-2418.

46. Brooks, M.A. & Hackman, M.R., *Anal. Chem. 47* (1975) 2059-2062.

47. Zuman, P., in *Substituent Effects in Organic Polarography,* Plenum, New York (1967).

48. Brooks, M.A., Bel Bruno, J.J., De Silva, J.A.F. & Hackman, M.R., *Anal. Chim. Acta 74* (1975) 367-385.

49. Streitwieser, A., in *Molecular Orbital Theory for Organic Chemists,* Wiley, New York (1966) pp. 173-187.

50. Bergman, I., *Trans. Faraday Soc. 50* (1954) 829-838.

51. Smyth, M.R., Smyth, W.Franklin & Barrett, J., *to be published.*

THE LUMINESCENCE ASSAY OF DRUGS

E-3

James W. Bridges
Department of Biochemistry
University of Surrey
Guildford, GU2 5XH, U.K.

Interference from light scattering materials and other luminescent substances, arising either from the biological sample itself or from the sample work-up procedure, is frequently the major limitation to the sensitivity of a luminescence assay rather than the intrinsic luminescence of the drug concerned. Some of the means by which this biological blank may be suppressed are discussed. Since quenching and photodecomposition may also affect analytical sensitivity and accuracy, methods of reducing these problems are considered. The various approaches to the fluorimetric assay of drugs, i.e. native fluorescence, chemically induced fluorescence, fluorescence derivatization, and enzyme-linked assays are reviewed, and examples of each given.

Phosphorescence assay methods should be regarded as complementary to fluorescence techniques. An appraisal is made of the types of drugs whose phosphorescence characteristics are appropriate for analytical purposes. Largely due to deficiencies in sample-handling procedures, phosphorescence analysis has had only extremely restricted use. Consideration is given to various new approaches to sample handling, such as the measurement of phosphorescence on TLC plates or in microcapillary tubes, which overcome most of these limitations.

The particular appeal of luminescence techniques to the analyst lies in their potentially high sensitivity and the wide range over which the emission intensity is linear with concentration. Commonly, however, the sensitivity achieved with pure drugs cannot be attained when the same drugs are extracted from biological fluids or tissues, because of the presence of light-scattering or luminescent contaminants ('biological blank').

'BIOLOGICAL BLANK'

Contaminants may stem from the biological material itself; but frequently they are added during the sample work-up procedure. Common sources of interference are from distilled water stored in plastic containers, partial degradation of ion-exchange resins, or the presence of traces of fluorescent detergents or stopcock grease. Many 'Analar' solvents and chemicals also contain considerable amounts of luminescent materials. Purity guarantees of 'less than 1 ppm' in the reagents involved in an assay are clearly unlikely to be always entirely adequate when drug detection limits at the ng or sub-ng level are sought. Spectroscopic-grade solvents, e.g. spectroscopic-grade ethanol, may also be quite inadequate for many luminescence assay purposes, particularly in the blue region of the emission spectrum. Some spectrofluorimetric grade solvents are available; but these are limited in range and are expensive. It is often possible, however, to remove the bulk of luminescence contaminants from water-immiscible solvents simply by shaking the solvent with 0.1 M HCl, then 0.1 M KOH and finally, with glass-distilled water.

Light-scattering is characterized by identical excitation and emission wave-lengths (i.e. $\lambda_{ex} \equiv \lambda_{em}$) and will interfere with fluorescence but not with time-resolved phosphorescence. Scattering by large particles may be exacerbated during sample preparation by contributions from chromatography columns or emulsions in organic solvents. Scattering of this type may either increase or decrease the light signal. Fortunately it can usually be largely removed by centrifugation. Scattering is particularly common in microcuvettes at the air-cuvette and cuvette-solution interfaces. Scattering by small molecules (Rayleigh scattering) is particularly a problem for compounds which fluorescence in the UV region, because the intensity of scatter α $1/\lambda_{ex}^6$, and the excitation and the emission wavelengths frequently overlap so that the exciting light interferes with the emission signal. Scatter disturbance of this type may be considerably reduced, albeit with some loss of sensitivity, if the wavelength of excitation is set below its maximum and the wavelength of emission above its maximum.

REDUCTION OF THE LUMINESCENT SIGNAL

In common with light absorption, interactions of the compound under study with other molecules in the ground state may alter the expected photodetector signal (static quenching). The luminescence process is considerably more vulnerable to changes in the environment (e.g. solvent, other solutes, temperature variation) surrounding the luminescing molecules than that of light absorption because it involves chemically highly reactive species (i.e., molecules in the excited state) which may undergo chemical change (photodecomposition) or may give up their energy in the form of heat (dynamic quenching). Dynamic quenching, which causes a decrease in the excited state lifetime, is related to the diffusion rate of the luminescent molecules; it is therefore experienced especially at high temperatures in low viscosity solvents. The use of high viscosity solvents or solid samples, or reduction in temperature of the sample, may largely circumvent dynamic quenching. This may also improve the sensitivity of the assay by imposing rigidity and/or planarity on the luminescent species *(see below)*. The entrapment of air bubbles in viscous solvents may, however, exacerbate light-scatter problems.

In general, large temperature changes are required to significantly affect the signal ($\sim 1\%$ for a 1° change in temperature); however a few compounds are notably temperature-sensitive ($\sim 5\%$ for a 1° change, e.g. *p*-anisidine) and a quick check on the temperature dependence of luminescence may prove useful in developing an assay [1, 2].

With compounds containing a large aromatic nucleus, although not with most other substances, quenching by dissolved oxygen may occur. It is often encountered in the assay of polycyclic hydrocarbons, and can be avoided merely by bubbling solutions with oxygen-free nitrogen for a few minutes. Some fluorescent molecules are quenched either by electron-donating anions, e.g. Cl^-, Br^-, or by electron-donating anions, e.g. NO_3^- (depending on the redox potential of the molecule's excited state). This type of quenching appears to be a relatively specific process which is clearly of analytical potential for selectively surpressing the luminescence of one molecular apecies in a mixture of luminescing materials. Unfortunately its application has been very limited. Tryptophan has been identified in biological mixtures by the fact that bisulphate ions quench its luminescence but not that of most other luminescing species likely to be present [3]. Certain aromatic hydrocarbons have been specifically determined in complex mixtures by the selective quenching effects of nitromethane [4], and oxygen has been determined in air by the quenching of the luminescence of a borate-benzoin mixture [5].

Loss of fluorescence may also occur as a consequence of the presence in its vicinity of other molecular species (acceptors) which have appropriate absorption characteristics to enable the transfer to them of the excited state energy. Energy transfer (resonance transfer) is a relatively specific process, being critically dependent on the distance and orientation of the donor and acceptor molecules [α $1/(\text{distance})^6$] although they do not need to actually come into contact. This process is independent of solvent viscosity, and has found its greatest application as a 'spectroscopic ruler' to determine the distance between donor and acceptor molecules [6]. The fluorescence of the cofactor $NADH_2$ is thought to be a result of intramolecular energy transfer from its purine to its *N*-substituted pyridine nucleus [7].

As yet the energy transfer phenomenon has not been used for analytical purposes although it has some interesting possible applications. For example, the binding of molecules with an appropriate fluorescence (acceptors) to fluorescent macromolecules (donors) such as fluorescent-tagged immunoabsorbents could be measured directly by simply setting the fluorimeter excitation wavelength to that of the donor and the emission wavelength to that characteristic of the acceptor, and observing the photodetector signal.

Quenching may also occur through the luminescence emitted by a donor compound being re-absorbed by an acceptor substance (radiative transfer). The extent of this type of quenching is dependent on the degree of overlap between the emission spectrum of the donor and the excitation spectrum of the acceptor. The use of light-absorbing solvents or the presence of dicromate due to its inadequate removal from glassware often leads to such interference with UV fluorescence. At high concentrations of drug its luminescence may be self-quenched (if there is overlap of its excitation and emission wavelengths) by the high preponderance of unexcited drug molecules leading to a loss of linearity of signal with concentration. (Commonly this occurs above 5 µg/ml of compounds and can be avoided simply by diluting the sample. *See* [1]). The problem, which is much more common in fluorescence than phosphorescence, can be largely avoided by using microcells rather than the more conventional 1 cm² cell (*N.B.* it is not the width of cuvette but the distance through which the light beam travels that is important), or by employing front surface geometry in the fluorimeter cell compartment instead of the more usual right-angle system. Below 1-10 µg/ml linearity with signal is often experienced over a 100-fold to 10,000-fold concentration range.

Photodecomposition is often experienced on assaying very dilute solutions of drugs which have excitation maxima below 350 nm, i.e. high-energy wavelengths. The usual consequence of photodecomposition is a reduction in the luminescence signal, although occasionally a higher signal is observed. If an enhanced signal is observed it may be used to analytical advantage, for example in the assay of coumarin and of some flavin and 4-aminoquinoline derivatives [10, 11].

Photodecomposition effects are especially observed when the whole of the sample is exposed to the exciting light beam, as in the case of microcuvettes. Where photodecomposition causes significant interference in an assay it can be lessened by keeping a closed shutter between the light source and the cell until the actual moment of reading the sample. Photodecomposition effects may sometimes be reduced by changing the solvent (Fig. 1) or by bubbling the sample with oxygen-free nitrogen.

INSTRUMENTAL VARIABILITY

The great majority of commercially available instruments are not capable of directly giving absolute intensity and wavelengths readings; hence the results recorded on a particular machine may differ from those obtained on an apparently identical piece of equipment. In addition, most instruments show both short-term and long-term fluctuations in lamp intensity and hence in the strength of the emission signal. For the most accurate results it is therefore essential to make regular checks, during an assay, on instrumental response using standards of know luminescence intensity. Quinine sulphate (1 µg/ml) in 0.1 M H_2SO_4, fluorescein in 0.1 M NaOH, Rhodamine B in 0.1 M NaOH, anthracene in ethanol (after flushing with nitrogen), and tryptophan in

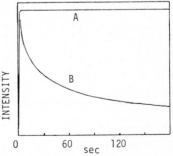

Fig. 1. Photodecomposition of chlorpromazine in (A) ethanol, and (B) water, as shown by the effect of UV irradiation (320 nm) on the phosphorescence emission. *From ref. [12]; acknowledgement to American Chemical Society.*

Table 1. Native fluorescence of some drugs.

Compound	λ_{ex}	λ_{fl}	Conditions	Sensitivity limit, µg/ml	Ref.
Acridine	358	475	trifluoracetic acid	good	8
p-Amino-salicylate	300	405	pH 11	good	8
Barbiturates	278	420	alkaline pH	0.1	9
Desipramine	295	415	alkaline pH	fair	8
L-Domoran	275	320	pH 1	poor	8
Griseofulvin	295	450	pH 7	good	8
Harmine	300	400	pH 1	good	8
Imipramine	295	415	pH 14	fair	8
Indomethacin	300	410	alkaline pH	good	9
LSD	325	445	acid pH	good	9
Menadione	335	480	ethanol	fair	8
Methapyrilene	238	363	neutral pH	good	9
Morphine	285	350	pH 7	poor	8
Nalidixic acid	330	370	pH <0	fair	8
Pamaquine	370	530	pH <0	fair	8
Quinacrine	285	420	pH 1	good	8
Quinine	350	450	acid pH	good	9
Salicylates	310	400	chloroform-acetic acid	good	9
Stilbamidine	~365	blue	pH <0	good	8
Sulphonamides	275	350	neutral pH	0.02	9
Trimethoprin	370	460	on TLC plate	good	9
Warfarin	290	385	methanol	fair	8
Yohimbine	270	360	pH 1	fair	8
Zoxazolamine	280	320	pH 11	good	8

water at pH 7.4 are widely accepted fluorescent standards. For phosphorescence, p-nitrophenol may be used. Recently a number of fluorescent plastic standards have become commercially available which are rather more convenient to use than liquid standards. As an alternative to these approaches, the Raman spectrum of the solvent may provide a very quick and reliable means of checking instrumental performance. In reporting fluorescence data it would be helpful if intensity data were always related to those of an accepted fluorescent standard.

METHODS FOR DRUG ASSAY

a) Fluorescence methods

i) Native fluorescence

For a drug to display appreciable fluorescence it must possess a conjugated system of double bonds held in a planar and preferably rigid form. The fluorescence process is usually facilitated if one or more -OH,-NH$_2$ or -CN groups are directly attached to the π-electron system. Ionization of -OH groups to -O$^-$ often encourages fluorescence, whereas ionization of -NH$_2$ groups to -NH$_3$ usually detracts from it. The presence of -NO$_2$, -Br or -I groups also generally tends to lessen fluorescence.

Molecules possessing these appropriate features may be assayed directly either in aqueous solution in an organic solvent or in a solid matrix (Table I). For drugs incorporating ionizable groups attached to the π-electron system, careful selection of pH conditions may bolster the sensitivity and selectivity of an assay. For example, barbiturates can be assayed as their di-anions in alkali, whereas the mono-anion and unionized forms of these molecules are only very weakly fluorescent [13].

Many of the pH effects on fluorescence intensity are predictable from consideration of the ground states of the molecules concerned. — Indeed, fluorescence changes may be used to determine pK_a's at very low concentrations of compounds. Thus drugs

$$\text{unionized} \quad \underset{pH\ 7}{\longleftrightarrow} \quad \text{mono-anion} \quad \underset{pH\ 10\text{-}11}{\longleftrightarrow} \quad \text{di-anion}$$

containing a quinoline nucleus which are poorly fluorescent at neutral pH are often more fluorescent in weak acid where the pyridine nitrogen is protonated, and phenolic materials which are poorly fluorescent in acid usually fluoresce much better in alkali. Many drugs exist as anions or cations but do not display appreciable fluorescence. They may be estimated fluorimetrically by combining them with a fluorescent ion of the opposite charge to form an ion pair. Provided that the solvent extraction conditions are carefully chosen, considerable selectivity can also be achieved. For example, 8-methoxyanthracenesulphonate has successfully been used as the fluorescent counter-ion to estimate propantheline bromide [14, 15]. Sometimes information on ground state pK_a's is not a true guide to fluorescence characteristics, due to molecules becoming ionized subsequent to their excitation (termed 'excited state ionization'). Under these conditions the observed fluorescence will be characteristic of the ionized form, while the excitation is that of the unionized species. It is commonly observed among closely related compounds that one will show excited state ionization whereas the other will not, e.g. naphthols. The phenonomenon has been used analytically to measure 2-hydroxybiphenyl (which shows excited state ionization) and 4-hydroxybiphenyl (which shows normal fluorescence) in mixtures. This assay provides the end-point in a new technique for assessing the carcinogenic potential of chemicals [16].

Investigation of fluorescence at extremes of pH has yielded a number of surprisingly sensitive and specific assays. This type of fluorescence appears to defy the rules cited above. An illustration of the analytical application of this approach is the direct fluorimetric assay of small amounts of benzoic acid and its conjugates in urine to which 70% sulphuric acid has been added. Under these conditions closely related materials are almost non-fluorescent [17]. Similarly 5-hydroxyindoles can be distinguished from other indoles by their fluorescence in 3 M sulphuric acid [18]. Because the fluorescence process is environmentally dependent, changing the solvent may have a dramatic effect on luminescence characteristics. Often addition of a less polar solvent leads to a changed fluorescence intensity and a hypochromic shift (i.e. to lower wavelength) in the emission maximum. Selection of the appropriate solvent may enable the fluorescence intensity to be maximized and/or a shift in the emission wavelength away from that of interfering substances to be achieved. For example (Fig. 2), warfarin shows a fluorescence at 386 nm at pH 7.4 and a relative intensity of 17; in n-butanol it emits at 383 nm with a relative intensity of 37, while in n-hexane the fluorescence maximum is 354 nm and the relative fluorescence intensity is reduced to 2 [19]. When warfarin binds to serum albumin it also shows a marked change in its fluorescence characteristics compared with those in aqueous solution (λ_{fl} 374, relative intensity 100). This effect permits a rapid assessment of warfarin binding to serum albumin and the identification of drugs which displace warfarin from plasma proteins, as shown by Bridges and Wilson [20]. This approach, which is known as 'fluorescence probing', is widely employed in biochemistry for investigating membranes [21]. Increasing the viscosity or lowering the sample temperature will frequently enhance the fluorescence of conjugated non-rigid molecules (as well as diminishing collisional quenching - *see above*) by increasing molecular rigidity and/or planarity. For example, 5-phenyl-substituted barbiturates and those substituted with an unsaturated group show marked enhancement of fluorescence at low temperatures [2]. In solid matrices, e.g. on TLC plates, fluorescence is often seen whereas no fluorescence is observed in solution. Thus, the compound 2-toluidinonaphthalene-6-sulphonate which is weakly fluorescent in water shows a 1,000-fold increase in fluorescence intensity in ice [22].

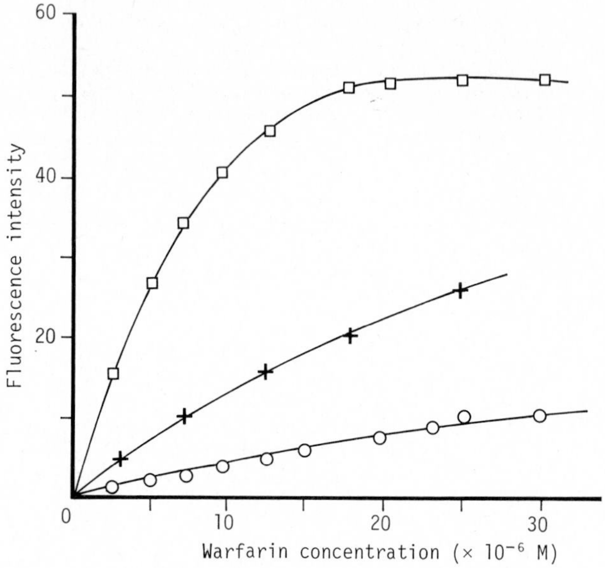

Fig. 2.   Fluorescence of warfarin, in phosphate buffer (o), and bound to human serum albumin in the presence (+) or absence (□) of phenylbutazone, 2×10^{-5} M. $\lambda_{ex} = 320$ nm. $\lambda_{fl} = 374$ or, in phosphate (o), 386 nm.

ii)   Chemically induced fluorescence

By simple chemical manipulation, increases in the π-electron system and in molecular planarity and rigidity can often be achieved, and groupings favourable to fluorescence inserted and those which detract from fluorescence removed or modified. Apart from enhancing the intensity of the emission, this approach may also be used by careful selection of the reaction conditions to increase the selectivity of an assay method, to increase the separation between the excitation and the emission wavelength maxima, and to shift the fluorescence maximum into the blue spectral region where optimal photomultiplier sensitivity occurs. A good illustration of this is the fluorimetric assay of adrenaline.

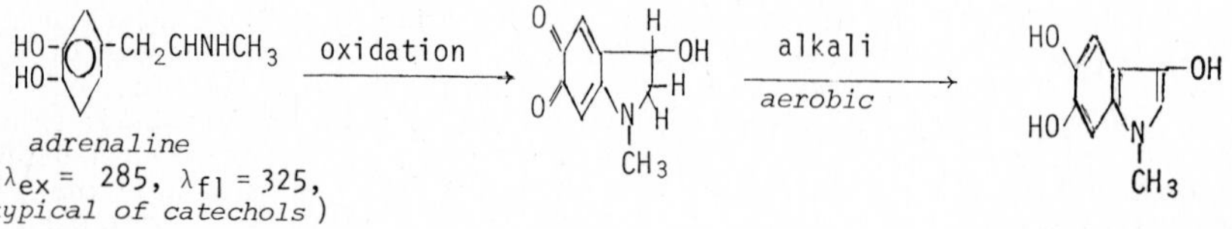

adrenaline
($\lambda_{ex} = 285$, $\lambda_{fl} = 325$, *typical of catechols*)

trihydroxyindole
($\lambda_{ex} = 436$, $\lambda_{fl} = 540$) *using reaction conditions at pH 6.5 specific for adrenaline*

A very wide variety of assays based on chemically induced fluorescence have been developed for drugs. The great majority of these assays have arisen randomly by mere trial of a number of chemical treatments on a drug and careful observation of their effects on the fluorescence process. In many cases the

Table 2. Examples of assay of drugs by chemically induced fluorescence.

Compound	Method	Sensitivity limit, μg	Ref.
Acetylcholine	reduction to ethanol & estimation by ADH	fair	8
Adrenaline	oxidation to trihydroxyindole	good	8
Amprolium	alkaline oxidation	fair	8
Chloroquine	photochemical induction	good	8
Chlortetracycline	heating with alkali	fair	8
Gitoxigenin	heating with strong acid	fair	8
Heroin	heating with strong acid	good	8
Hydrocortisone	heating with strong acid and ethanol	good	8
Imipramine	reaction with formaldehyde and acetyl-acetone	0.15	24
Isoniazid	coupling with salicylaldehyde and reduction	good	8
Librium	formation of lactam	good	25
6-Mercaptopurine	oxidation with $KMnO_4$	fair	8
Metaraminol	condensation with *o*-phthaldehyde	good	8
Methotrexate	oxidation with $KMnO_4$	fair	8
Morphine	conversion to pseudomorphine	good	26
Oxytetracycline	complexing with Mg^{2+} and EDTA	fair	8
ditto	alkaline degradation	0.1	27
Pheniramine	coupling with cyanogen bromide	fair	8
Phenothiazines	oxidation with H_2O_2	good	28
Quercetin	complexing with tetraphenylboron	1.0	29
Reserpine	oxidation	good	8
ditto	treatment with HNO_2	0.2	30
Streptomycin	coupling with β-naphthoquinone-4-sulphonate	good	8
Thiohydantoin	coupling with 2,6-dichloroquinone-chloroimide	good	8

chemistry has not been fully worked out. For example, atropine may be assayed by heating it with concentrated nitric acid, making alkaline, adding zinc dust and estimating the fluorescence after 30 min. The mechanism of the reaction is unclear, but presumably involves nitration of the benzene ring followed by reduction to form a fluorescent amino compound [23]. Reduction of nitro groups, condensation of π-electron systems together (e.g. estimation of morphine by formation of pseudomorphine) and cleavage of halogen residues represent logical approaches to enhancing fluorescence. Some examples of drug assay by chemically induced fluorescence are given in Table 2.

iii) Fluorescent derivatives

An alternative approach to chemically induced fluorescence that is very rapidly gaining in popularity is the tagging of particular functional groups in a drug with a fluorescent label. A variety of such labels are available for primary amino groups (Table 3) Coupling primary amines with fluorescamine (fluoram) has gained particular acceptance because the reaction can be carried out rapidly at room temperature in aqueous solution at pH 8-9 and the reagent itself and its degradation products are almost non-fluorescent [42]. The quantum yield of the product is poor and the reagent too rapidly hydrolyzes in aqueous solution for fluorescamine to be regarded as the ideal reagent for primary amines. Improved reagents based on the same reaction principle are already being devised.

Table 3. Examples of assay of drugs by fluorescence derivatization.

Derivatization method	Compound	Ref.
4-Bromomethyl-7-methoxy-coumarin	Fatty acids	31
4-Chloro-7-nitro-2,1,3-benzoxadiazole	N-Methylcarbamates	32
	Propoxyphene	33
Dansyl chloride	Barbiturates	34
	Hashish	35
o-Diacetylbenzene	Aminomethylphosphinic acids	36
4-(Dichloro-s-triazinyl)-1-ethoxynaphthalene	Tolamolol	37
Fluorescamine	Aminomethylphosphinic acids	36
	Substituted hydrazines	38
	Sulphonamides	39
9-Isothiocyanatoacridine	Amphetamine	40
o-Phthaldehyde	Aminomethylphosphinic acids	36
	Substituted hydrazines	38
Pyrene aldehyde	Amphetamine	41

The development of fluorescent labels for other groupings is so far less well developed. The use of the reagent 4-dichloro-s-triazinyl-1-ethoxynaphthalene for hydroxyl groups appears to be a most useful development. It has been used successfully to assay the β-blocking drug tolamolol [37]. Dunges [31] has proposed the use of 4-bromomethyl-7-methoxy-coumarin for assaying compounds containing carboxylic acid groups. It is to be hoped that a number of suitable fluorescent labels will be available before long. As it is unlikely that they will all be capable of reacting under very mild conditions, the parallel development of

fluorescamine   a pyrrolinone

micro-sample techniques for derivatization, probably along the lines described by Dunges [31], will be necessary.

Fluorescence derivatization alone generally gives a rather poor specificity compared with chemically induced fluorescence methods, thus putting great onus on separation techniques either prior or subsequent to the derivatization reaction. Separation is usually achieved by TLC followed by direct measurement of the fluorescence intensity on the plate, although HPLC separation with use of a fluorescence detector may provide a most attractive alternative. Devices for measuring fluorescence on TLC plates are available as attachments for the majority of commercially available spectrophotometers. Many of these devices unfortunately make very inefficient use of the emitted light, and most scanning densitometers are generally equally useful or better for estimating fluorescence intensity on plates. In order to achieve the best results a fluorescent standard should be run on each plate. Considerable improvements in sensitivity can often be achieved by wetting the plate with triethanolamine, liquid paraffin, or buffer, to make it more transparent just prior to estimating the fluorescence intensity.

iv) Enzyme-linked assays

Drugs which are substrates for dehydrogenase enzymes can be assayed by determining the fluorescence of the cofactors $NADH_2$ or $NADPH_2$. Very high sensitivities can be obtained in this manner. Guilbault [43] has suggested that this approach could provided a basis for many drug

$$NAD \qquad NADH_2$$
$$non\text{-}fluorescent \quad (\lambda_{ex} \ 340, \ \lambda_{fl} \ 460)$$
$$AH_2 \rightleftharpoons \underset{dehydrogenase}{\rightleftharpoons} A$$

assays. Drugs which inhibit dehydrogenases could also be estimated using the above principle. Similarly, drugs which inhibit hydrolytic enzymes could be estimated by their effects on the reaction:-

The enzymes concerned in drug metabolism may be measured fluorimetrically using similar techniques [44].

$$conjugate\text{-}O \overset{hydrolytic}{\underset{enzyme}{\longrightarrow}} \ ^-O \quad + \ conjugate$$

very weak fluorescence *strongly fluorescent*

b) Phosphorescence assay methods

The structural requirements for a molecule to phosphoresce are somewhat different from those for fluorescence, although many molecules display both fluorescence and phosphorescence. Excitation from a lone pair of electrons (rather than π-electrons) favours phosphorescence. Halogens and heavy metal ions, wherever substituted, and nitro groups if inserted close to the electrons being excited, also enhance phosphorescence by encouraging inter-system crossing from the excited singlet state (from which fluorescence normally occurs) to the excited triplet state which is the prerequisite to phosphorescence. The excited triplet is far more stable (msec to sec) than the excited singlet state (10^{-8}-10^{-9} sec) and is therefore much more vulnerable to collisional quenching. As a consequence, phosphorescence is seldom observed in solution while it may be intense in a solid matrix. The most effective means of sample preparation for phosphorescence is to freeze the material being assayed to 77°K with liquid nitrogen. Normally this is achieved by placing a solution of the material in a thin round quartz sample tube which is then immersed in liquid nitrogen contained in a Dewar flask bearing an optically transparent window (Fig. 3).

A solvent which forms a clear glass on freezing is needed to obtain reliable results: ethanol, diethyl ether, isopentane or a mixture of these is commonly employed. In order to study the phosphorescence of ionized molecules, ethanolic hydrochloric acid or ethanolic potassium hydroxide can be used. Although this approach is useful, it suffers from the drawbacks of severely restricting the solvent choice and of bubbles in the liquid nitrogen around the sample causing interference with the phosphorescence signal. Considerable improvements in reproducibility over that of commercially available equipment are achieved by rapid rotation of the sample tube. The recent introduction of microcapillary tubes now permits aqueous solutions to be assayed [45]. Gifford and co-workers [46] have developed an attachment for spectrofluorimeters which enables phosphorescence to be measured directly on TLC plates. The device (Fig. 4) consists of a metal- or plastic-backed TLC plate wrapped around a copper drum containing the liquid nitrogen. Interestingly, spraying the TLC plate with a solvent such as ethanol just prior to placing it around the drum usually produces a dramatic increase in both sensitivity and reproducibility, as found in TLC fluorimetry [47]. Considerable qualitative use has been made of

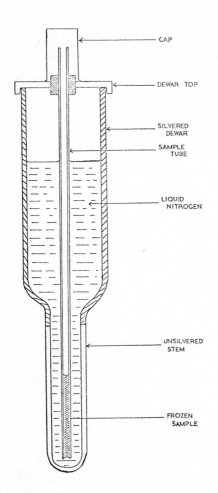

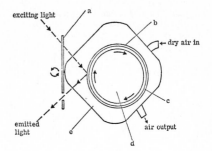

Fig. 4 *(above)*. TLC phosphorimeter, enabling fluorimetry or phosphorimetry to be performed directly on plastic- or metal-backed TLC plates or on other surfaces such as cellulose acetate strips. *From ref. [9], with acknowledgement to Ciba Foundation.*
a, Single-disc phosphoroscope, rotating in the direction shown by *arrows*;
b, TLC plate, wrapped round a slowly rotating motor-driven copper drum, c, containing liquid nitrogen d; e is a dry airtight box which prevents water condensation on the plate.

Fig. 3 *(left)*. Phosphorescence attachment for a spectrofluorimeter, consisting of a Dewar/sample-tube assembly.

TLC phosphorimetry, usually by merely dipping TLC plates into liquid nitrogen. For example, it has been used to detect purine antimetabolites in ng amounts [48]. Its value as a qualitative technique is a clear pointer to its potential quantitative application. The half-lives of phosphorescence emissions range from msec to sec. It is therefore possible to ascertain the half-lives of phosphorescence of many drugs by means of a simple mechanical light chopper which alternately allows light to reach the sample, then interrupts the exciting light path and permits any emitted light to reach the photodetector. By carefully selecting the chopper speed it is often possible to determine the phosphorescence of a particular component in a drug mixture. The potential of this approach can be realized by examining the phosphorescence lifetimes of some drugs as cited in Table 4. Half-lives are valuable criteria for identification, particularly when used in conjunction with λ_{ex}, λ_{fl}, λ_p and the ratio of fluorescence intensity to phosphorescence intensity. Employing a light chopper also eliminates interference from scatter and fluorescence (which are prompt emissions). Spurious phosphorescence from solvents and reagents involved in the work-up procedure is often the factor which imposes limitations on the sensitivity obtained. Precautions such as pre-washing of TLC plates can reduce this interference.

Table 4. Native phosphorescence of some drugs.

Compound	λ_{ex}	λ_p	Decay time	Conditions*	Sensitivity limit,μg/ml	Ref.
Amphetamine	270,335	385	10.6	EW	-	9
Aspirin	240	380	2.1	EPA	0.1	24
Atropine		410	1.4	ethanol	0.1	24
Benzocaine	310	430	3.4	ethanol	0.007	24
Chlordiazepoxide	310,320	450,470	0.16	EW	-	9
Chlorpromazine	335	495	0.072	EW	-	9
Chlorprothixene	260,310,385	470	0.2	EW		9
Cocaine	240	400	2.7	ethanol	0.01	24
Codeine	275	505	0.3	ethanol	0.01	24
Diazepam	290, 325	440,470,510	0.070	EW	-	9
Dicumarol	305	475	0.6	ethanol	0.001	24
Dopamine	270	420	0.4	ethanol	1.0	24
Ephedrine	225	390	3.6	ethanol	0.2	24
Iprindole	310	425,450,485	5.3	EW	-	9
Iproniazid	300,370	440		EW	-	9
Lidocaine	2.5	400	1.1	ethanol	1.2	24
Morphine	285	500	0.3	ethanol	0.01	24
Papaverine	260	480	1.5	ethanol	0.0005	24
Phenacetin	410	499	-	EPA	0.002	24
Phenobarbitone	240	380	1.	ethanol	0.10	24
Procaine-HCl	310	430	3.5	ethanol	0.01	24
Quinine-HCl	340	500	1.3	ethanol	0.04	24
Strychnine phosphate	290	440	1.2	ethanol	0.05	24
Sulphacetamide	280	410	1.3	ethanol	0.0001	24
Triflupromazine	345	510,520	0.072	EW	-	9
Thioridazine	335	500	0.066	EW	-	9
Warfarin	305	460	0.8	ethanol	0.01	9

* EW is 50% ethanediol-water.
EPA is diethyl ether : isopentane : ethanol (5 : 5 : 2 by vol.)

Aspirin was one of the first drugs to be assayed phosphorimetrically following its chloroform extraction from plasma. Background interference in this case was found to be mainly from tyrosine and tryptophan [49]. Maximum phosphorescence backgrounds of ether extracts from blood are found at pH 5, as compared with pH 6-7 from urine extracts [50].

Many widely used drugs are phosphorescent. Assays for a number of drugs have already been devised. At present all of these assays are based on the estimation of native phosphorescence. In some instances (such as those in which large quantities of scatter materials are unavoidably present) derivatization with a phosphor such as *p*-nitrophenol to produce a more strongly phosphorescent molecule could be of considerable value. The complementary nature of phosphorimetry and fluorimetry is nicely illustrated by the luminescence analysis of the anticoagulants. For diphenadine, phenindione, tromexan and dicoumarol, phosphorimetry was found to be most sensitive, with detection limits of 1.0, 1.0, 0.01 and 0.001 µg/ml respectively, whereas for warfarin fluorimetry was the most sensitive with a detection limit of 1.0 ng/ml [51].

Fluorescence and phosphorescence may also be used effectively in conjunction with each other. For example, the characterization and determination of the cannabinols and their metabolites has been achieved by a study of the absorption, fluorescence and phosphorescence spectra. Detection limits were of the order of 10 ng/ml [52].

An indication of the potential scope of phosphorimetry may be gleaned from a study of the phosphorescence of 37 antimetabolites. Analytically useful phosphorescence was displayed by 17 of the drugs, and in each case the sensitivity compared favourably with that obtained by colorimetric and enzymic assay methods [53]. Compounds bearing a purine nucleus frequently display a particularly impressive phosphorescence, with detection limits in the sub-nanogram range. These sensitivities could probably be further improved by employing a signal accumulation device.

OTHER APPLICATIONS OF LUMINESCENCE PROPERTIES OF DRUGS

Fluorescence methods may be used to assess the binding of drugs to macromolecules. In addition to the probe approach cited for warfarin *(see above)*, light polarizers may also be employed effectively for studying macromolecular interactions. Free molecules of a fluorescent drug will be able to rotate about their axes between absorbing polarized light and giving up their energy; therefore the emitted fluorescence will be non-polarized. In contrast, when they are bound to macromolecules the rotation will be comparatively slow and the fluorescence will therefore remain polarized. An interesting possible application of this approach is for drug immunoassay by a non-RIA method. On adding a specific antiserum which is saturated with the fluorescent-tagged drug to a biological sample containing the untagged drug, and determining the reduction in polarized fluorescence, the amount of drug present may be measured.

References

1. Williams, R.T. & Bridges, J.W., *J. Clin. Path. 17* (1964) 371-394.

2. King, L.A., Miller, J.N., Thorburn-Burns, D. & Bridges, J.W., *Anal. Chim. Acta 68* (1974) 205-206.

3. Duggan, D.E. & Udenfriend, S., *J. Biol. Chem. 223* (1956) 313-319.

4. Sawicki, E., Stanley, T.W. & Elbert, W.C., *Talanta 11* (1964) 1433-1441.

5. Parker, C.A. & Barnes, W.J. *Analyst 82* (1967) 606-618.

6. Stryer, L., *Science, 162* (1968) 526-533.

7. Weber, G., *Nature 180* (1957) 1409.

8. Bridges, J.W., in *Handbook of Analytical Toxicology* (Sunshine, I., ed.), CRC, Ohio (1969) pp. 909-930.

9. Bridges, J.W., in *The Poisoned Patient: the Role of the Laboratory, Ciba Found. Symp. 26* [ASP/Elsevier, Amsterdam] (1974) 171-187.

10. Feigl, F., Feigl, H.E. & Goldstein, D., *J. Amer. Chem. Soc. 77* (1955) 4162-4163.

11. Brodie, B.B., Udenfriend, S., Dill, W. & Chenkil, T., *J. Biol. Chem. 168* (1947) 319-325.

12. Gifford, L.A., Miller, J.N., Phillips, D.L., Thorburn-Burns, D. & Bridges, J.W., *Anal. Chem. 47* (1975) 1699-1701.

13. Gifford, L.A., Hayes, W.P., King, L.A., Miller, J.N., Thorburn-Burns, D. & Bridges, J.W., *Anal. Chem. 46* (1974) 94-99.

14. Westlund, D. & Borg, K.O., *Anal. Chim. Acta 67* (1973) 89-98.

15. Westlund, D. & Borg, K.O., *Anal. Chim. Acta 67* (1973) 99-106.

16. McPherson, F.J., Bridges, J.W. & Parke, D.V., *Nature 252* (1974) 488-489.

17. Adamson, R.H., Bridges, J.W., Evans, M.E. & Williams, R.T., *Biochem. J. 116* (1970) 437-443.

18. Bridges, J.W. & Williams, R.T., *Biochem. J. 107* (1968) 225-237.

19. Al Gailany, K.A.S., Wilson, A.G.E. & Bridges, J.W., *Trans. Biochem. Soc. 2* (1974) 113-117.

20. Bridges, J.W. & Wilson, A.G.E., in *Progress in Drug Metabolism, Vol. 1* (Bridges, J.W. & Chasseaud, L.F., eds.), Wiley, London (1976) pp. 193-247.

21. Azzi, A., *Quart. Rev. Biophys. 8* (1975) 237-316.

22. McClure, W.O. & Edelman, G.M., *Biochemistry 5* (1966) 1908-1918.

23. Udenfriend, S., *Fluorescent Assay in Biology and Medicine, Vol. 2,* Academic Press, New York (1969) 660 pp.

24. Hayes, T.S., *Clin. Chem. 19* (1973) 390-394.

25. Koechlin, B.A. & D'Ardonte, L., *Anal. Biochem. 5* (1963) 195-207.

26. Nadeau, G. & Sobolewski, G., *Canad. J. Biochem. Physiol. 36* (1958) 625-631.

27. Scales, B. & Assinder, D.A., *J. Pharm. Sci. 62* (1973) 913-917.

28. Ragland, J.W., Kinross-Wright, V.J. & Ragland, R.S., *Anal. Biochem. 12* (1965) 60-69.

29. Gugler, R. & Dengler, H.J., *Clin. Chem. 19* (1973) 36-37.

30. Haycock, R.P., Sheth, P.B., Connolly, R.J. & Mander, W.J., *J. Agric. Food Chem. 14* (1966) 437-440.

31. Dunges, W., *Anal. Chem.* (1976) *in press.*

32. Lawrence, J.F. & Frei, R.W., *Anal. Chem. 44* (1972) 2046-2049.

33. Valentour, J.C., Monforte, J.R. & Sunshine, I. (1974) *Clin. Chem. 20* (1974) 275-277.

34. Dunges, W. & Peter, H.W., in *Methods of Analysis of Anti-epileptic Drugs (ICS No. 286)* (Meijer, J.W.A., Meinardi, H., Gardner-Thorpe, C. & Van der Kleyn, E., eds.), Excerpta Medica, Amsterdam, pp. 126-133.

35. Just, W.W., Werner, G. & Weichmann, M., *Naturwiss. 59* (1972) 222.

36. Fourche, J., Jensen, H., Neuzil,E., *Anal. Chem. 48* (1976) 159-161.

37. Stopher, D.A., *J. Pharm. Pharmac. 27* (1975) 133-134.

38. Weeks, R.W., Yasuda, S.K. & Dean, B.J., *Anal. Chem. 48* (1976) 159-161.

39. De Silva, J.A.F., *Anal. Chem. 47* (1975) 714-718.

40. DeLeenheer, A., Sinsheimer, J.E. & Burckhalter, J.H., *J. Pharm. Sci. 62* (1973) 1370-1371.

41. Huang, K., Miller, J.N., Thorburn-Burns, D. & Bridges, J.W., *unpublished work.*

42. Udenfriend, S., Stein, S., Bohlem, P., Dairman, W., Leimgruber, W. & Weigele, M., *Science* 178 (1972) 871-872.

43. Guilbault, G.G., *Enzymatic Methods of Analysis,* Pergamon, Oxford (1970).

44. Bridges, J.W., in *The Fluorimetric Estimation of Enzymes* (Leaback, D., ed.), Elsevier, Amsterdam (1976) *in press.*

45. Lukasiewicz, R.F., Rozymes, R.A., Sanders, L.B. & Wineferdner, J.D., *Anal. Chem.* 44 (1972) 237-240.

46. Gifford, L.A., Miller, J.N., Thorburn-Burns, D. & Bridges, J.W., *J. Chromatog.* 103 (1975) 15-23.

47. Phillips, D., Gifford,L.A.,Miller, J.N. & Bridges, J.W., *unpublished work.*

48. Maddocks, J.L. & Davidson, G.C., *Brit. J. Clin. Pharmacol.* 2 (1975) 359-360.

49. Latz, H.W., *Ph.D. thesis,* Univ. of Florida, Gainesville (1963)..

50. McCarthy, W.J. & Winefordner, J.D., *Anal. Chim.* Acta 35 (1966) 120-123.

51. Hollifield, H.C. & Weinfordner, J.D., *Talanta* 14 (1967) 103-107.

52. Bowd, A., Bryom, P., Hudson, J.B. & Turnbull, J.H., *Talanta* 18 (1971) 697-705.

53. Sanders, L.B., Ceterelli, J.J. & Winefordner, J.D., *Talanta* 16 (1969) 407-408.

E-4   QUANTITATIVE TLC DETERMINATION OF DRUGS IN BIOLOGICAL FLUIDS

D.B. Faber
Laboratory of Toxicology & Biopharmacy, Dept. of Pharmacy,
Academic Hospital of the Free University,
De Boelelaan 1117, Amsterdam, The Netherlands

Achievement of optimal and safe dosage regimens for drugs calls for assay methods that are sensitive, rapid, specific, and not over-expensive. A special difficulty is that most drugs are extensively metabolized, so that the method must reveal the drug in the presence of structurally very similar compounds. The use of a radioisotopically labelled drug is helpful but is usually precluded in man. Classical bioanalytical methods have been reinforced by methods such as GC, densitometry, immunoassay, spectrofluorimetry, isotope-dilution techniques, HPLC, and stable-isotope techniques.

Quantitative TLC, whilst not universally applicable, ranks well by the various criteria. It can be performed semi-quantitatively, in an elution mode, or densitometrically. Each mode can vary widely in sensitivity and precision, as is discussed. Densitometry offers accuracy and precision that may be limited only by sample/application errors, and simplicity approaching that of visual methods. For selectivity and sensitivity, besides speed and simplicity, fluorodensitometry excels, and is more flexible than HPLC or GC. Its scope and limitations are indicated below. Only recently has attention been paid to improving TLC materials, sample application, running conditions, fluorescence strength of compounds, and precision of detection. Densitometry is coming to the forefront in quantitative TLC, and will undergo further improvement.

New therapeutic agents, especially if chemically similar to natural bioconstituents, can entail problems with interfering substances. Differences among patients in dosage regimen, metabolism and interactions call for improvements in sample preparation and separation, and also in detection and data-handling to increase sensitivity, specificity and precision. Amongst systems that can cope with sub-nanogram levels (Table 1), immunoassay, HPLC, GC and TLC densitometry offer the requisite sensitivity and/or specificity due to the separation capability. Such methods are becoming more widely applied to pharmaceutical and pharmacological problems. The micro-assay of drugs in biological materials has been well reviewed [1].

As instanced by digitoxine (p.247; cf. [2]), endogenous counterparts of drugs not only may be structurally similar but are fairly constant in concentration, hence their ratio to the drug may vary with time from 10^{-3} to 10^3 or even more. A further problem arises from possible chemical or biological degradation of the drug during storage, besides the presence of biological material in the sample.

Scheme 1 summarizes possible improvements in separation-detection methods, e.g. in the sensitivity of TLC-densitometry through new chemical reagents capable of converting various drugs into fluorophors [3-5] and reagents labelled with [^{3}H] of high specific activity. In RIA, more specific antigens are desirable.

Table 1. Usual sensitivities of measurement procedures.

PROCEDURE	DETECTION LIMIT, g
Absorption spectrophotometry	
IR	10^{-5}
NMR	10^{-6}
Visible	10^{-7}
UV	10^{-7}
Spectrofluorimetry	10^{-9}
GC	
Thermal conductivity det'r	10^{-5}
FID	10^{-8}
ECD	10^{-11}
Radioisotope procedures	
Chromatogram scanning	10^{-9}
Liquid scintillation	10^{-11}
Scintillation counting, γ	10^{-9}
Enzyme assay	10^{-12}
Bioassay	10^{-12}
RIA	10^{-12}

QUANTITATIVE TLC

Most methods fall into one of three categories.

(1) 'Semi-quantitative' methods. These involve visual comparison with standards or, less frequently, correlations between spot area and amount.

(2) 'Elution' methods. Quantitation is 'off-line'.

(3) 'Densitometric' methods. Instrumental quantitation is performed directly on the plate.

Sensitivity and precision vary widely within each category, being determined largely by the properties of the compounds and the means of detection. They are poor, as is accuracy, for *(1)*; but the simplicity of operation lends itself to multi-sample screening, where generally a 'yes/no' decision is required. Approach *(2)* ranks well except for convenience, and the risk of incomplete recovery can be minimized by eluting without scraping the layer off the plate [6]. Approach *(3)* likewise ranks well, for convenience also; sensitivity is especially good with fluorodensitometry.

With both *(1)* and *(3)* the concentration of molecules per unit area of surface is measured. Through concentrating a given amount of material into a smaller spot, there is a gain in sensitivity and precision, these being limited by the ability to detect small amounts and to differentiate from the TLC-plate background.

Scheme 1. Sub-nanogram assays.

In the performance of —

∿ TLC densitometry
∿ HPLC
∿ GC-MS
∿ RIA

separation/detection may be improved by —

∿ new reagents to convert drugs into fluorophors
∿ specific detectors
∿ suitable detecting systems
∿ suitable quantitation methods.

TLC-DENSITOMETRY

Quantitation *in situ* is well established [7, 8], and when greatly improved chromatogram spectrophotometers came on the market about 15 years ago it became possible to determine substances absorbing in the range ∿200-800 nm or emitting visible light with UV excitation [9, 10, *inter alia*]. Improved conditions for sample application, TLC development and optical evaluation eventually allowed measurement of substances of average absorptivity down to 100 ng and of fluorescent substances down to ∿10 ng [11-14]. Variations in layer thickness affect quantitation, especially by transmittance [11, 12]. In the visible range, reflectance is the preferred approach, or simultaneous measurement by the two approaches [15].

Fluorescence measurement has the advantages that the reading is independent of spot area and is linearly related to concentration. Although no method is of universal application, fluorodensitometry warranted development because of its various advantages including the possibility of multi-sample work.

THEORETICAL ASPECTS OF IMPROVING TLC-DENSITOMETRY

For the sake of sensitivity and reliability especially, improvements are needed in:
— sample preparation, e.g. clean-up on the thin layer after initial extraction;
— liquid-liquid extraction, as affected by pH, electrolyte concentration, or use of mixed solvents;
— TLC material, through micro-particles and uniform particle size;
— sample application, of as much as 25-50 µl in therapy control or pharmacokinetic studies, or of only 50-500 nl to allow more standards and 'clean' extracts of samples to be run;
— running techniques insofar as they affect separation, sensitivity and spot shape;
— fluorogens, with due regard to intensity, specificity, excitation/emission properties, linearity, and detection limit;
— detection systems, entailing micro-scale approaches and micro-optics;
— data handling, to allow integration and faster and better calculation of peak areas, the calibration graph, and external/internal standards.

To achieve the foregoing, we have used the 'HPTLC' and 'PMD' approaches as now described.

HIGH-PERFORMANCE TLC (HPTLC)

The silica gel 60 HPTLC plates (Merck, Darmstadt) differ from conventional plates in having a reduced and more homogeneous particle size and a somewhat thinner layer, giving a packing which in terms of density compares with a well packed HPLC column. Scaled-down TLC with these features brings 'high performance': resolution is high through the very small plate height; small application volumes allow multi-sample running; detection sensitivity is high; proper exploitation of the technique can keep spot travel to only a few cm, with shortened analysis times. Only 10-100 nl need be applied, suitably by micro-capillaries with a Merck applicator and with a lower volume for standards than for biological samples. Streaks may be applied, say 1 µl along 80 mm. Spots of <1 mm usually diffuse to no more than 3 mm when run. An eluent migration distance of 30-60 mm suffices, entailing a much shorter running time than with comparable non-HPTLC pre-coated plates [Ripphahn, 16] although there is a lowering by $\sim\frac{1}{3}$ of the velocity coefficient κ (mm²/sec) = (distance from solvent front to solvent surface in the trough)²/running time for this distance.

PROGRAMMED MULTIPLE DEVELOPMENT (PMD)

PMD, which we used to improve sensitivity and precision, is an automatic cyclic method entailing repeated development of a conventional TLC plate with the same solvent in the same direction, with intervening controlled evaporation (Fig. 1). The development time is 'programmed' to increase with successive development cycles (Fig. 2), whereas it is fixed in conventional multiple development. Fig. 3 shows 'spot re-

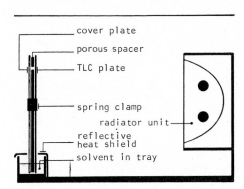

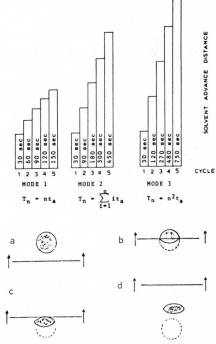

Fig. 1. Solvent removal from the TLC plate, still in the reservoir and $\sim$12 cm distant from and centered with respect to the radiator.

Fig. 2 *(top right)*. The development time may be programmed to increase as a function of cycle number *(see text)* in one of 3 modes. T_n = development time during the nth cycle; t_a = a user-selected unit time. Between developments the plate is either heated or 'blown' down with nitrogen till the solvent front recedes past the origin.

Fig. 3 *(right)*. Spot re-concentration in each of the brief development steps, without sacrifice of centre-to-centre separation between spots. As the advancing solvent, a, traverses a spot, the bottom molecules begin to move, b, while the top molecules remain in place. By the time the front has traversed the spot, c, it has been reduced to $(1-R_f)$ of its former width, d.

concentration', this being the most important feature of PMD. It occurs twice during each development cycle — during solvent advance and then during solvent removal,with shrinkages of comparable magnitude (Fig. 3, *Legend*) in the two solvent movements. Many cycles can be programmed within a reasonable time, usually 30 min, without sacrifice of the centre-to-centre separation between spots; hence the top-to-bottom width of spots is typically as little as 1-2 mm [17].

Since conventional TLC plates are used in PMD, essentially any technique that is applicable to concentional TLC will serve also for PMD. For quantitative work the main advantages of PMD are:
1. Better signal-to-noise (S/N) ratio due to the re-concentration and narrower spots.
2. High resolution over a small separation distance: cis/trans isomers and positional isomers are routinely separable.
3. Feasibility of ultra-low level assay with semi-micro technology.
4. Smaller sample size.
5. Less sample preparation.
6. Multi-sample analysis.
7. External standards usually suffice and can be the actual test compounds.
8. Saving of time.
9. Other savings - reagents, solvents, man-hours: e.g. in tissue furazolidone analyses, 6 persons can assay 36 samples per day including sample preparation, compared with 40 samples assayed by 30 persons in a week without PMD [18].

PRACTICAL ASPECTS OF IMPROVING TLC-DENSITOMETRY

Both the HPTLC and the PMD techniques can improve the S/N ratio, with benefit to sensitivity as well as to separation. With HPTLC, the smaller the amount applied, the better is the resolution. With PMD, spot re-concentration is the most important feature. Micro-HP-TLC plates combined with PMD may give the best results, especially with diluted biological material such as serum or extracts that needs large application volumes. With properly performed application [Kaiser, 16] and data handling [Hezel, 16], fluorimetry allows even 10 pg or lower to be detected. Thereby it will be possible to analyze biological material, especially serum/plasma or CSF, directly without sample preparation at the level of 0.1-10 µg/ml serum, and after sample preparation in the 0.1-100 ng range.

Taking account of the good linearity and reproducibility of TLC as reflected in the low S.D. for the overall process (application, development and fluorimetry), 8 or more samples (X) depending on the spot size can be run on one 10 × 20 cm plate with an external standard (S), e.g.: X_1, S_1, X_2, X_3, X_4, S_2, X_5, X_6, X_7, X_8. In TLC it is always better to measure in the direction of the solvent flow when non-resolved substances are likewise similar in absorption or fluorescence maxima. With sufficiently great resolution, $R_s \gg 1.5$, then measurement at right angles to the solvent flow has some advantages: a better blank correction is obtained in the direct surroundings of the spot and more spots can be measured per unit time with only one instrument setting, giving higher statistical assurance, and moreover the use of the optimal wavelength for each substance increases sensitivity. However, in PMD the re-concentration of the spots into narrow bands entails measuring in the direction of solvent flow. TLC-densitometry contrasts with GC in that the sample can be applied directly, and with HPLC in that there is less decrease in sensitivity.

ILLUSTRATIVE EXPERIMENTS: CARBAMAZEPINE IN SERUM

Amongst the many reported approaches to the assay of carbamazepine in body fluids are GC [e.g. 19], spectrophotometry [e.g. 20], TLC [e.g. 21], HPLC [22] and GC-MS [23]. Generally some procedure has to be employed for extracting the drug,from serum or plasma volumes of at least 0.5 ml. Occasionally a direct application of serum (1 µl) to a TLC plate has been performed [e.g. 24]. Recent progress in TLC-densitometry of the drug can be taken further by use of HPTLC and/or PMD, through lowering of the detection limit, better separation, and direct application of diluted serum or CSF to the plate.

An impression is now given of results obtained both with HP-TLC using the micro material with with PMD, for serum carbamazepine as an example. Measurement was performed with a Zeiss Chromatogram Spectrophotometer (KM3) and Autolab Computing Integrator. Fluorescence was generated by treatment with HCl vapour under the influence of UV light.

Firstly we used normal pre-coated thin layers on either glass or aluminium and compared PMD with conventional TLC (single development). PMD on aluminium gave the best separation of carbamazepine and its metabolites and the highest S/N ratio (Fig. 4). Linearity was good. Then we compared PMD with conventional TLC using micro-thin layers on glass (Fig. 5) or aluminium, applying 1-5 ng (0.2 or 2 µl). It appeared that PMD with the high-performance material on aluminium gave especially concentrated spots as needed for a good S/N ratio.

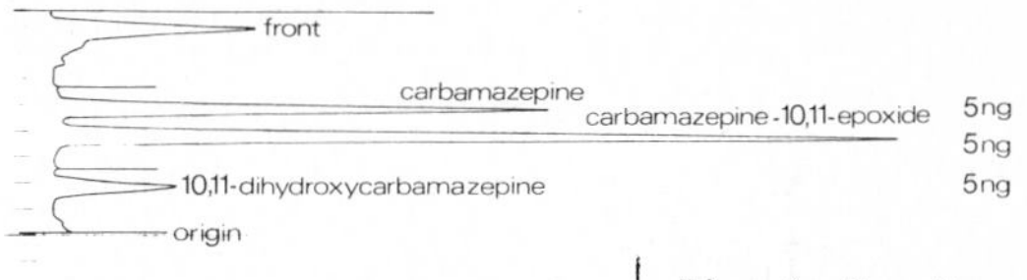

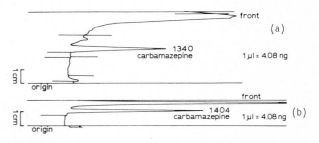

Fig. 4. Densitogram showing PMD separation of carbamazepine and its metabolites with a normal thin layer on aluminium. *The load volumes were 1-5 µl.*

In the PMD runs the chosen operating conditions [25] entailed use of chloroform : acetone (80 : 60) as solvent. For normal thin-layer aluminium, and for the micro material on glass (*in parentheses if different*), the conditions were:
MODE I: cycles 6, 30 (50) sec advance, power 0%
                      30 (40) sec removal, power 40% (60%).
MODE III: cycles 3, 50 sec advance, power 0%
                      40 sec removal, power 50% (60%).
These conditions may be especially suitable for some biological material but need further exploration. PMD allows a higher application volume and a better clean-up on the TLC plate. Direct application of 1 µl of an unknown serum dilu-

---

Fig. 5. Densitogram showing the separation of carbamazepine by HPTLC on glass, (a) with conventional development, (b) with PMD.

Fig.7 *(bottom right)*. Densitogram showing the separation of carbamazepine and its metabolites by normal TLC on aluminium.
(a) Standard.
(b) Serum.

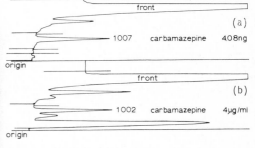

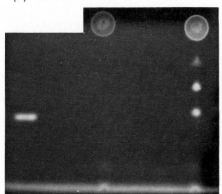

Fig. 6 *(left)*. Separation of carbamazepine and its metabolites after direct application of serum; normal thin-layer on aluminium.

diluted with 2 μl of distilled water gives a separation (Figs. 6 & 7) as good as after application of the serum extract. This TLC approach for carbamazepine can become a sensitive, rapid, selective and simple assay for routine serial analyses [26].

CONCLUSIONS

TLC-densitometry is becoming the commonest quantitative approach. TLC-fluorodensitometry can furnish a really specific and sensitive assay method, with good precision and accuracy; unlike GC and HPLC, it enables the serum to be loaded directly, subject to the detection limit. This could be improved 1,000-fold, down to ≪10^{-12} g, by use of extraction and by combining HPTLC with PMD, if the physical properties are favourable. Densitometric methods being specific and flexible, they facilitate drug interaction studies in adults and very small children given more than one drug.

References

1. Maickel, R.P., *Critical Revs. in Clin. Lab. Sciences 4* (1973) 383-420.

2. Faber, D.B. & Kok, A. de, *submitted for publication*.

3. Ackerman, H.S. & Udenfriend, S., *Fluorimetry*, in *Handbook of Experimental Pharmacology 28, Pt. 2* (Brodie, B.B. & Gilette, J.K., eds.), Springer-Verlag, Berlin (1971) 21-41.

4. Udenfriend, S., *Fluorescence Assay in Biology and Medicine, Vol. 2*, Academic Press, New York (1969), 660 pp.

5. Udenfriend, S., Stein, S., Böhlen, P., Dawman, W., Leimgruber, W. & Neigele, M., *Science 178* (1972) 871-872.

6. Falk, H. & Krummen, K., *J. Chromatog. 103* (1975) 279-288.

7. Stahl, E. (ed.), *Dünnschicht-Chromatographie*, 2nd edn., Springer, Berlin (1967).

8. Jork, H., *Z. Anal. Chem. 221* (1966) 17-32.

9. Goodall, R.R., *J. Chromatog. 103* (1975) 265-278.

10. Ebel, S. & Herold, G., *Chromatographia 8* (1975) 35-37.

11. Seiler, N. & Möller, H. *Chromatographia 2* (1969) 273-280, 319-324, 470-475.

12. Jork, H., *J. Chromatog. 82* (1973) 85-94.

13. Faber, D.B., Mulder, C. & Man in't Veld, W.A., *J. Chromatog. 100* (1974) 55-61.

14. MacNeil, J.D. & Hikichi, M., *J. Chromatog. 101* (1974) 33-37.

15. Hezel, U., *Chimia 28* (1974) 407-410.

16. Kaiser, R.E. (ed.), *Einführung in die Hochleistungs-Dunnschicht-Chromatographie* Inst. für Chromatographie, Bad Dürkheim (1976).   *Includes articles by:* Ripphahn, J.; Kaiser, E.; Hezel, U.; pp. 182-207, 12-49 & 117-181 respectively.

17. Perry, J.A., Jupille, T.H. & Curtice, A., *Separation Sci. 10* (1975) 571-591.

18. Hiotis, J.P. *(Norwich Pharmaceutical Co., New York), Personal communication.*

19. Mashford, M.L., Ryan, P.L. & Thomson, W.A., *J. Chromatog. 89* (1974) 11-15.

20. Beyer, K.H. & Klinge, D., *Arzneim.-Forsch. 19* (1969) 1759-1760.

21. Breyer, U., *J. Chromatog. 108* (1975) 370-374.

22. Gauchel, G., Gauchel, F.D. & Birkhofer, L., *Z. Klin. Chem. Klin. Biochem. 6* (1973) 127-131.

23. Palmer, L., Bertilsson, L., Collste, P. & Rawlins, M., *Clin. Pharmacol. Ther. 14* (1973) 827-832.

24. Hundt, H.K.L. & Clark, E.C., *J. Chromatog. 107* (1975) 149-154.

25. Perry, J.A., Haag, K.W. & Glunz, L.J., *J. Chromatog. Sci. 11* (1973) 447-453.

26. Faber, D.B. & Koster, J., *unpublished work*.

E-5 HPLC CAPABILITIES AS EXEMPLIFIED BY PORPHYRIN ESTER ASSAY

S.A. Matlin[*], A.H. Jackson and N. Evans
Chemistry Department, University College, Cardiff CF11XL.

Attention has been focused on factors affecting HPLC detection and resolution, in connection with separating porphyrin esters. The design of a low-cost and reproducible gradient-elution system has enabled porphyrins to be quantitated in the urine of normal and porphyric humans. In conjunction with field-desorption MS, HPLC constitutes a powerful and rapid tool for analysis. Preparative applications and the use of fluorimetric detectors and ion-exchange chromatography have also been examined.

The objective was to develop a rapid, quantitative assay of the porphyrins present in urine. There are a number of conditions, including hereditary porphyrias and alcohol poisoning, in which excretion of porphyrins is greatly increased and the establishment of the porphyrin patterns characteristic of each condition is of diagnostic value [1].

Protoporphyrin IX (3) is a tetrapyrrolic, macrocyclic pigment which serves as the iron-carrying group in haemoglobin. Its biosynthesis involves the condensation of four units of a precursor pyrrole (porphobilinogen) to form uroporphyrin III (1). The acetate side-chains of the latter are enzymatically decarboxylated in a sequential fashion [2] to give coproporphyrin III (2) which then suffers a further oxidative decarboxylation of two of the four propionate side-chains to furnish protoporphyrin IX. *(The double arrows signify a reaction sequence.)*

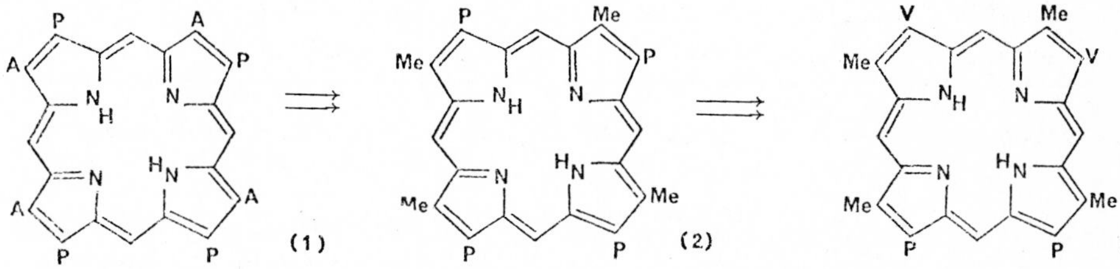

A = CH₂COOH

P = CH₂CH₂COOH

V = CH₂=CH₂

APPROACHES

Porphyrins have an intense UV absorption maximum at around 400 nm (Soret band) with an extinction coefficient in excess of 100,000. In developing an HPLC analysis of porphyrins a Cecil variable-wavelength UV detector was selected to take advantage of this. For convenience of handling and analysis the porphyrins were separated adsorptively as their methyl esters. Isocratic (i.e. non-gradient) elution (Fig.1) gave a good separation, the polarity of the compounds varying with the number of ester groups attached. However, this analysis suffers from the disadvantage that an increase in flow rate is required to elute the more polar components in a reasonably short time and to reduce peak broadening; a concomitant decrease in sensitivity of detection results for the later peaks. To overcome this problem, a gradient elution analysis was developed.

[*]
Present address: Chemistry Department, The City University, London EC1V 4PB.

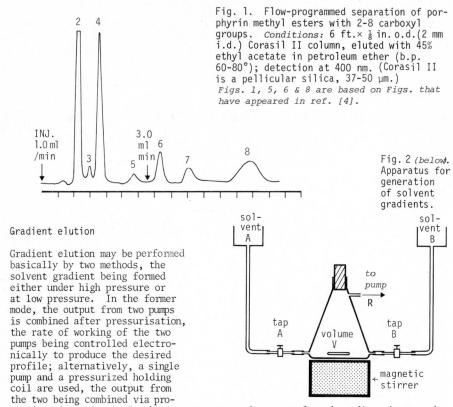

Fig. 1. Flow-programmed separation of porphyrin methyl esters with 2-8 carboxyl
groups. *Conditions:* 6 ft.× ⅛ in.o.d.(2 mm
i.d.) Corasil II column, eluted with 45%
ethyl acetate in petroleum ether (b.p.
60-80°); detection at 400 nm. (Corasil II
is a pellicular silica, 37-50 μm.)
*Figs. 1, 5, 6 & 8 are based on Figs. that
have appeared in ref. [4].*

Fig. 2 *(below)*.
Apparatus for
generation
of solvent
gradients.

Gradient elution

Gradient elution may be performed
basically by two methods, the
solvent gradient being formed
either under high pressure or
at low pressure. In the former
mode, the output from two pumps
is combined after pressurisation,
the rate of working of the two
pumps being controlled electro-
nically to produce the desired
profile; alternatively, a single
pump and a pressurized holding
coil are used, the output from
the two being combined via pro-
portionating valves. In the low-pressure mode, a pre-formed gradient is passed
through a single pump, which must hence be of low internal volume. The gradient
may be generated with the aid of programmed flow valves which supply separate solvents to a low-volume mixing chamber before the pump, or by using arrangements of
simple glass mixing vessels and reservoirs.

In view of the availability of a Waters 6000M pump, which is of the low
internal volume reciprocating type, an exploration was made of the last-named of
these methods, which is also the cheapest.

The mixing chamber (Fig. 2) consists [3] of a stoppered conical flask to
which three side-arms have been joined. Reservoirs of solvents A and B are connected to the two lower side-arms via glass taps and PTFE tubing, and the mixing chamber is filled initially with solvent A. Elution is commenced with tap A open and
tap B closed, the stirred contents of the flask being drawn directly into the pump.
When it is desired to commence the gradient, tap A is closed and tap B immediately
opened. The concentration of solvent B in the mixture then emerging from the mixing
vessel increases with time (t) in an exponential manner, depending on the volume (V)
of the mixing chamber and the flow rate (R) according to the equation:

$$\% \text{ B in mixture} = 100(1 - e^{-\frac{Rt}{V}}) \qquad \textit{(Equation 1)}$$

Examples of gradients are shown in Fig. 3. Agreement between calculated and
experimental gradients was found to be very good (within 1% at all points), giving
highly reproducible analyses of mixtures on chromatography. Alterations in gradient

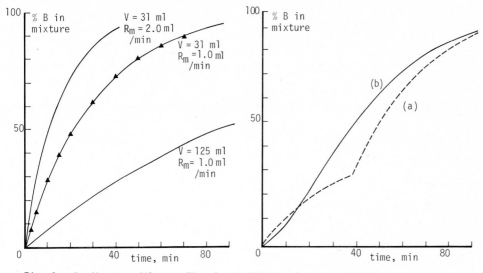

Fig. 3. Gradient profiles produced by mixing vessel. ——, calculated gradients; ▲, experimental points.

Fig. 4. Modified solvent gradients. (a) ————, consecutive use of two solvent mixtures: with pure A in the mixing flask a 4:1 mixture of A & B is added, followed after 37 min by pure B; flow rate 1.0 ml/min. (b) ——, two mixing flasks in series, vols. 16 and 32 ml; flow rate 1.0 ml/min.

profile (Fig. 4) can readily be made, making the system versatile as well as reliable and cheap.

Application of this gradient-forming system to a mixture of standard porphyrin esters gave rapid and complete resolution, with full sensitivity of detection maintained throughout (Fig. 5).

ANALYSES ON URINE, WITH FIELD-DESORPTION MS TO CHECK IDENTITIES

In carrying out chromatographic analysis of mixtures from natural sources, it is always advantageous to have available independent evidence of the identity of components present, so that total reliance is not placed on chromatographic retention data alone. A particularly valuable technique in the present case, where the compounds present are non-volatile and of relatively high molecular mass, is field desorption (FD) mass spectrometry, a 'soft' ionisation technique which produces little or no fragmentation, making it very easy to identify molecular ion groupings in complex mixtures. The FD spectrum of porphyrin methyl esters from the urine of a human porphyric patient [4] is given in Fig. 6 and shows the characteristic pattern for porphyrins with 4-8 carboxymethyl groups, the molecular ions being separated by intervals of 58 mass units.

An internal standard was required for absolute quantitation in the urine analyses, and as protoporphyrin IX is not present in urine a closely related compound, mesoporphyrin IX (4), as the dimethyl ester, was an appropriate choice. This has the merits that it elutes before all other components, is readily available, is stable, and has the characteristic intense Soret band in its

P = CH₂CH₂COOH

(4)

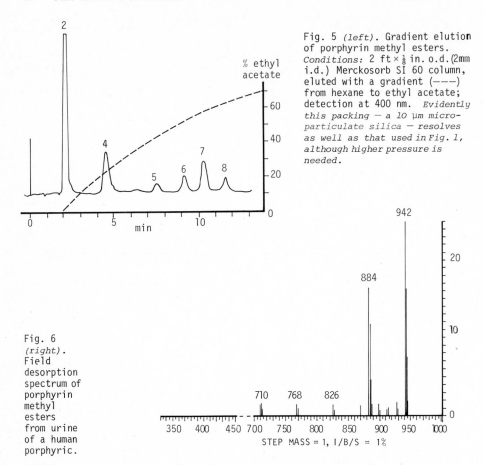

Fig. 5 *(left).* Gradient elution of porphyrin methyl esters. *Conditions:* 2 ft × ⅛ in. o.d. (2mm i.d.) Merckosorb SI 60 column, eluted with a gradient (———) from hexane to ethyl acetate; detection at 400 nm. *Evidently this packing — a 10 μm microparticulate silica — resolves as well as that used in Fig. 1, although higher pressure is needed.*

Fig. 6 (right). Field desorption spectrum of porphyrin methyl esters from urine of a human porphyric.

STEP MASS = 1, I/B/S = 1%

UV spectrum. Calibration graphs of mole ratio porphyrin/mesoporphyrin IX *versus* area ratio porphyrin/mesoporphyrin IX were obtained (Fig. 7), giving straight line plots in all cases.

Urine samples (50 ml) were extracted by a modification of a published proce-dure [5]. The sample was adjusted to pH 3.0, extracted once with Et acetate : *n*-BuOH (1:1) and then with further portions of *n*-BuOH until neither phase showed any fluo-rescence. The combined organic extracts were evaporated, esterified with 5% H_2SO_4 in methanol, and analyzed by HPLC.

Results obtained for urine samples obtained from four patients presenting clinical symptoms of porphyria are shown in Table 1. Patients 1-3 all have similar porphyrin patterns associated with symptomatic porphyria, whereas patient 4 exhibits an entirely different pattern and is believed to be suffering from a different complaint. Work is still in progress on the characterisation of porphyrin excretion patterns.

During the development of the above method, a number of variations in the chromatographic system were examined. The possibility of direct analysis of por-phyrin-free acids without esterification was explored, and Fig. 8 shows a separa-tion obtained by ion exchange. The mobile phase was chosen specifically to enable

HV 8078
73.L72

HF 5549.5→2

KF 9434.R5

RM 315.P62

RS 189.G83

QS 36.854 #28

LB840.A8

HF 5549.5.D7

G#V944

samples collected from the HPLC to be easily evaporated for further MS examination.

Fig. 9 shows an isocratic separation of porphyrin methyl esters with a fluorimetric detector coupled in sequence with the UV detector, both operating at maximum sensitivity. Porphyrins exhibit intense fluorescence in the visible region, which should in principle permit greater sensitivity than is obtainable with UV detection, but

Table 1. Analysis of urine samples from porphyric patients (designated *1-4*)

Porphyrin (cf. Fig.5)	Constituent as % of total, in 4 patients			
	1	2	3	4
8	65	57	57	11
7	27	31	36	3
6	3	2	4	1
5	2	4	2	9
4	3	6	1	76

in this case much of the potential improvement is lost owing to quenching by the organic mobile phase. This latter effect is also partly responsible for the unacceptably large solvent peak in the fluorescence trace, and presents problems in attempting to carry out gradient elution. These disadvantages should be avoided, and maximum benefit obtained, in the ion-exchange, fluorimeter-monitored analysis of porphyrin-free acids.

Fig. 7. Calibration graphs for porphyrin methyl esters, in different mole ratios to mesoporphyrin IX methyl ester as internal standard.

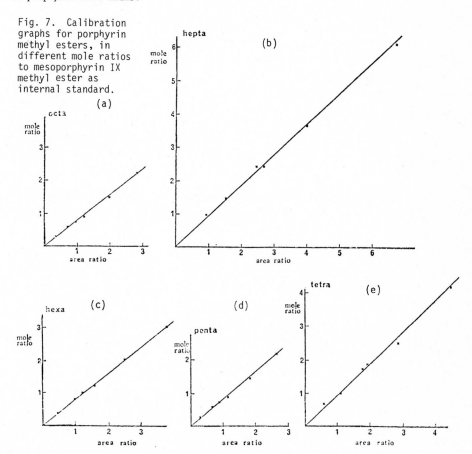

Other HPLC studies on urinary porphyrins include those in Gray's laboratory [6], where urinary porphyrins have been separated on microparticulate silica as methyl esters (or sometimes by reverse-phase HPLC), using a flow programming technique with isocratic elution similar to that described in the foregoing account and in an account appearing elsewhere [7].

Acknowledgements

We thank the Medical Research Council for financial support (to N.E.) and Dr. D. Dean (Department of Dermatology, Liverpool Royal Infirmary) for providing the urine samples. A grant from the Royal Society towards purchase of the HPLC equipment is gratefully acknowledged.

References

1. *"Porphyria - A Royal Malady"*. British Medical Association, London (1968).

2. Jackson, A.H., Sancovich, H.A., Ferramola, A.M., Evans, N., Games, D.E., Matlin, S.A., Elder, G.H. & Smith, S.G., *Phil. Trans. Roy. Soc. 273 B* (1975) 191-206.

3. Matlin, S.A. & Evans, N., *Chem. and Ind., submitted* (1975).

4. Evans, N., Games, D.E., Jackson, A.H. & Matlin, S.A., *J. Chromatog. 115* (1975) 325-333.

5. Fernandez, A.A., Henry, R.J. & Goldenberg, H., *Clin. Chem. 12* (1966) 463.

6. Gray, C.H., Lim, C.K. & Nicholson, D.C., in *High Pressure Liquid Chromatography in Clinical Chemistry* (Dixon, P.F., Gray, C.H., Lim, C.K. & Stoll, M.S., eds.), Academic Press, London (1976) 76-85.

7. Evans, N., Jackson, A.H., Matlin, S.A. & Towill, R. *As for* ref. 6.

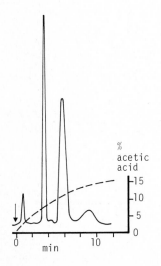

Fig. 8. Ion-exchange analysis of porphyrin di-, tetra- and penta-carboxylic acids. *Conditions:* 3 ft × ⅛ in. o.d. AS Pellionex SAX (a pellicular anion-exchanger) with a gradient (———) from methanol to acetic acid; detection at 400 nm.

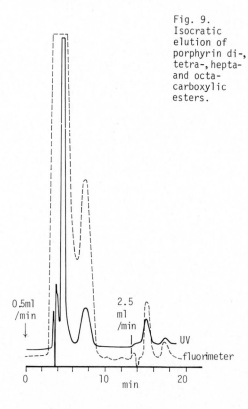

Fig. 9. Isocratic elution of porphyrin di-, tetra-, hepta- and octa-carboxylic esters.

E-NC$_{2-5}$ NOTES AND COMMENTS RELATING TO INSTRUMENTAL TECHNIQUES
(Arts. 2-5; for GC and GC/MS, see p. 9)

POLAROGRAPHIC TECHNIQUES

Polarographic assay - Art. 2 (W. Franklin Smyth & M.R. Smyth)

Remark by L.E. Martin.— The sensitivity of the anodic oxidation technique for catecholamines can be 100 pg/ml. *To* F. Battig *and* R.G. Muusze, *the authors answered:* We have no experience of the use of electrochemical detectors in HPLC. However, various workers *(cf. end of Art. T-2, and see ref. [7] cited in Art. G-1.—ED.)* including B. Fleet (Imperial College, London) and P.T. Kissinger (Purdue University, Indiana) and their collaborators have used solid indicator electrodes (e.g. glassy carbon) very effectively in conjunction with HPLC. These electrodes can detect many more oxidation processes than conventional mercury electrodes, and if surface contamination problems can be solved (particularly at the trace level), relatively low limits of detection will be feasible for assaying organic molecules in biological fluids.

Modes of polarographic/voltammetric analysis - *Editorial Note*

The incipient revival of polarographic methods for quantitative analysis [1] arises from technical advances which, seemingly, few practitioners have set down in plain, unambiguous language for the benefit of uninitiated persons such as the Editor. In a better-than-average exposition, Zuman [2] writes concerning classical *D.C. polarography*: "mean currents during the life of each [mercury] drop have been recorded and measured ... [but] at the 10^{-6} level, the capacity current becomes larger than the faradaic [diffusion-controlled] current and hence the determination of concentration became difficult." This problem is minimized in 'DPP', viz. the *differential* (as distinct from integral) mode of *pulse polarography*, which is explained in Art. E-2. During each operating interval in the DPP mode, the current is sampled twice: prior to applying a sudden burst of potential, and sufficiently late during the pulse "to allow the capacitive current to decay to a low value, [whereas] the faradaic current, although it also decays somewhat, still does not reach the diffusion-controlled level, [the outcome being a] difference current-curve, which is proportional to the concentration of material ... [and] has the appearance of a peak rather than the ususal polarographic step" [3].

In *A.C. polarography,* the signal due to capacitive current is suppressed not by letting it decay but by an alternative means which need not be considered here. This mode is advantageous where many electroactive species are present but, unlike DPP, is not equally sensitive to reversible and irreversible processes. Other modes to be noted merely in passing are *fast linear sweep voltammetry*, a D.C. polarography variant in which a single mercury drop is subjected to an unmodulated potential change, and *stripping voltammetry,* a technique relevant to metals rather than to drugs. (For amplied notes on pulse and other modes, see [1], e.g. Jee.)

The term 'voltammetry' (a 'voltammogram' is really a current *versus* voltage curve !) is not restricted to the use of the dropping mercury electrode that is usually connoted by the term 'polarography'. Stationary electrodes may be employed, as in a simplified D.C. voltammetry instrument (Bioanalytical Systems Inc.) suitable for many screening or assay applications. It incorporates 3 operational amplifiers, viz. a 'sweep generator', a 'potentiostat', and a 'current-to-voltage converter'. "Modern instruments incorporate a potentiostat which controls the potential right at the working electrode/solution interface, eliminating errors owing to solution resistance ... by making use of a three-electrode system" [3]: the key feature is a reference electrode, situated as close as possible to the working electrode.

Electrochemical detectors for flowing liquids such as HPLC effluents usually entail *hydrodynamic chronoamperometry*, with a fixed applied potential appropriate for the compound to be measured [4]. A thin-layer cell with a carbonaceous working electrode [1] is suitable. The current remains constant as long as the solute concentration, solution velocity, and other factors remain constant. Coulometric detectors, where there is complete electrochemical conversion of the compound, offer an alternative but entail complications which may outweigh their analytical advantages [4].

1. Barker, G.C., *& others, Proc. Analyt. Div. Chem. Soc. 12* (1975) 179-191.

2. Zuman, P., *Proc. Analyt. Div. Chem. Soc. 12* (1975) 199-208.

3. Flato, J.B., *Anal. Chem. 44* (1972) 75A-87A.

4. Riggin, R.M. & Kissinger, P.T., in *Laboratory Techniques in Electroanalytical Chemistry* (Kissinger, P.T., ed.), Dekker, New York, *in press*.

LUMINESCENCE TECHNIQUES - Art. E-3 (J.W. Bridges)

Replies to questions by J.V. Jackson: Have you striven to elucidate the nature of the compounds that give the so-called biological blank ? — Unfortunately, different components of a biological sample interfere in different assays; it appears that a cholesterol-like material may produce some of the biological blank fluorescence in the 'blue region'. Doesn't the universal nature of the 'biological blank' contradict your statement that only about 2% of compounds have a native luminescence ? — Not really; many compounds are present in extracts of biological material but only very few of these fluoresce.

Reply to J.S. Cridland.— De-gassing of solvent doesn't result in any major improvement in the 'cracking' of most solvents, although it does help with ethanol.   *Remark by* D.A. Stopher.— I have tried dansyl chloride for making a fluorescent derivative but without success due to formation of fluorescent breakdown products. 1-Ethoxy-4-(dichloro-s-triazinyl)naphthalene was found to be more useful.

QUANTITATIVE TLC - Art. E-4 (D.B. Faber; *see also* T-NC, p.246)

C.R. Jones *commented thus:* You have mentioned advantages of Programmed Multiple Development (PMD). Some of the disadvantages are worth mentioning:

a) Only single solvents are useful, because when running up a hot plate the more volatile constituents of a mixture tend to evaporate.
b) Many of the usual TLC solvents are too slow-running to be amenable to PMD.
c) The compounds must be stable to heat, unless gas drying is used.
d) Compounds of low R_f and of high R_f are difficult to deal with together on the same plate.
e) There may be a fire risk with some solvents.
f) It takes much effort to establish working systems.
g) The price is very high (£3,000).

Reply by D.B. Faber:
a) There is no restriction to single solvents; as in conventional TLC, reproducible results are obtained by discarding the solvent mixture remaining in the trough following each run and replacing it with fresh mixture stored in a capped container.
b) Solvent travel distance from origin to solvent front is approximately proportional to the square of elapsed time ($d \propto t^2$). With the high resolution of PMD, 5-8 cm usually suffices; ∿30 min is allowed for development - cf. the 45-60 min in conventional TLC.
c) PMD apparatus allows solvent removal with nitrogen in the case of heat-sensitive substances. Many compounds hitherto considered unstable have survived the PMD process (ref. [18] in Art. E-4), possibly due to the protective effect of the solvent vapour in the sandwich in tempering the effect of heat on the compounds *(personal communication)*. One should keep in mind that only a minority of compounds are thermostable and suitable for GC analysis; PMD with nitrogen aids quantitative TLC.

d) Compounds of high and low R_f present no problems, because after some pilot separations you can choose your optimal program for a solvent system. Firstly one experiments with the solvent system itself, both in conventional TLC and in PMD. It is worth consulting the work of Perry *et al.* (as cited) to get a true impression of the aim and basis of the separation technique.

e) This indeed needs to be considered. Since February 1974 Dr. J.P. Heotis and associates ([18] in Art. E-4) have processed >3,000 plates in the PMD mode without incident, using the following solvents (usually as combinations) with the developer placed in the hood: acetone, acetonitrile, benzene, chloroform, dichloroethane, ethyl acetate, hexane, cyclohexane, nitromethane, and also small amounts of formic or acetic acid or ammonia in some studies; diethyl ether was never used, as a matter of policy.

f) The extent of one's knowledge of the principles and practice of both conventional TLC and PMD, and of the physicochemical properties of the compounds to be analyzed, determines how long it will take to develop a suitable working system. Moreover, the flexibility of PMD programming allows rapid exploration of solvent/ program parameters and the solvent selection is not so critical as it is in conventional TLC.

g) The price is indeed £3,000, but another TLC unit can be connected to the same programmer as was bought in the first instance. Cost elements in analysis include manpower, time per analysis (real time), overheads, and solvents and reagents; cost falls with a rise in the number of assays, as where carbamazepine in diluted serum is determined directly on the plate (Art. E-4), and only the equipment cost at the outset is high.

B. Scales *enquired* whether, when using the PMD system, the line of 12 samples remains perfectly horizontal ? Is this an essential requirement when scanning from one side of the plate to the other ? *Reply by* D.B. Faber.— Reading from left to right on the plate discards the crucial advantage of PMD-TLC, viz. the tremendous enhancement of the signal/noise ratio caused by the spot re-concentration and high-resolution separation (over a short range) of similar compounds. With the narrow bands instead of spots in PMD, you always have to measure in the solvent direction. With suitable densitometric and data-handling equipment, drugs in biological media can be specifically determined at ultra-low levels with relatively small sample sizes, as instanced by carbamazepine (Art. E-4). *Reply to a further question by* B. Scales.— The choice amongst commercial aluminium-backed plates is not so important when using PMD, due to the markedly enhanced signal/noise ratio. The multiple sweeping of the plate moves impurities to the solvent front, preventing their interfering with the determination.

TLC quantitation by fluorimetry

Remarks by J.G. Allen (cf. D.B. Faber's contribution, Art. E-4): As compared with elution and off-line fluorimetry, direct scanning of TLC plates has both advantages and disadvantages, but can give reliable results with proper precautions. *Answer to* C.R. Jones: We do find it advantageous to use a densitometer slit-width similar in size to the diameter of the spot being measured, although some workers prefer the slit to be narrower than the spot. *Answer to* J.W. Bridges: We scan spots dry rather than wet because in actual analyses (where we spot 4 standards and 8 unknowns on the plate) it is difficult to maintain the better sensitivity that is obtainable by wet scanning. *Comment by* B.G. Muusze: In wet scanning, the amount of fluid on the silica layer can be stabilized merely by putting a quartz or glass plate on top of it.

HPLC AS AN ANALYTICAL TOOL *(See also Art. G-1 — ED.)*

HPLC, and field-desorption MS, as applied to porphyrins (S.A. Matlin, Art. E-5)

Question by F. Battig: Insofar as you stressed that the internal volume of the Waters M6000 pump is low, but we found it to be ∿2.5 µl such that trouble could arise with narrow-bore columns, what was the i.d. of the columns you used ? *Reply by* S.A. Matlin: For analytical work the i.d. was 2 mm. As we showed (Art. E-5), passage through the Waters pump does not spoil the gradient profiles as obtained by coupling the pump directly to a monitor (Cecil Insts.) which served to plot out automatically the gradient profile resulting from mixing a UV-absorbing solvent with a UV-transparent one in the apparatus illustrated.

Enquiry by B. Scales: Whilst the use of 400 nm for detection confers reasonable specificity to the assay, the use of ethyl acetate and butanol must extract very much extraneous material.— What happens to it ? Does it remain on the column and change the column characteristics, or does it elute because of the preliminary methylation procedure ? *Reply by* S.A. Matlin: Routinely we flush occasionally with an alcohol solvent, e.g. isopropranol. Because of the methylation step and of a gradient elution which finishes with a quite polar solvent, very little column contamination occurs, and we find column life to be very good. *Question by* J. Chamberlain: Insofar as porphyrins have a high molar absorption, and use of 400 nm solves many problems due to impurities, has any attempt been made to link porphyrins to other compounds for the assay of the latter ? *Reply:* I know of no attempts to use porphyrins as chromophoric groups in the assay of other materials. The idea is interesting, but many problems could arise because porphyrins are not very stable and suitable derivatives would be difficult to prepare.

Reply to D. Dell: In collecting samples for field desorption (FD) we did not usually find it necessary to purify normal laboratory-grade solvents. We generally obtained very clean spectra, and it is obviously advantageous that porphyrins are of relatively high molecular mass: for compounds where this is lower, we often re-distil solvents before use. *Question by* R.E. Majors: What is the limit of sensitivity of the FD-MS method when used with analytical HPLC columns ? *Reply:* The FD-MS spectrum shown (Art. E-5) was performed on a sample before HPLC injection, and served to indicate the range of compounds present, by virtue of the molecular ions that predominate in the FD spectrum. HPLC eluates must be evaporated down to a small volume ($\sim$10 µl); thereby, typical sample loads (e.g. 10 µg) can be detected.

HPLC analysis of biological samples *(See also Arts. G-1 & S-5 — ED.)*

Discussion following a paper by R.E. Majors *(Varian Associates; no publication text)* With UV detection, the best sensitivity obtained with a *non*-extracted standard without out running into 'noise' problems has been 10 ng per peak (R.E. Majors, *answering* A. Bye). *Remark by* R.G. Muusze: With biological samples in comparison with standards the larger injection volumes make a serious contribution to peak broadening. *Remark by* J.J. de Ridder: Crude plasma extracts prepared with hexane or ethyl acetate have caused us no trouble with 'Corasil II' (40-50 µm) columns, but only hexane extracts could be used with 'µ-Porasil' (5-10 µm) columns.

Section on General
Analytical strategy

G-1   CHROMATOGRAPHIC AND OTHER ASSAY APPROACHES

Eric Reid
Wolfson Bioanalytical Centre
University of Surrey, Guildford GU2 5XH, U.K.

*Complementing the preceding articles, some thoughts on the state of the chromato-
graphic art are now put forward, commencing with HPLC. Bonded-phase packings represent a major advance, especially the microparticulate totally porous type; yet they
may contribute to the frustrations of the investigator seeking to apply HPLC to the
analysis of trace compounds in body fluids. GC-ECD will hold its own as a notably
powerful approach; but instrumental advances may restore TLC to favour for assays
where high sensitivity and precision are not vital.*

*A strategy is put forward for method development, with consideration of approaches
to sample preparation and to assessing inadvertent losses. In anticipation of the
following Section, some comments are made on the possible usefulness of a chromatographic approach in the work-up procedure, and on other sample-preparation aspects.*

Whereas the Techniques Forum which generated this book was essentially an exchange
of experiences amongst 'old hands', the main purpose of this specially written
article is to help the novice by putting possible approaches in perspective, whilst
leaving it to the reader's initiative to look up tactics elsewhere in the book
(with the aid of the Contents list and the Index). The strategy put forward near
the end of the article is concerned largely with the bewildering variety of options
available for preparing the sample, some of which are then commented upon (and are
more fully considered elsewhere [1]). Unlike most books and reviews written by
analysts, a recent book [2] aimed at undergraduates (while hardly concerned with
body fluids) does give some attention to sample preparation, besides tersely sur-
veying measurement methods with the curious exception of fluorimetry. Choice of a
suitable end-step is cardinal to the development of an assay procedure, as was the
consensus of opinion in a 'chicken-or-egg?' discussion summarized later (p. 103).

A chromatographic procedure is commonly employed as the end-step and may
also be helpful in sample preparation. Chromatographic and other separation
methods are considered in depth elsewhere [3, 4]. The following jottings may
help knit together the chromatographic presentations elsewhere in the book. HPLC
will first be considered.

THE STATE OF THE HPLC ART

In the page on Abbreviations early in this book, the terminology jungle is outlined
and 'high-pressure liquid chromatography' is adopted as the least objectionable
term. The novice may be bewildered by the variety of terms and, moreover, by expo-
sitions of the technique which, with a few exceptions [e.g. 5, 6], give a somewhat
blurred picture of the nature, scope and execution of the technique. Well-intentioned
literature from manufacturers, and some 'academic' literature, are marred by such 'rough
spots' and also by illustrative separations which give no inkling of the 'noise'
associated with biological samples. Fortunately for this author's equanimity, a book
indexer's error accounted for a curiosity in the array of synonyms invented for
'HPLC', insofar as the text of the book [2] does not really refer to "high-speed
liquidation"!

As amplified elsewhere [7], the development of HPLC seems to have reached or,
in the case of packings, be nearing a temporary plateau, uncongenial in some respects.

HPLC hardware

An excellent appraisal ("A Consolidation Phase ?") has been made by Bristow [8], with whose views the following remarks partly agree. Instrumentation is showing a welcome trend towards falling costs, e.g. through omission of luxuries such as column thermostatting. It may, however, be a false economy to buy a constant-pressure rather than a constant-flow pump, if ever the user might have occasion to characterize by retentions, or to quantitate peaks on an area rather than a height basis, or to collect fractions for off-line examination. — Complications would clearly result from a change in flow rate due to a change in resistance within the column.

A gradient-making facility, usually entailing the costly purchase of a second pump although Matlin (Art. E-5) circumvented this, is an asset to method-development studies. Solvent gradients (or even abrupt steps) are, however, a handicap in routine assay work because of the slow turn-around associated with the recommended 'purge' with pure second solvent (Art. T-2) and with reversion to the first solvent and re-attainment of equilibrium. (From his ion-exchange experience, Dr. A. Bye shares the author's view of the importance of purging for preserving resolution, even in reverse-phase systems.) Moreover, an injudiciously steep gradient can mask heterogeneity that an isocratic system would show up (Art. T-2). Yet a gradient is helpful where components differing widely in retentivity are being looked for.

In choosing hardware, a decision has to be made on column dimensions. The use of short columns, say 250 rather than 500 mm, economizes on packing materials and operating time, but may jeopardize difficult separations. Elimination of wall effects is reckoned to be a benefit from using 'infinite diameter' columns, say 4.4 mm i.d. (unhelpfully designated $\frac{1}{4}$" on the basis of o.d.) [8]. However, in comparison with 2.2 mm i.d. columns they entail a dramatic drop in sensitivity of detection and rise in the cost of packings and solvents; moreover, design constraints in particular HPLC apparatus such as the Varian 4200 may entail poor flow rates per mm^2 cross-section and frequent topping-up of solvents with loss of operating time. A narrow (2.2 mm) column does not preclude use of a loop injector, if an injection volume of 10 µl is considered sufficiently small; the reproducibility achievable with such an injector has to be weighed up against its incompatibility with 'infinite diameter' operation whatever the column diameter.

Detection sensitivity is a notorious weak spot in the HPLC analysis of body-fluid constituents, particularly where the compound has poor UV absorbance. Alternatives to classical UV detection, summarized elsewhere [7, 8], offer no panacoea but could give advantages in selectivity, e.g. through polarography [9].

HPLC packings

Table 1 summarizes the options available when a packing is to be bought (loose or as a pre-packed column) or made in one's own laboratory. Steric exclusion (a term preferable to 'gel permeation' [7]) is an approach seldom applicable to small molecules such as drugs. For other modes, there is a trend away from pellicular packings back to totally porous packings, but of reduced diameter

Table 1. Types of HPLC packing.

Classified according to assumed separation principle:

Steric exclusion (Molecular size exclusion, Gel permeation)

Adsorption (Liquid-solid) ⎫
Partition (Liquid-liquid) ⎬ *may be* bonded phase: *termed* reverse phase *if mobile phase aqueous*
Ion-exchange ⎭

Classifications according to physical form:

Totally porous *(say 20-40 µm diam.)*   ⎫ Regular
Pellicular (Superficially porous, Porous layer)   ⎬ Irregular
Totally porous, micro-particulate

Table 2. HPLC approaches for particular types of molecule: a simplified strategy.

NATURE OF MOLECULE	TYPE OF PACKING	MOBILE PHASE aq = mainly aqueous, org = organic, non-polar
Large molecules	STERIC EXCLUSION	aq. *or* org.
Small molecules		
SOL. IN ORG. SOLVENTS		
∿ feebly or non-polar	ADSORPTION	org.
∿ quite polar	PARTITION/BONDED PHASE	org.
	or REVERSE PHASE	aq.
SOL. IN WATER		
∿ non-ionic	REVERSE PHASE	aq.
∿ ionic	ION-EXCHANGE	aq. (ionic)

(say 10 μm) in the interests of resolving power. Partition systems with a liquid stationary phase can be temperamental, and are being largely superseded (except for ion-pair systems, Art. G-3) by bonded-phase packings which are commonly of 're-verse-phase' type, i.e. the mobile phase is the more polar. However, bonded-phase columns including those of the cation-exchange type have often been short-lived in our laboratory because of spontaneous 'stripping' of the bonded phase (Art.T-2), which is a saddening experience when £115 has perforce been expended on a factory-packed column. Manufacturers now seem aware of the need to find a remedy, which may lie in choosing a core material more stable than silica. They may also come to close a gap in the range of commercial packings: weak cation-exchangers are lacking. For the range available, the diverse trade names can be perplexing.

Aspects of HPLC practice

With biological samples it is particularly desirable that the main column be pro-tected by a pre-column (Art. S-5), ideally of the same packing material if purcha-sable in loose form. If the 'nearest equivalent' has perforce to be used, there is a risk of over-retentivity as encountered in a cation-exchange study (Art.T-2). Glass beads are of some help (Art.T-7), but will not meet the possible need to hold back some unwanted bioconstituents in the sample.

    Some practitioners of HPLC boldly apply unprocessed plasma or urine, with satisfactory analytical results if the concentration of the constituent is well above (say) 1 μg/ml. Often, however, a sample-preparation procedure is obliga-tory, at least to obtain a concentrate [1, 6, 7]. To help the latter aim in the HPLC analysis of urine (with an electrochemical detector) for catecholamines, Kissi-nger *et al.* [9] vacuum-dried the alumina onto which the catecholamines had been adsorbed, and thereby managed to keep the volume of acidic eluent low. For anti-convulsants in serum, a simple charcoal-adsorption step has been advocated [10]. A cation-exchanger may be helpful (Art. T-2).

    There is no easy path for the novice faced with choosing a packing and solvent system. Table 2 gives simplified guidance on the basis of the extent to which the molecule is polar (ionic ?). By this criterion, a reverse-phase packing such as 'C$_{18}$' or 'ODS' will be the first choice for many drugs, with an aqueous eluting solvent containing acetonitrile (and possible methanol; cf. Arts. T-2 & T-7). It must be remembered that acetonitrile is toxic, the threshold limiting value (time-weighted average) being 70 mg/m^3 of air in the U.K. safety code. For ionic compounds an ion-exchange system will be the first candidate, with careful choice of pH. An alkaline pH, albeit below the pK$_a$, was the key to separating two amines (metadrenalines; Art. T-2) on an 'ODS' column, but such columns are stated to be more suitable for acidic or neutral compounds than for bases [11], which may respond better to ion-exchange.

Many practitioners of HPLC have been plagued at times with bumpy baselines and spurious peaks, suggestive of 'creepage' of material out of the packing. The purging procedure mentioned above may flush out lingering bioconstituents or solvent impurities. In respect of the latter, prevention is of course better than cure. The need for pure solvents is especially great in the 'trace enrichment' procedure, which entails passing a very dilute sample (e.g. drinking water) through the column so as to accumulate the constituents of interest prior to the chromatographic separation. With electrochemical detection, a false "irreproducible peak" unconnected with the sample has been observed in the cation-exchange separation of urinary catecholamines: it was observed even in mock injections (as if the needle were responsible) and was eliminated by use of a non-metallic rotary valve for sample injection [9]. An interesting cause of spurious peaks, or of other troubles such as obstructed flow, is deposition of solvent constituents (particularly dissolved salts, where applicable) when columns are stored wet, especially if slow evaporation occurs. As is recommended in this connection (by G. Smith, in a Spectra-Physics leaflet), it is advisable to blow the column dry before storage, by passing nitrogen through for a few minutes at 100-200 psi; but a swellable packing (e.g. polystyrene-based) is a contra-indication to use of this stratagem. We have not tried it.

With some types of sample, even 'optimized' conditions may furnish rather squat peaks with a long (and perhaps variable) retention time. Peak area rather than peak height is then likely to be obligatory as the means of quantitation. For a range of anticonvulsants, either height or area could be used, expressed as ratios relative to an internal standard added to the injection mixture; the concentration relationship had to be verified with any change of column or reagents [10]. However, "poor resolution has a much greater effect on peak area than on band height", as Kirkland [6] remarks in an article which gives valuable guidance on the practice and interpretation of HPLC runs. One expedient which he advocates is 'back-flushing' as a means of purging columns between runs.

ASPECTS OF GC

Investigators faced with choosing or using GC equipment to assay trace compounds in biological samples are well served with sources of guidance [e.g. 2, 12, 13]. GC is well surveyed from the column viewpoint in a book published by a company [14]. Only certain aspects are briefly considered below and elsewhere in this book (e.g. derivatization; p. 11 *et seq.*).

In an issue of *Journal of Chromatographic Sciences* devoted to pesticides, there is an excellent survey of GC detectors [15]. It rightly stresses the importance of detector cleanliness: ".... much of what passes as detector performance may originate outside the detector. Septum and column bleed, impurities in the carrier gas, flow and temperature control can all have a profound influence, and of course different detectors vary greatly in susceptibility to these disturbances." This applies especially to ECD, which is prone to engender a love-hate relationship as a favoured contender when GC assay is to be performed with a concentration below 0.1 µg/ml in the raw sample. In principle, the sample preparation procedure can be simpler when ECD rather than FID is to be used, but in practice this may be fallacious because of the risk of detector contamination. With MS detection (cf. Art. 1), the analysis of charcoal-concentrated trace constituents of drinking water was complicated by spurious peaks which turned out to be attributable to PTFE components in the equipment [16]. An uncoated glass vessel is safest for derivatization, risking adsorptive losses.

In a useful appraisal of the GC assay of drugs [17], eight types of GC column differing in polarity were examined, and the SE-30 and OV-17 types were found to be particularly versatile. Correct choice of column and operating temperature will be in vain if the injection conditions are unsatisfactory. Thus there may be peak tailing unless a needle dwell time of 5-10 sec is allowed in the hot zone of the injector (B. Welton & M. Arnold, *Perkin-Elmer Analytical News, 9*). Optimization may not be easy with automatic injectors (e.g. squat peaks suggest maladjustment); also, re-cycling may be futile because the puncturing of the vial septum may let water vapour enter (with detriment to derivatized solutes) or volatile contents escape. An impediment to accuracy in automatic injection, not obviated by between-sample rinsing, may be carry-over due to hold-up in the syringe and needle. Yet an automatic injector is a good investment, since manual runs tend to anchor the operator to the instrument.

QUANTITATIVE TLC

A revival in the use of TLC for quantitative repetitive work [18] has long seemed to be round the corner. Systems are available which allow of automatic operation with little operator attention, but are inevitably elaborate and costly. The TLC process does, however, lend itself to automatic or work-simplified performance of particular steps. The application of the samples is an especially tedious and error-prone step if each has to be loaded as repetitive aliquots so as to get enough solute onto the TLC plate. Syringe-type automatic applicators are of some help, but are less convenient than a type based on loops [18-20].

Elution of separated spots for off-line measurement can be facilitated by a 'vacuum cleaner' device or precision scraper, or by flexible TLC plates that can be cut with scissors. Measurement *in situ* is advantageous in principle, as shown elsewhere in this book by practitioners of fluorodensitometry, but calls for a costly instrument and for patient validation. An alternative to densitometry, with a potentially simple instrument which has yet to be commercially developed, is assessment of spot area as a measure of the amount of the substance [19, 21], entailing a decision as to whether the relationship originally published [21] is the right one for the analyst's particular system. This approach, even with manual measurement of areas, deserves wider adoption where high precision is not needed.

A radical departure from conventional TLC conditions is the replacement of the plate by individual coated rods, each of which is finally passed through an FID device so as to quantitate the separated rings of material [22]. This approach, with ceramic-coated rods that can be re-used repeatedly, has been pursued in Japan, and an instrument ('Iatroscan') put on the market. Reports of its applicability to trace components of body fluids will be awaited with interest; it will call for thorough clean-up of the sample.

CHOICE OF CHROMATOGRAPHIC ASSAY PROCEDURE

The following remarks apply particularly to the proposed use of a chromatographic end-step for the sake of sensitivity and/or specificity or of multi-component assay. A survey by Moffat [17] is especially useful for weighing up the possible usefulness of GC or TLC and for choosing conditions suitable for drugs. Table 3 may be helpful as a check-list, in the context of assaying trace components without recourse to techniques such as TLC fluoroden-

Table 3. Rough appraisal of chromatographic end-steps. *Rating ± means 'fair' or 'it depends'.*

DESIRABLE FEATURE	Classical LC	HPLC	TLC, PC	GC
Convenience and speed	-	+	±	+
Aq. samples with salts O.K.	±	±	-	-
Load vol. can be large	+	-	-	-
Derivatization unnecessary	+	+	+	-
Samples run side-by-side	-	-	+	-
Good assay sensitivity *without special approaches*	-	±	-	+

sitometry. GC-ECD ranks as the leading contender; but the relative ease of performing the actual GC run has usually to be weighed up against the inconvenience and possible trickiness of derivative formation. The need to keep the load volume down to a few µl in most chromatographic procedures entails either the inconvenience of preparing a concentrate (usually in an organic solvent) or the acceptance of sensitivity much poorer than is suggested by claims of an instrument response with a few ng. TLC and PC are facilitated by availability of an automatic applicator *(see above)*, but it may be hard to achieve low and consistent blanks. HPLC sensitivity can sometimes be improved by generating a fluorescent product before or after the separation [7].

LIGHTENING THE ANALYST'S TASK

For short but diverse work-runs, automatic equipment is likely to be uneconomic and, in any case, unavailable except for certain operations such as TLC loading and GC sample injection. Automatic HPLC is already feasible. In conventional column chromatography with a mobile liquid phase, an elution program can be run automatically, with constant [23] or diverse [24] solvent volumes, but the initial and final manipulations may remain time-consuming, even if disposable packed columns are used. At least the labour of off-line colorimetry or UV spectrophotometry can be lightened by various types of automatic equipment [19].

As reviewed elsewhere [1], limited possibilities exist for lightening the tedium of solvent extraction, but with a constraint which may be unacceptable — that the phases cannot be centrifuged automatically: even if there is no emulsion problem, there may be a risk of carry-through of interface solids (possibly with ultimate contamination of an ECD system) if centrifugation is not performed. To collated lore [1] on obviating or breaking emulsions, the following example [25] is added.— "Sometimes an emulsion forms during extraction [of serum by chloroform, for methaqualone assay] and persists after centrifugation. It can be broken by hitting the base of the tube against the palm of the hand and rolling the tube on its side, allowing the solid material to stick to the sides of the tube while the liquid falls to the bottom of the centrifuge tube." Analysis is indeed an art.

Phase-separating paper may help where an underlying organic solvent phase has to be harvested. This is an example of 'work-simplification' — an approach which can lighten the task of multi-sample analysis through common-sense plus inexpensive devices such as dispensers which eliminate meniscus-watching [19]. Examples of the use of different types of manually operated dispensers are given later (Scheme 2). For convenient and safe dispensing of plasma or serum, the type which draws the aliquot only into a detachable plastic tip is especially useful; a 'reverse' mode of operation may improve accuracy in the case of whole blood [26]. This type of dispenser may also be useful in place of the traditional bulb-operated pipette where one phase in a solvent extraction has to be sampled or completely removed. If there might be solvent attack on the plastic tip, a detachable glass tip could be used although it is expensive. Analysts seem not to have come to grips with simplifying phase removal. To preserve an undisturbed interface during withdrawal, the tip could usefully be bent at right-angles, as when subcellular biochemists seek to remove a supernatant without disturbing a pellet.

PRE-MEASUREMENT IMPEDIMENTS TO GETTING THE RIGHT ANSWER

In the working up of biological samples for measurement of a trace constituent, there are many possible pitfalls. The following remarks concern losses, rather than interfering substances which should be removed during sample preparation lest, for example, spuriously high or low values be obtained in a final fluorimetric assay. If there is an intermediate chromatographic step in the sample preparation procedure, there might be a small absolute loss of the test substance due, for example, to irreversible adsorption onto 'hyper-active sites' on the solid medium. A more common cause of a small absolute loss is inadvertent adsorption onto glass surfaces [1], as touched on by several contributors to this book. This may be minimized by silanization or, where the test substance is in a nonpolar solvent, by adding an alcohol in small amount. The problem may be particularly serious with basic substances, insofar as glass surfaces may have cation-exchange properties. A related trouble is 'creepage', reduced by silanization [27].

Incomplete recoveries may be due not merely to 'losses' such as the above, but to discarding some of the test substance, either deliberately as when only an aliquot is taken from a solvent layer, or willy-nilly as when the partition coefficient in a solvent extraction is not heavily weighted in favour of the desired phase. Liquid hold-up in a protein precipitate is another example.

'Spiking' to correct for variations, especially in work-up recovery

A method in which satisfactory clean-up is achieved at the expense of recovery can be perfectly acceptable, and in principle it is not even necessary to know the recovery since the calculations are based on identically processed 'calibration standards'. In practice, recoveries often vary from one tube to another within an assay run, not due to carelessness. A particular biological sample might, for instance, contain an odd protein which sabotages solvent extraction of a drug, as revealed by spiking with the drug. To save proliferation of assay tubes and to allow for 'rogue' behaviour not associated with particular samples, it has become the custom to spike each sample 'internally' as expounded in Scheme 1. An actual example, in a GC-ECD assay, is shown in Schemes 2 & 3 with some important practical points.

Scheme 1. Possible spiking strategies, in the assay of serum samples for 'X'.

In each assay run, samples of normal serum (free from the compound 'X') are set up as BLANKS and, after spiking with different amounts of 'X', as CALIBRATION STANDARDS. These, with *constant* recovery, suffice for calculation.

Problem: possible sample-to-sample *differences* in analytical recovery.

Classical remedy: divide each test sample into two, and spike one portion with a fixed amount of the authentic compound 'X'; finally determine ΔX value for each sample, and adjust results accordingly.

Work-saving remedies, depending on the availability of —

*X = radio-labelled 'X' of high enough s.a. to allow mass to be neglected,
or Y = a compound which behaves like X during extraction etc. but is distinguishable from X in the final estimation - 'INTERNAL STANDARD'.
or Z = a compound which behaves like X in the final steps (following sample preparation) except that it is separable for estimation.
or DX = deuterium-substituted X (or other heavy isotope)

Their application:-

POSSIBLE SPIKING OF EACH TEST SAMPLE *and* EACH CALIBRATION STANDARD
governed by the feasibility of measuring the spike
in the final step

FINAL ANALYTICAL STEP	POSSIBLE INITIAL SPIKE	PROCEDURE FOLLOWING SAMPLE PREPARATION
Photometric estimation (e.g. fluorimetry)	*X	Measure *X - *no losses are anticipated in the photometry*
TLC (or PC, but not HPLC unless fractions collected, nor GC)	*X	Measure *X once separated chromatographically
Any form of chromatography	Y *(preferred spike)*	Measure the chromatographically separated Y
GC, if search unsuccessful for an X-like cpd. (Y) - also applicable to HPLC	*X	Before derivatization (if any) & GC, measure *X and *spike with* Z - *i.e. 2-stage recovery correction*
Mass spectrometry (with or without GC)	DX	Measure deuteriated ion(s) whilst measuring the normal ions from X

NOTE: Except for photometric estimations, spiking serves to correct not only for variable preparative losses but also for loading errors or instrumental variations in the final step. 'Classical' spiking, with X itself, corrects only for any loss systematically occurring with a particular test sample.

Scheme 2. Hypothetical 'belt-and-braces' scheme *(cf. 'protocol' opposite)* to assay plasma samples for a drug (practolol [28]; can be whole blood or serum, rather than plasma) which has an acetylamino group but no halogen atoms.— A trifluoroacetyl (TFA) derivative is prepared for GC-ECD. *In a routine method one would hope to confine 'recovery spiking' to a valid, unlabelled internal standard (oxprenolol ?). As a last resort, one may put drug-spiked duplicates throughout, for losses correction.*

STEP	TEST (POST-DOSE) SAMPLES	NORMAL (PRE-DOSE ?) SAMPLES			NOTES ON MANIPULATIVE ASPECTS *esp. to get reliable % recoveries*
		CAL. STD.	*BLANK*	*GC SPIKE*	
Dispense aliquots (1 or 0.5 ml)	Suitably 15 ml tubes, ∿15mm i.d.; stoppered type *Treat blood-derived samples as a HAZARD*		unnecessary	'CHROMA-TOGRAPHY STD.'-No action	*Add by Eppendorf-type dispenser* [19] *perhaps in 'reverse mode'* [26] *if whole blood.*
Set up cal(ibration) standards		Say 0.2-1 µg of drug. Equilibrate.		*till deri-vatization stage*	*Conceivable causes of 'rogue' low recs. include adsorption on to tube wall if delivery not below liquid surface (esp.*
Spike with counts	Add, say, 1 nCi (20 ng?) [^{14}C]-drug with silanized syringe.				*if isotope < 0.1µg) & local pptn. if MeOH for the additions. Use*
Spike with int. std.	Add, say, 1 µg of oxprenolol *(will it mimic practolol ?).*				*aq. MeOH; add by syringe with immersed needle & 'Whirlimixing'*
Deprotein-ize	Add, with 'Whirlimixing', the reagents - Na$_2$SO$_4$, tungstate, acid; pause, & spin.				*'Reservoir' dispensers* [19]. *Inevitable liquid hold-up in protein pellet.*
Deacetylate	Heat acidic supernatant 1 h at 85-90° & cool; in stoppered tubes.				*Eppendorf-type dispenser suitable for taking the aliquot to heat.*
Solvent-extract	Add acid-washed cyclohexane + chloroform; 10 min in oscillating shaker, & spin.				*All-glass reservoir dispenser; to remove, Eppendorf type (glass tips ?).*
Solvent dried down (& isotope rec. as-certained)	In tubes with tapered bottom gently heated in block, with gentle stream of dry N$_2$ over surface & with heated collar round top of tube. Residue & tube wall can usefully be desiccated (P$_2$O$_5$?) overnight to ensure no water.				*An alcohol added to, say, 2% may reduce any adsorption on tube wall. Swill contents occasionally. When dry, Whirlimix with small vol. of methanol, sample for [^{14}C] counts, & re-dry. (Risk of spurious GC peaks if silanized tube used.)*
Set up 'chr-omat. std.'	*(If oxprenolol does NOT ex-tract like the drug, add NOW.)*			Add drug & int. std.	*Use deacetylated drug, added to tapered tube.*
Derivatize & dry down	Et$_2$O (dry) soln. of res., say 0.5 ml (mix well, in capped tube) treated with TFA, then dried as above, ∿r.t. initially, then higher to remove TFA.				*[Logical to sample for counts at this stage, but Et$_2$O aliquot would be unreliable (& the MeOH effects a useful rinse-down)] Shun old TFA !*
GC analysis	Res. (can be kept 1 night, dry & cold) shaken with dry Et acetate (kept away from air/light, say 0.5 ml); 1 µl aliquot(s) taken.				*TFA derivative is NOT stable for several days. To check GC perfor-mance, a halogen compound may be run.*
Calculation	Correct all deacetylated practolol GC peak heights to refer to a constant % rec., based on initially added ox-prenolol or, if erratic extraction, on isotope rec. and on rec. of int. std. added at derivatization stage. Test values are calculated from the 'cal(ibration) standard' values by a factor or, if non-linearity, a curve.				*The 'GC spike', in which the drug (deacetylated) and internal standard ('hydrolyzed') are added at the deri-vatization stage to an extract from unspiked normal plasma or merely to a mock-extract, serves merely to in-dicate the extent of extraction losses, complementing the isotopic values. BLANK peak= only [^{14}C] drug ?*

Scheme 3. A work-sheet for planning and recording multi-sample assay runs having a chromatographic end-point, with a specimen fill-in for a notional 'mini-run'. In this run, practolol was supposedly assayed in blood specimens, by GC-ECD following work-up steps ('sample preparation'; cf. Scheme 2); the specimens were supposedly spiked with [^{14}C]practolol and, as a hopefully suitable internal standard, atenolol (which in practice is *not* very suitable). The sheet could also serve for TLC or HPLC assays. *The sheet concerns assays where there are inadvertent sample-preparation losses and possibly instrumental variations. These are allowed for by the* 'int(ernal) std.'— *a reference compound resembling the test substance in extraction behaviour but not in chromatographic position. Both substances are put in* 'cal(ibration) stds.' *initially (zero-time or normal blood), and in* 'chr(omatography) stds.' *when derivatizing.- See Scheme 2. For '% taken through', see foot of p.60.*

UNIVERSITY OF SURREY
Wolfson Bioanalytical Centre
PROJECT....'7'....

BATCH SHEET FOR CHROMATOGRAPHIC ASSAY

SHEET REF. *1st Mar.'76*
(usually the setting-up date for sample preparation)

Operator's/checker's
INITIALS

Practolol ....in BLOOD / SERUM / PLASMA / URINE /..........

GENERAL PROCEDURES: intended; actual (if different); comments

BB #Sample (history? @ 3°) (handling?):.1 ml, spiked with 20 µl of *Atenolol*.... (int. std.) from 0.1 mg/ml soln., i.e. 2 ng
[GENERALLY calcu-late back to 1 ml] Spiking with authentic, as tabulated (only exceptions: 1 ml → test samples): from 0.1 mg/ml soln.
Spiking with isotope: 10 µl from 0.1 µCi/ml soln., i.e. 2 nCi, giving 5680 ......cts/min
(plus 10% = aliquot to be counted, as tabulated)

#Work-up (Att/-40% taken through): method ref.: Sheet P3 (50%, 1/5 th)

BB #Derivatization: on 0.2 ml ex ....ml (=100%,'D') of worked-up sample, with TFA ....(date:3rd)
on 0.2 ml ex 0.4 ml(=0.25%,'C') of derivative soln. unless tabulated otherwise

KJM #Chromatography: on .1 µl ex 0.4 ml(=0.25%,'C') of derivative soln....: Sheet P3; detector at 270°
(date:4th); method outline & ref.: Sheet P3; detector at 270°

BB #Calculation & transcription: on basis of PEAK HEIGHT, cm/PEAK AREA, cm², adjusted (after deducting sample blank) to the int.std. value indicated below as typical

#Recovery assessment: on basis of 'chr. stds', usually 0.2 ng of authentic, 0.2 ng of 'int.std.' [expressed as wt. of un-modified cpd. if (e.g.) deacetylated in work-up]

RT's ~ 4.3 (*deacetyl'd practolol*) & 5.1 (*processed atenolol*)

Supplementary info. & comments:
Continue on back of sheet

[The 0.2 ng practolol (actually deacetylated) & 0.2 ng atenolol (actually 'hydrolysed') were the amts. put on GC column]

#Factor 'F' for recovery assessment: reciprocal of proportion of original sample actually chromatographed, viz.
$$\frac{10^6}{T \times D \times C} = 100.0$$

'R' below DENOTES REPEAT of an analysis done on a previous day (if on left) or REPEAT NEEDED (if on right)

SAMPLE with ref. & comments, e.g. haemolysis	CAL. STD.: No. in chromato-graphic sequence	VARIATIONS in above quantities, e.g. & REMARKS	(if re-run: COMMA, or put at end)	Indi-vidual measure-ment(s) peak(s)	Ditto satel-lite INT. STD. measure-ment(s) peak(s)	Accepted NET MEAN, with BL.	Ditto, corr. to INT.STD. value deducted but uncorr.	TEST ng/ml, calc. from CAL.STD.	Other data: satellite pks./iso-tope cts.	OVERALL % REC. from INT.CAL.STD.	Work-up % rec. by isotope, AND REMARKS
CHR. STD.	—		C3, C7	none	11.4,12.4	8.0		—	—	—	—
PL.: Only 1 bl. run	—		C1	0.1	0.1	Mean 0.1 BL.	0.1		—	—	—
CAL. STD.	10	=1µg→CC t/s 100% rec.	C2	18.0	5.1	17.9	17.7	1750	/284	43 44	50
CAL. STD.	20		C6	34.7	5.0	34.6	34.6	Δ for 1µg/ml -use graph?	/295	42 46	52
TEST:171(R)	—		C4	28.1	5.4	28.0	26.0	14.8	/256	45	45
172	—		C5	40.2	5.1	40.1	39.3	22.4	/250	43	44 R₁

Normal serum

The application of the 'spiking philo-
sophy' set down in Scheme 1 is not without its
problems, one possible constraint being the
specific activity of the labelled compound (if
procurable) as is discussed below. Merely to
achieve reliable spiking is not easy, even in
setting up calibration standards with the
authentic compound. Scheme 2 indicates some
precautions, together with tactical tips for
the various manipulations in a method development exercise concerned with assaying blood
for practolol (eraldin) with a deacetylation
step [28]. There has been no report of a
satisfactory internal standard that could be
taken right through the sample preparation,
derivatization and GC steps. Whilst still
hoping to find one (not necessarily exactly
similar to practolol in extractability etc.),
we were resigned to the possible expedient of
dual internal standards — initial spiking with
labelled drug, to be measured prior to derivatization, and spiking with an unlabelled compound at the latter stage; contingency provision is made for the latter in Scheme 2. The
precautions are concerned partly with possible
adsorptive losses — a risk which led Curry (Art.
T-4) to use polycarbonate tubes in the initial
stages of a sample preparation scheme.

One peril in complex assays is confusion
in procedure or in calculation of results.
A standard work-sheet as shown in Scheme 3 can
repay the trouble of devising it, and soon
comes to be appreciated by the bench worker
even though it may seem complicated at first
sight. The specimen entries relate to Scheme
2, i.e. to a method-development exercise, but
the sheet was devised primarily for routine
assays. If the end-step were of conventional
photometric type rather than chromatographic,
a different version of the sheet would be
needed.

APPLICABILITY OF RADIOISOTOPES, AND THE
RADIODERIVATIZATION APPROACH

One possible constraint in the use of a radioisotopically labelled compound for assessing
recovery is that, if the concentration of the
unlabelled compound in the test sample is well
below, say, 1 µg/ml, 'trace'-spiking may
entail adding a significant weight quantity
so as to get enough counts in the aliquot
measured later. For a [^{14}C] compound, 1 nCi
would be a bare minimum and would, if the
specific activity were only 10 µCi/mg, entail
adding 0.1 µg, manifest in the reagent blank.

A related difficulty can arise where
very low levels are measured by radioderivatization, enzymatic (Scheme 4) or chemical. With the double-isotope approach shown, a spike with the [^{3}H] compound could

PLASMA
for estimation of adrenaline (A)
and noradrenaline (NA); *may also
contain dopamine & other catecholamines*

SET UP	[*Me*-^{14}C]-*s*-adenosyl
INCUBATION	methionine *(excess)*
MEDIUM	and, *to assess recove-*
(with app-	*ries, tracer amounts*
ropriate	*of* [^{3}H]A *and* [^{3}H]NA;
blanks),	*incubate with excess*
pH 8.4;	catechol-*o*-methyl-
1 h at 37°;	transferase (COMT);
then ADD	*finally add* unlabelled
CARRIERS	M & NM *(carriers)*

INCUBATED REACTION MIXTURE
containing 3- (& some 4-)-*o*-[^{14}C]-
methyl-A *and* -NA, *i.e.* metadrenaline (M) & normetadrenaline (NM)

DESTROY	briefly heat at
EXCESS	alkaline pH, then
REACTANTS	put through cation-
& ISOLATE	exchange column *(or*
M + NM	*solvent-extract)*

DRIED-DOWN ELUATE
containing M *and* NM

SEPARATE	TLC; locate M & NM
M AND NM	and elute each

M- AND NM-CONTAINING FRACTIONS

FINAL	Oxidize to vanillin,
WORK-UP OF	which is extracted
EACH	into toluene

M AND NM IN SCINTILLANT
for double-isotope counting

The [^{14}C] *counts, related to s.a. of
the methyl donor and corrected for
assay losses from the* [^{3}H] *counts,
give the values for A or NA in
the original plasma sample.*

Scheme 4. Radioderivatization
method of Engelman *et al.* [29].
*This double-isotope approach obviates
the need for a parallel set of samples
spiked with A & NA (unlabelled) as
standards. Assay losses are ∼90%, this
being acceptable to ensure specificity.
Sensitivity is limited by the s.a. of
the* [^{14}C] *methyl donor: A in normal
plasma (50 pg/ml) is just detectable.*

furnish a recovery figure for each catecholamine (A and NA), and it is not essential that the weight of [^{3}H]-A or -NA added be 'infinitely small' compared with the endogenous amount that is being assayed. The amounts of the respective radioderivatization products (M and NM) that come through to the final measurement step are ascertained from the [^{14}C] counts in relation to the molar specific activity of the [^{14}C] methyl donor. However, even if the latter is used as bought, undiluted by unlabelled donor, the final [^{14}C] counts may be so low, because of the low levels of the catecholamines, that the plasma sample may have to be as large as 5 ml [29]. The sample can, however, be under 1 ml if [^{3}H] methyl donor is used [30], insofar as [^{3}H] compounds are commonly available with much higher specific activities than [^{14}C] compounds — a point which is not always appreciated. The penalty is that recovery cannot be ascertained by use of [^{14}C]-A and -NA in view of their low specific activity; the classical procedure of running parallel test sample aliquots spiked with unlabelled A and NA has to be used (cf. Scheme 1), the abandonment of the double-isotope approach being justified by the gain in sensitivity and precision [30]. (Problems with isotopes, e.g. low s.a., are also considered in Art. G-2.)

Even if used in the single-isotope mode, radioderivatization can be advantageous because of its sensitivity, notwithstanding the inevitable need to free the derivative from other compounds which have likewise become labelled by virtue of non-specificity in the derivatization. As exemplified in Scheme 4, the purification may be tedious, yet less rigorous than for the classical isotope dilution approach. Whatever the connection in which use is made of a radioisotope, there should be awareness of the risk of inadvertent adsorption on to glass and also, in the case of [^{3}H], of possible instability of the stock material unless stored in liquid nitrogen (Art. T-2).

GENERAL STRATEGY FOR DEVELOPING AN ASSAY

Since assay experts faced with training novices often depend more on an apprenticeship system than on guided reading, the literature being scanty, some systematization has now been attempted. With some diffidence, a strategy is now suggested (Scheme 5) in which the central feature is the choice of end-step, whereupon the choice of sample-preparation is considered. Firstly, however, the Scheme deals with the initial treatment of the sample so as to get a solution suitable for work-up. The option of initial freeze-drying is an example of an approach which is considered elsewhere in this Volume (by R.A. Chalmers), as can be ascertained from the Contents list or the Index.— *There is little cross-referencing in the present Article*. There are examples elsewhere of extracting solid samples, e.g. pig-feed.

The commonest starting-material in the present context is plasma or serum (the distinction between which is usually irrelevant) or, at least where the constituent is disproportionately distributed, whole blood containing an agent such as oxalate. Exceptionally, there may be an urgent need to remove formed elements including platelets at the time of collection [30]. Storage for more than a few days can be at -20° unless stability is better just above 0°, as is sometimes the case for drugs. When the samples come to be processed, the inconvenience of a deproteinization step may have to be accepted (even with urine) if, for example, its omission leads to high GC or colorimetric blanks. Whether blood proteins have to be removed, and how, is decided empirically, and little guidance comes from protein-binding information. Thus, B. Scales and colleagues found with practolol that only by a tungstate protein-precipitation procedure [28] was the drug obtained in a 'clean' state, unassociated with the denatured protein. Protein binding *in vivo* is a distinct, important field, to which analysts must be alert. Drug-assay methods may, in years to come, have to take cognizance of free as well as total drug levels; but this subtlety is beyond the scope of the present Volume.

Some deproteinization procedures have been listed elsewhere [1], with mention of the desirability of first diluting the sample — likewise for solvent extraction, where the further precaution of pre-acidifying is advisable to release basic drugs, whose salts are solvent-soluble [31]. With perchloric acid as sometimes used

Scheme 5. Principles of assay design for a trace compound. — A 'catechism'.

1. Is the sample in a suitable form for work-up ?

  1a. If a liquid: Dry down, with a view to selective extraction ? *Not commonly done.*
      If a solid: What extraction method will give a suitable solution ?

  1b. Is deproteinization necessary ? *Will any protein-bound compound be released ?*

  1c. Is hydrolysis necessary ? *Conjugated compound (usually glucuronide or sul-*
      phate) may have to be released, especially with urine.

  1d. Would chemical modification be helpful ? *Possibly an isotopic derivative (for*
      radioderivatization approach), or a fluorescent derivative, or a 'complex' to
      aid extraction. Modification might be deferred till a later stage.

  1e. Should some labelled compound, or an internal standard, be added ? *For % recovery.*

  1f. Is de-salting necessary ? *Salt could sabotage an ion-exchange step.*

2. Which analytical criteria are especially important ?

  2a. Accuracy (specificity) ? *Any metabolites that should be included or excluded?*
      Any sample constituent that could lead to a false answer ? Any systematic error?

  2b. Precision (reproducibility) ? *A reproducible but false answer is a possible*
      pitfall. Non-reproducibility of % recovery can be circumvented (cf. 1e).

  2c. Detection limit (sensitivity) ? *'Noise' sources: the sample/reagents / the measu-*
      ring instrument! Suitable BLANKS are vital.

  2d. Convenience and cost of assay ? *Aspects to be considered in routine multi-*
      sample assay include productivity and instrumentation cost. Devise work-
      simplification for each step, if feasible; can any step be automatic ?

3.   Which end-step is preferable in terms of the criteria and of available instruments ?

  3a. Colorimetry, spectrophotometry or (sensitive !) fluorimetry may suffice; or pola-
      rography? *Suitable conditions can give specificity, even where two components*
      have to be assayed (e.g. by differential fluorimetry).

  3b. A chromatographic method (with on-line measurement ?) is inherently discriminatory.
      More than one component can be estimated, including any internal standard (cf. 1e).
      Insensitivity of UV detection may preclude HPLC. Remarkable sensitivity is
      attainable by GC-ECD (need to introduce halogen atoms ?).

  3c. A 'non-classical' approach (no sample preparation?) may be feasible or obligatory.

      ∿ Mass spectrometry (MS). *Often coupled to GC. Deuterium analogues are helpful.*
      ∿ Affinity, commonly radioimmunoassay (RIA). *RIA hinges on a good antiserum.*
      ∿ Microbiological assay. *Especially for antibiotics; usually on crude sample.*
      ∿ Isotope dilution. *Sample preparation may need heroic effort.*

4. What scheme, leading to the end-step, would suit for sample preparation (work-up) ?

  4a. Is the object (or one object) to obtain a salt-free concentrate ? - *E.g. for TLC.*

  4b. Is some separation (or at least 'clean-up') necessary ? *In end-step also ? - cf.* 3b.
  -
  [∿CONVERT INTO VAPOUR ? - Steam-distil? *Seldom done.* GC ? *Only as the end-step.*]
  Or, either for the DESIRED COMPOUND(S) or for UNWANTED CONSTITUENTS, at suitable pH:-
  ∿TRANSFER TO AN IMMISCIBLE LIQUID ? - Solvent extraction *or variant. Ion-pair ?*
  ∿TRANSFER TO A SOLID PHASE ? *Batchwise or chromatographic procedure.*
      # Adsorption ? *= liquid-liquid*   # Ion-exchange ? - *Allows of selectivity.*
  ∿SEGREGATE IN A SINGLE-PHASE MODE ? *Traditional for macromolecules.*
      # Steric exclusion ? - *E.g. 'gel filtration' (lipophilic?).* # Electrophoresis ? - *>1000 V ?*

5. If a chromatographic step with liquid mobile phase, what physical mode ?
      # Paper ? Thin-layer? *Automatic applicator ? Measure* in situ? # Column? + *collector ?*

to precipitate plasma proteins, use of KOH for neutralization has the advantage of furnishing a $KClO_4$ precipitate, leaving the desired compound in solution; a subsequent ion-exchange step would thereby be facilitated.

Aspects of conjugate hydrolysis and 'chemical modification' (1c and 1d, Scheme 5) are considered elsewhere in the Volume. Selective derivatization may be adopted for the purpose of 'chemical masking'. One context in which chemical modification might be practised, either initially or later in the procedure, is HPLC as the final step: a group with strong UV absorbance or with native fluorescence can be introduced to achieve a good detector response, with the minor penalty that the desired separation may be harder to achieve where molecular dissimilarities have been reduced through introduction of a common group into several of the constituents of the sample.

The question of initial spiking has already been considered. The question of interference by electrolytes in sample preparation arises especially with urinary hydrolysates. Electrodialytic de-salting would be troublesome in multi-sample assay work; but even a cation-exchange step can be designed to tolerate salts (Art.T-2).

Metabolites and other 'framework' features in assay design

The framework to this book as a whole is the design of assay methods for trace constituents *the identity of which is already known*. It is especially important that metabolic pathways (besides conjugation) should have been delineated, to furnish briefing on metabolites which should be excluded from or included in the measurement and which are commonly more polar than the parent compound (this being relevant to solvent extraction). Guidance on such delineation is to be found elsewhere [e.g. 17, 32, 33, & a pharmacology handbook cited in Art.S-1]. One example is a practolol study [28].

Amongst other aspects of the framework for assay design (2 in Scheme 5), it is cardinal to know *the lowest concentration that will have to be determined in test samples*. A useful list of therapeutic and toxicological levels of drugs has been compiled [34]. This and other literature [e.g. 33] should of course be scrutinized in case there already exists a satisfactory assay for the compound and *milieu* in question. Attainment of the desired accuracy and sensitivity may have to be at the expense of precision and convenience (2b and 2d in Scheme 5). In weighing up costs, one has to consider not only instrument choice but also staff time (and equanimity, which influences precision), with due regard to work-simplification possibilities outlined above.

An inspired guess has to be made about the most appropriate end-step and mode of measurement, with constraints which include equipment availability (3 in Scheme 5; also 5). Once it has been decided in principle to have a chromatographic end-step or intermediate step, its tactics have to be decided (cf. Table 3). There is, of course, the possibility that one of the 'non-classical' approaches shown in Scheme 5 (3c) may be advantageous, or even necessary because of sensitivity or specificity requirements; these approaches call for experience and skill, as well as equipment, that many laboratories do not possess.

Both for measurement approaches and for sample-preparation options now to be considered, ideas and information abound in the pages of *Clinical Chemistry* (two issues in particular [35]) and of *Journal of Pharmaceutical Sciences*. An important reservation concerns papers devoted to multi-drug investigation, especially for drugs of abuse: the multi-purpose methodology entails compromises that may be disadvantageous where only a single drug has to be measured and 'screening' is unnecessary.

Sample preparation principles

It is helpful to consider possible strategies according to the phase transfer involved in each type of approach (4 in Scheme 5). A volatilization step, as often applied to solvents, is inconvenient for test compounds, although preparative GC could be applicable in principle. Steric or electrophoretic separations, without phase transfer, have their respective weaknesses when applied to small molecules, viz. indiscriminate entry of small molecules into the pores, and diffusion problems (minimized with high voltages) besides the constraint of a low load volume. Yet the use of lipophilic gels such as 'LH-Sephadex' can allow the discriminatory separation of molecules of low polarity, although the mechanism seems to be partly adsorptive, i.e. two-phase [36].

The most widely practised approaches entail transferring the test compound (or unwanted constituents) to a second liquid phase, or to a solid phase which in some instances acts by virtue of an associated film of liquid immiscible with the bulk liquid phase (as when silica gel is used in a non-polar *milieu*). Operationally the two approaches are best distinguished merely by whether or not an agent insoluble in the bulk liquid phase is added. The following notes on the two approaches, with a few examples of their application, are intended mainly to complement other articles in this Volume. A survey [1] which includes other approaches to sample preparation may be consulted for amplification, and it should be kept in mind that individual separatory procedures may well have to be selected with a view to building up a multi-step separation scheme in which different properties of the test compound are exploited in turn [3, 4].

Solvent extraction

The basic strategy and tactics of solvent extraction — which still holds first place in the array of sample-preparation approaches — are considered in Art. S-1 [see also 37]. For charged or dissociable molecules, the pH must be chosen carefully even if subtle separations (Art. S-2) are not sought. However, where a base is to be extracted from plasma an acidic pH rather than the customary alkaline pH may be desirable [31], as mentioned above. Sometimes, as when the organic solvent has some water-miscibility or is being kept to a relatively small volume, addition of an inorganic salt in high concentration may be obligatory. Such a system, which may minimize emulsion formation as an incidental benefit, sometimes carries the unfortunate term 'salt-solvent pair [38]. It is not to be confused with the highly efficacious ion-pair approach which G. Schill describes in Art. G-3 [cf. 37].

The principle that the organic solvent to be selected should be *just* polar enough to extract the test compound efficiently is applied by S.H. Curry in Art. F-4, concerned with chlorpromazine and its metabolites in plasma, where the GC estimation (by ECD, without derivatization) was performed after *n*-heptane extraction and subsequent back-extraction steps to concentrate the drug. Inadvertent interaction between solvent and test compound can occur [A.H. Beckett, 17], as stressed by J.J. Pisano in a thoughtful article [13] centred on GC analysis and the requisite sample preparation: ketonic constituents are especially prone to react with amines. Amines are also susceptible to traces of peroxides in diethyl ether. In the GC assay of codeine and norcodeine [39], the latter was hard to measure unless, as occurred inadvertently with some batches of chloroform, it were converted into norcodeine carbamate: this conversion was due to ethyl chloroformate that arose from the ethanol present in the chloroform (as a preservative) by the action of phosgene formed through exposure of the chloroform to air.

Ethanol in chloroform turned out to be the key to getting acetylamino acids to move down a silica gel column with 'chloroform' as eluent, as A.J.P. Martin reminisces [13]. In solvent extraction, supplementation of weakly polar solvents with an alcohol (e.g. iso-amyl) can be a useful stratagem, to minimize adsorptive losses [31] and/or improve extractability. Such observations reinforce rather than detract from the need to purify solvents in assay work. Impurities such as peroxides may be removable by alumina treatment, as well described in company literature (Woelm). Prior to extraction of aqueous solutions, organic solvents (especially chlorinated) should be washed with water, *before* any mixture is made up.

Exposure to a solid phase

Alumina is commonly employed [9, 40] to isolate compounds with vicinal hydroxyl groups. Its use in the catecholamine field is indicated in Scheme 1 of Art.T-2, as is the applicability of strong or weak cation-exchange resins. These, although rather neglected elsewhere in the Volume, deserve to be more widely used for isolating basic substances. Even the electrolytes in a urinary hydrolysate can be tolerated by a sulphonic cation-exchanger under suitable conditions (Art.T-2), although a weak cation-exchanger should be considered as an alternative or subsequent step if a 'clean' eluate is needed [40]: for *strong* bases it may be vital. The scope of anion-exchangers [41] is outlined in Art.S-6. In general the use of ion-exchangers calls for a grasp of principles [cf. 2-4] and for meticulous operation. It must be remembered that non-volatile salts in an eluate could jeopardize subsequent chromatography (cf. Table 3, *above*); ammonium formate can be useful since small amounts can be removed by a desiccator method [41]. The efficacy of ion-exchangers when applied direct to undeproteinized plasma [cf. 40, 42] cannot be taken on trust.

As indicated in Art.T-2, there has been some revival of interest in charcoal, either 'active' or 'pre-coated'. On occasion it has been used, e.g. as charcoal-impregnated filter paper, to remove unwanted substances. Conveniently (and, in 'cartridge' form, expeditiously [43]), it allows adsorption and subsequent elution of the desired substance. It does display some selectivity, such that it serves to clean up, as well as to concentrate [e.g. 10, 16; cf. 4, Scheme 5]. This also holds for the non-ionic resin 'XAD-2' (Amberlite' series) as applied, for example, in the isolation of aldosterone from plasma for RIA [44] or steroid conjugates from urine for subsequent hydrolysis and GC [45]. Its capabilities and limitations [1] are exemplified later in this Volume, notably in Art. T-2. Its advent may account for the lull in the use of charcoal in the 1960's. Conditions for XAD-2 must be optimized (e.g. [46]-urinary morphine).

CONCLUDING COMMENTS

Guide-books such as the present one need to be reinforced by experience. The mark of the 'old hand' is the knack of picking a good route amongst the trees so as to emerge from the wood with minimum trouble. Various articles in Section 'T' tell a salutary tale of difficulties and remedies. Especially challenging was the problem of setting up a reproducible GC-ECD method for chlorpromazine in S.H. Curry's laboratory (ref. [14] in Art. T-4). Troubles are not confined to basic compounds. Thus, chloroform extraction of succinimide anticonvulsants for GC-FID demands ingenuity [47].

References

1. Reid, E., *Analyst 101* (1976) 1-18.

2. Fifield, F.W. & Kealey, D., *Principles and Practice of Analytical Chemistry,* International Textbook Co., London (1975), 378 pp.

3. Morris, C.J.O.R. & Morris, P., *Separation Methods in Biochemistry,* 2nd edn., Pitman Medical, London (1976), 1045 pp.

4. Karger, B.L., Snyder, L.R. & Horvath, C., *An Introduction to Separation Science,* Wiley, New York (1973).

5. Fallick, G.J., *Adv. Chromatog. 12* (1975) 62-97.

6. Kirkland, J.J., *Analyst 99* (1974) 859-885.

7. Leppard, J.P. & Reid, E., *Annu. Rep. Prog. Chem. 71B* (1974) 44-55.

8. Bristow, P.A., *Trans. Biochem. Soc. 3* (1975) 858-860.

9. Kissinger, P.T., R.M. Riggin, R.L. Alcorn & L.-D. Rau, *Biochem. Med. 13* (1975) 299-306.

10. Adams, R.F. & Vandemark, F.L., *Clin. Chem. 22* (1976) 25-31.

11. Twitchett, P.J. & Moffat, A.C., *J. Chromatog. 111* (1975) 149-157.

12. Riedmann, M., *Xenobiotica 3* (1973) 411-434.

13. Kroman, H.S. & Bender, S.R. (eds.), *Theory and Applications of Gas-Liquid Chromatography in Industry and Medicine,* Grune & Stratton, New York (1968).— *Includes relevant articles by:* Martin, A.J.P. (p. 1); Pisano, J.J. (p. 147); de Silva, J.A.F. (p. 252).

14. Supina, W.R., *The Packed Column in Gas Chromatography,* Supelco, Bellefonte, Pa. (1974), 166 pp.
15. Aue, W.A., *J. Chromatog. Sci. 13* (1975) 330-333. *[Pesticide issue: starts p.301.]*
16. Grob, K., *J. Chromatog. 84* (1973) 255-273.
17. Papers in *The Poisoned Patient, Ciba Found. Symp. 26* (1974), *including* Beckett, A.H. (p. 57); Moffat, A.C. (p. 83). *[The Discussion summaries are illuminating.]*
18. Shellard, E.J. (ed.), *Quantitative Paper and Thin-Layer Chromatography,* Academic Press, London (1968), 140 pp.
19. Reid, E., *Multi-Sample Analysis,* in *Industrial Aspects of Biochemistry* [Spencer, B., ed.], North-Holland, Amsterdam (1974) 913-932.
20. Leppard, J.P., Harrison, A.D.R. & Nicholas, J.D., *J. Chromatog. Sci.* (1976) *in press.*
21. Purdy, S.J. & Truter, E.V., *Analyst 87* (1962) 802-809.
22. Padley, F.G. (1969). *J. Chromatog. 39* (1969) 37-46.
23. Barlow, G.B. & Ersser, R.S., *Lab. Pract. 24* (1975) 163-164.
24. Horn, Von K., Henner, J., Müller & Scriba, P.C., *Z. Klin. Chem. Klin. Biochem. 13* (1975) 173-178.
25. Evanson, M.A. & Lensmeyer, G.L., *Clin. Chem. 20* (1974) 249-254.
26. Pinchin, M.J., *Lab. Pract. 24* (1975) 811.
27. Kushinsky, S. & Anderson, M., *Clin. Chem. 20* (1974) 1528-1534.
28. Scales, B. & Cosgrove, M.B., *J. Pharmac. Exp. Ther. 175* (1970) 338-347.
29. Engelman, K. & Portnoy, B., *Circulation Res. 26* (1970) 53-57.
30. Passon, P.G. & Peuler, J.D., *Anal. Biochem. 51* (1973) 618-631.
31. Brodie, B.B., Udenfriend, S. & Baer, J.E., *J. Biol. Chem. 168* (1947) 299-309.
32. Curry, S.H., *Drug Disposition and Pharmacokinetics with a Consideration of Pharmacological and Clinical Relationships,* Blackwell, Oxford (1974), 224 pp.
33. Hirtz, J.L., *Analytical Metabolic Chemistry of Drugs,* Dekker, New York (1971), 395 pp.
34. Baselt, R.C., Wright, J.A. & Cravey, R.H., *Clin. Chem. 21* (1975) 44-62.
35. Papers in *Clin. Chem. 20* (1974) 111-311 [March]; also *22* (1976) [June].
36. Sjövall, J., Nyström, E. & Haahti, E., *Adv. Chromatog. 6* (1968) 119-170.
37. Lyle, S.J., *Selected Annu. Rev. Anal. Sci. 3* (1973) 1-57. *[Inorganic 'slant'.]*
38. Horning, M.G., Gregory, P., Nowlin, J., Stafford, M., Laetratanangkoon, K., Butler, C., Stillwell, W.G. & Hill, R.M., *Clin. Chem. 20* (1974) 282-287.
39. Brunson, M.K. & Nash, J.F., *Clin. Chem. 21* (1995) 1956-1960.
40. Weil-Malherbe, H., in *Analysis of the Biogenic Amines and Their Related Enzymes* (Glick, D., ed.), Wiley-Interscience, New York (1971) 119-152. *[Citations of use of cation-exchangers on plasma:* Häggendahl, J.; Steinsland, O.S.*]*
41. Hurlbert, R.B., Schmitz, H., Brumm, A.F. & Potter, V.R., *J. Biol. Chem. 209* (1954) 23-39.
42. Ratcliffe,W.A., Challand, G.S. & Ratcliffe,J.G., *Ann. Clin. Biochem.11* (1974) 224-229.
43. Hindmarsh, K.W., Hamon, N.W. & LeGatt, D.F., *Clin. Chem. 21* (1975) 1852-1853.
44. Roginsky, M.S., Panetz, A.I. & Gordon, R.D., *Clin. Chim. Acta 63* (1975) 303-308.
45. Moore, J.C., *Clin. Chim. Acta 39* (1972) 532-538.
46. Miller, W.L., Kullberg, M.P., Banning, M.E., Brown, L.D. & Doctor, B.P., *Biochem. Med. 7* (1973) 145-158.
47. Bonitati, J., *Clin. Chem. 22* (1976) 341-345.

G-2

AFFINITY METHODS FOR DRUG ASSAY[†]

Vincent P. Butler, Jr.
Department of Medicine, College of Physicians & Surgeons,
Columbia University, 630 W. 168th St.,
New York, N.Y. 10032, U.S.A.

Because of their sensitivity, specificity, precision, rapidity, and convenience,
drug-specific immunoassay and competitive protein-binding assay methods are now*
widely used both in clinical and investigative laboratories. This review deals
with the synthesis and characterization of drug-protein conjugates, immunization
with drug-protein conjugates, the detection and immunological characterization of
drug-specific antibodies, the use of drug-specific antibodies in the development
of immunoassays and, finally, the development of competitive protein-binding assay
methods for the measurement of drug concentrations in human or animal serum.

The introduction of immunoassay methods into clinical and investigative medicine by Berson and Yalow [e.g. 1-3] and the subsequent extension of the basic principles of immunoassay to the development of competitive protein-binding assay methods [4-7] have added a new dimension to the identification and measurement of pharmacologically active substances in the plasma and tissues of man and experimental animals [8-13].

Immunoassay and competitive protein-binding assay methods often provide the sensitivity, specificity, precision, rapidity and convenience needed for the daily performance of large numbers of drug analyses on small volumes of serum in clinical laboratories. Thus, one technician can perform blood drug level determinations on microlitre volumes of unextracted serum from 40 patients within a few hours; automation could readily increase the number of analyses performed daily to 200 or more. For example, at my own institution, the clinical laboratory under the direction of Dr. S. Raymond Gambino will perform, on a same-day basis, 10,000 individual serum digoxin determinations by radioimmunoassay (RIA) on blood specimens from patients during this calendar year. Such assays aid physicians in properly individualizing digoxin dosage schedules [14-16] and appear to have helped decrease the incidence of digoxin toxicity in digoxin-treated patients [17]. Another example of the convenience and rapidity of immunoassay methods as employed in our hospital is that blood levels of anticonvulsant drugs are measured within an hour by a portable instrument while patients wait to see their physicians in the seizure disorder clinic [18]. The simplicity and convenience of immunoassay and competitive protein-binding assay methods also renders them highly suitable for large-scale studies of drug bioavailability [19-22], pharmacokinetics [23], compliance [24], and abuse [11].

PHARMACOLOGICAL APPLICATION OF IMMUNOASSAY AND COMPETITIVE PROTEIN-BINDING ASSAY METHODS

To illustrate the broad pharmacological applicability of immunoassay methods, Table 1 lists some drugs and toxins for which immunoassay methods have already been developed. These include a variety of narcotic and analgesic agents, several antibiotics, certain anticonvulsants, anti-inflammatory drugs, antineoplastic agents, many cardiac glycosides and other cardiovascular drugs, CNS stimulants, hallucinogenic drugs, oral hypoglycaemic agents, several insecticides, various sedatives and tranquillizers (notably the barbiturates), D-tubocurarine, more than a dozen synthetic steroid drugs (including oral progestins), and finally,

---

* *General term that can also be used: 'saturation analysis'.- EDITOR.*
   [†] *For ACKNOWLEDGEMENTS see p. 85.*

several toxins. Table 2 lists other immunoassays of pharmacological interest. These include assays for conjugated bile acids, catecholamines, serotonin and melatonin, insect and plant hormones, nucleosides and nucleotides, numerous mammalian peptide hormones, spermine, prostaglandins, numerous steroid hormones, thyroid hormones and Vitamin B_{12}.

In Table 3 are listed some drugs and other substances for which competitive protein-binding assay methods have been described. It is apparent that these methods have not yet been used as extensively as immunoassay methods for drug measurements, but several new assays are currently being developed. I am confident that the number of drugs for which such assay methods are available will increase significantly in the next few years.

In view of the wide applicability and utility of drug immunoassay and competitive protein-binding assay methods, it seems appropriate to review the principles, development, application, and limitations of these methods.

DRUG IMMUNOASSAYS

General principles

Table 1. Immunoassays for drugs and toxins.

Analgesics and Narcotics	Hypoglycaemic Agents
.Anileridine	.Butylbiguanide
.Codeine	.Glibenclamid
.Etorphine	**Insecticides**
.Fentanyl	.Aldrin
.Meperidine	.DDT
.Methadone	.Dieldrin
.Morphine	.Malathion
Antibiotics	**Sedatives and Tranquilizers**
.Amikacin	.Barbiturates
.Chloramphenicol	Barbital
.Gentamicin	Pentobarbital
.Isoniazid	Phenobarbital
.Penicillin	.Chlordiazepoxide
Anticonvulsants	.Chlorpromazine
.Clonazepam	.Cyclazocine
.Phenytoin	.Desmethylimipramine
Anti-inflammatory Agents	.Diazepam and N-desmethyldiazepam
.Colchicine	.Glutethimide
.Indomethacin	.Pentazocine
.Phenylbutazone	**Skeletal Muscle Relaxants**
Antineoplastic Agents	. D-Tubocurarine
.Adriamycin	**Synthetic Peptides**
.Daunomycin	.Saralasin
.Methotrexate	**Synthetic Steroids**
Cardiovascular Drugs	.Androgens
.Cardiac glycosides	Fluoxymesterone
Acetylstrophanthidin	.Oestrogens
Cedilanid	Diethylstilboestrol
Deslanoside	Ethinyloestradiol
Digitoxin	Mestranol
Digoxin	.Glucocorticoids
Gitoxin	Dexamethasone
Methyl digoxin	Methylprednisolone
Ouabain	Prednisolone
Proscillaridin	Prednisone
.Propranolol	.Metyrapone
.Quinidine	.Progestins
CNS Stimulants	Medroxyprogesterone
.Amphetamine	Norethindrone [acetate
.Benzoyl ecgonine	Norethisterone
(cocaine metabolite)	Norgestrel
.Methamphetamine	**Toxins**
.Pimozide	.Aflatoxin B_1
Hallucinogenic Drugs	.Genistein
.Lysergic acid diethylamide (LSD)	.Nicotine and metabolites
.Mescaline	.Paralytic shellfish poison
.Tetrahydrocannabinol	.Tartrazine

As with all immunoassays, the development of a drug immunoassay requires the availability of antibodies capable of binding the substance being assayed. As most drugs are of relatively low molecular mass (<1,000), they are usually not antigenic, and thus repeated injections of a drug into an experimental animal will not ordinarily elicit antibody formation. To obtain antibodies specific for a drug, it is therefore usually necessary to conjugate the drug (or a chemical derivative of the drug) covalently as a hapten to an antigenic protein or synthetic polypeptide carrier prior to immunization [25, 26]. A hapten may be defined as a small molecule, too small to be antigenic by itself, but which, when covalently coupled to a large antigenic protein or polypeptide carrier and injected into an animal, will

cause the formation of antibodies specific for the
chemically coupled small
molecule.

For proper apprecia-
tion of this phenomenon, one
must be aware of one important property of the immune
response, namely that, while
the antigen recognition and
processing system is stimu-
lated only by large mole-
cules such as proteins or
hapten-protein conjugates,
antibodies formed in res-
ponse to this stimulation
recognize only small parts
of the antigenic molecule.
Therefore, if a given anti-
body-forming cell forms
antibodies to a portion of
a hapten-protein conjugate
not containing hapten,
these antibodies will re-
act only with the protein
carrier, while cells for-
ming antibodies to areas
occupied by haptenic groups
produce the anti-hapten
antibodies used in drug
immunoassays. Fortunately,
antibodies to protein
carriers do not interfere
with properly designed

Table 2. Other immunoassays of pharmacological interest.

Bile Acid Conjugates	Peptide Hormones
.Cholylglycine	.Angiotensin
.Cholyltaurine	.Anterior pituitary
	.Bradykinin
Catecholamines	.Gastric
	.Hypothalamic
.Epinephrine	.Intestinal
.Norepinephrine	.Pancreatic
.Tyramine	.Parathyroid
	.Posterior pituitary
Fibrinopeptides	.Thyroid (calcitonin)
.Fibrinopeptide A	
.Fibrinopeptide B	Plant Hormones
Indolealkylamines	.Indole-3-acetic acid
	.Gibberellic acid
.Melatonin	
.Serotonin	Polyamines
Insect Hormones	.Spermine
	Prostaglandins
.Ecdysterone	Steroid Hormones
Nucleosides and Nucleotides	Thyroid Hormones
.Cyclic AMP	
.Cyclic GMP	.Thyroxine
$.N^2$-Dimethylguanosine	.Triiodithyronine
.7-Methylguanosine	
.Pseudouridine	Vitamins
.Thymidine	
	.Vitamin B_{12}

Table 3. Competitive protein-binding (CPB) assays for drugs.

	BINDING PROTEIN	
DRUG	Nature	Source
Antineoplastic Agents		
.Methotrexate	Dihydrofolate reductase	Mouse ascites tumor
Cardiac Glycosides		
.Digitoxin		
.Digoxin	Na^+,K^+-ATPase	Guinea pig brain
.Ouabain		
Synthetic Steroids		
.Danazol	Progesterone-binding	Pregnant guinea pig
.Medrogestone	globulin	serum
.Norethindrone		
	Corticosteroid-binding	Human (or canine)
.Prednisolone	globulin (CBG;	plasma
	transcortin)	
.Prednisolone	Cytoplasmic glucocorticoid	Rat hepatoma cells
	receptor	(tissue culture)
.Clogestone acetate	Cytoplasmic	Proestrus
	progesterone-binding	rat uterus
	tissue protein	

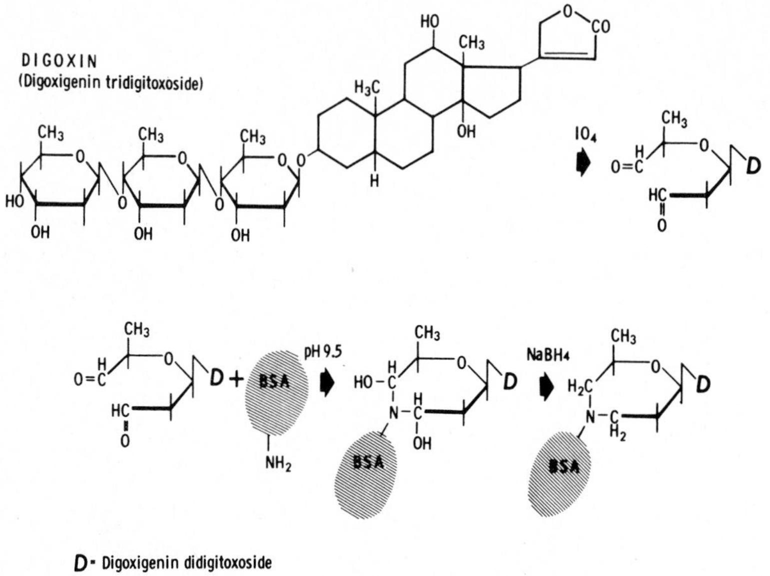

Fig. 1. Proposed scheme of conjugation of digoxin to bovine serum albumin (BSA) by the periodate oxidation method. *See text for explanation. Reprinted with permission from Butler* et al. [29]. *Courtesy of New York Academy of Sciences (likewise Fig. 3).*

drug immunoassays, but the possibility of such interference must always be considered in the development of any new drug immunoassay method.

The synthesis of digoxin-protein conjugates and the use of these conjugates to elicit, in rabbits, the formation of digoxin-specific antibodies [27] illustrate the general principles involved in the production of drug-specific antibodies. Digoxin is of too low molecular size (780) to be antigenic by itself. To elicit antibodies, the drug first had to be conjugated covalently to an antigenic protein carrier. This was accomplished by using the elegant but simple periodate oxidation method of Erlanger and Beiser [28]. Digoxin consists of the cardioactive aglycone, digoxigenin, and three inactive digitoxose residues (Fig. 1). Sodium periodate oxidizes the terminal digitoxose to form the dialdehyde derivative (Fig. 1, *upper portion*); then *(lower portion)* if the periodate-oxidized digoxin is added to bovine serum albumin at pH 9.5, the dialdehyde reacts with free amino groups of protein, derived principally from lysine residues, to form an unstable structure *(lower centre)*. This compound is then readily reduced with sodium borohydride, forming a stable structure *(lower right)* in which digoxin is covalently linked to the albumin carrier. As depicted schematically (Fig. 2, *top*), 3 to 8 molecules of digoxin are ordinarily incorporated into each molecule of albumin by this method. Then (Fig. 2, *bottom*) rabbits or sheep are repeatedly injected with this conjugate. Animals thus immunized form antibodies to the albumin carrier (which will not interfere with properly designed digoxin immunoassays) and, more importantly, they also form antibodies to digoxin, as depicted by the bivalent molecule *(lower right)* with two digoxin-binding sites.

Synthesis of drug-protein conjugates

In the synthesis of a drug-protein conjugate, a protein carrier first has to be chosen. Serum albumins of various species have been commonly used, for a number

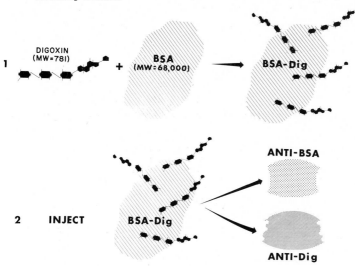

Fig. 2.
Schematic re-
presentation of
experimental
production of
antidigoxin
antibodies.
*See text for
explanation.
Reprinted with
permission from
Butler* [30].
*Courtesy of
Massachusetts
Medical Soci-
ety (likewise
Fig. 4).*

of reasons: their ready availability, low cost, high degree of immunogenicity, excellent solubility, and relative resistance to denaturation by the organic solvents and somewhat rigorous chemical conditions employed in some conjugation procedures. However, many other proteins and polypeptides (including homologous plasma proteins) have been used as carriers, and some may be superior to albumin in certain situations. The functional groups in albumins or other protein carriers to which haptenic drugs or drug derivatives may be conjugated include: free amino groups (ϵ-amino of lysine and NH_2-terminal residues); free carboxyl groups (aspartic acid, glutamic acid and $COOH$-terminal residues); and phenolic (tyrosine), sulphydryl (cysteine), imidazo (histidine), indolyl (tryptophan) and guanidino (arginine) functions. Most frequently the coupling has been to amino, carboxyl or phenolic groups [12, 26, 31 - 33].

In the method selected for conjugation of a haptenic drug or a drug derivative to a carrier, the chemical conditions must entail minimal structural alterations of the hapten and not cause sufficient denaturation of the carrier protein to render it insoluble. Many such relatively gentle methods have been described for coupling small molecules to protein carriers via carboxyl, hydroxyl, or amino groups in drugs or chemically related derivatives. For example, drugs or drug derivatives with free carboxyl groups can be coupled to amino groups of proteins by the mixed anhydride [34, 35] or carbodiimide [36] method. Numerous methods have been developed for coupling compounds with free hydroxyl groups to carrier proteins. The hydroxyl groups of steroids react with succinic anhydride to form the hemisuccinate [35] which, *via* its carboxyl group, can then be coupled to a protein, as just indicated. Phenols have been converted to active reagents by reaction with diazotized ρ-aminobenzoic acid [37]; such ρ-aminobenzoate derivatives, like hemisuccinate derivatives, can then be coupled to the amino groups of protein *via* their functional carboxyl group. Compounds with vicinal hydroxyl groups can conveniently be coupled to amino groups of protein carriers by the periodate oxidation method [28]. Aliphatic amines can be coupled to carriers using water-soluble carbodiimides [36] or bifunctional diisocyanates [38], or by conversion into ρ-nitrobenzoylamides followed by reduction to the ρ-aminobenzoyl derivative which, upon diazotization, can be coupled to the tyrosine residues of protein [39]. Aromatic amines can be diazotized and coupled directly to carriers [40]. These and other conjugation methods have been reviewed in detail recently [10, 12, 13, 31-33].

Characterization of drug-protein conjugates

Incorporation of too much, as well as too little, hapten into a hapten-protein conjugate may lead to a poor antibody response [10, 41]; in the experience of some workers [25, 32], 10 haptenic groups per molecule of carrier has seemed optimal when serum albumin was used. Hence, before one immunizes experimental animals with a newly synthesized drug-protein conjugate, it is usually desirable to determine the number of drug molecules one has conjugated to the protein (or polypeptide) carrier employed.

If the haptenic group has an absorption spectrum which can allow one to differentiate it from the protein carrier, the ratio between the molar extinction coefficient [42] of the conjugate and that of the hapten at an appropriate wavelength can be used to calculate the molar incorporation of hapten into protein carrier. However, even if there is overlap in spectra between hapten and carrier, reasonably accurate estimates of molar incorporation of hapten can be made by determining differences in molar extinction coefficients between conjugate and carrier, and then comparing the difference with the molar extinction coefficient of the hapten [35, 41, 43, 44, 47]. The extent of haptenic incorporation into a hapten-protein conjugate can also be determined by various chemical analyses of conjugates [36, 45], extent of incorporation of radiolabelled drug into conjugates [46-50], or by the decrease in free amino groups of carrier, following conjugation of a hapten to carrier by a method which utilizes the amino groups of the carrier [32, 35].

Immunization

Ordinarily, drug-protein conjugates are suspended in complete Freund's adjuvant mixture [51] at a final concentration of 1 mg/ml or less: usually 1 ml or less is injected into experimental animals, most often rabbits, sheep or goats, at intervals of 1 week or more. Longer periods of time (8-16 months, in some instances) than are employed for protein antigens may be required to obtain anti-hapten antibody of optimal titre, specificity, and affinity [44, 52]. Vaitukaitis *et al.* [53] have recently described a method which employs a small, divided primary immunizing dose together with *Bordetella pertussis* vaccine and which may be particularly useful when the quantity of hapten or conjugate is limited. These and other practical problems connected with raising antisera for use in immunoassays have been reviewed recently [31, 54, 55].

Antibody detection

Since most animals immunized with drug-protein conjugates form antibodies with specificity for the carrier protein, the method chosen for detection of antidrug antibodies must be one in which antibodies specific for the carrier will not also interact. The simplest and most direct methods for the detection of drug-specific antibodies without interference by carrier-specific antibodies involve the direct demonstration of binding of radioactively labelled drugs or drug derivatives by antibody. Such binding can be demonstrated directly by equilibrium dialysis [56] or indirectly by one of the many methods now available to separate antibody-bound drug from unbound drug [31, 57-60]. The modes by which antibody and antibody-bound radiolabelled drug are separated from unbound (free) radiolabelled drug when these separation methods are employed are indicated in Table 4. In addition to equilibrium dialysis, currently used methods include the dextran-coated charcoal technique [61], gel or membrane filtration [62-65], electrophoretic methods [66], and coprecipitation of radiolabelled drug with anti-immunoglobulin antibody by the so-called 'double-antibody' method [65, 67]. Since many drugs are bound to a significant degree by normal serum proteins (especially in undiluted serum), it is important to ascertain that binding of radiolabelled drug is not observed with appropriate dilutions of control sera from non-immunized animals and from animals immunized with unrelated antigens.

Table 4. Separation of unbound from antibody-bound radiolabelled drug in RIA procedures.

METHOD	MODE OF SEPARATION	
	Antibody & antibody-bound radioactivity	Unbound (free) radioactivity
Equilibrium dialysis	Retained inside sac	Equal concentration inside & outside sac
Dextran-coated charcoal	Not adsorbed to charcoal; in supernatant after centrifugation	Adsorbed to charcoal; in precipitate after centrifugation
Gel filtration	Eluted early	Eluted late
Membrane filtration	Bound to nitrocellulose membrane	Washed through membrane
Electrophoresis and chromatoelectrophoresis	In γ-globulin electrophoretic fraction	Migrates with its own electrophoretic mobility
Double antibody method	Precipitated by antibody to animal γ-globulin	In supernatant after centrifugation

The most useful methods for radiolabelling of drugs for use in the detection of drug-specific antibodies involve the incorporation of either tritium (^{3}H) or radio-iodine (^{125}I) into drugs or drug derivatives; [^{14}C]labelled drugs can also be used, but the specific activities thus achieved are relatively low. Methods employing ^{14}C labels are thus relatively insensitive both in the detection of antibodies and in the development of radioimmunoassays.

Tritium can readily be introduced into most drugs by the Wilzbach technique [68], followed by chromatographic purification. It has a long half-life of 12.3 years and it represents no major external radiation hazard. However, it is not ideal. Firstly, since tritium emits only β-particles, liquid scintillation counting of radioisotopic disintegration must be employed. This can be cumbersome, time-consuming and costly; quench corrections with the addition of internal standards may be necessary, and chemiluminescence can cause delays or misleading results unless proper control procedures are carried out [69]. Secondly, in the case of certain drugs, sufficient specific activity cannot be achieved to provide the sensitivity needed for the subsequent development of RIA procedures.

[^{125}I]labelled drugs have certain advantages over [^{3}H]labelled drugs. ^{125}I is a gamma-emitter, and gamma counting is faster, more convenient, and less expensive than liquid scintillation counting. In addition, higher specific activities can be achieved with ^{125}I than with ^{3}H, with resultant increases in sensitivity, both in antibody detection and in the subsequent development of RIA methods. However, to label with ^{125}I, one must first introduce a tyrosine or other phenolic group to which the iodine can be attached. Such coupling of a phenolic group to a drug may be chemically difficult and, moreover, the resultant change in drug structure may alter its immunological behaviour. Other disadvantages of ^{125}I include: a relatively short half-life of 60 days, possible chemical damage to the drug caused by radio-iodine, and the need for frequent iodination with purification and immunological assessment of each newly iodinated batch.

In the absence of radiolabelled drug, antibodies to drugs can be demonstrated by other methods, including inactivation of drug-enzyme conjugates [70-73] or of drug-bacteriophage conjugates [74-76]. It is also possible to employ classical precipitin, complement fixation or passive haemagglutination methods to demontrate the interaction of anti-drug antibody with conjugates in which the hapten is attached to a carrier antigenically unrelated to the carrier used for immunization. In this latter instance, it is particularly important to ascertain that the interaction with antiserum is specifically inhibited by free, unconjugated drug [26].

When antibodies to a carrier do interfere with the detection of anti-drug antibodies, such antibodies can usually be removed by prior absorption of anti-serum with unconjugated carrier protein or with an appropriate insoluble immunoad-sorbent containing the carrier protein [26]. If one wishes to avoid the formation of anti-protein antibodies almost completely, one may take advantage of the fact that, while haptens coupled to homologous albumins are immunogenic, such conju-gates usually do not elicit significant production of antibodies to the carrier [26].

Assessment of antibody specificity and affinity

Once it has been demonstrated that a radiolabelled drug or drug derivative is bound by an antiserum, it must be shown that this binding is specific. First, one must demonstrate that non-radioactive drug is an effective inhibitor of this binding. Then, one must proceed to assess the degree of inhibition caused by metabolic pro-ducts of the drug and by other structurally related molecules. To indicate the degree of specificity which can be achieved in selected anti-drug antisera, the structural formula of digoxin is compared in Fig. 3 with those of digitoxin, a closely related cardiac glycoside, and dihydrodigoxin, a pharmacologically ineffec-tive metabolic breakdown product of digoxin. Despite the minimal chemical diffe-rences between digoxin and these two closely related glycosides, it is possible to elicit antidigoxin antibodies which bind digoxin 20-30 times more effectively than they bind either digitoxin or dihydrodigoxin [28, 30, 45]. Finally, it is also necessary to demonstrate that structurally more distant compounds, notably other drugs or substances normally present in human plasma, do not inhibit the binding of drug by antibody. For example, antibodies to digitalis glycosides react with steroid hormones [27]; therefore, it was necessary to demonstrate that concentra-tions of steroid hormones encountered in human sera did not inhibit the binding of [^{3}H]digoxin by antidigoxin antibodies before the RIA method could be used clini-cally to measure serum digoxin concentrations [44, 77].

In connection with studies of antibody specificity, it is important to re-cognize that antibodies to a given drug will usually react with metabolites of that drug. It may occasionally be possible to remove some of the antibodies which cross-react in this manner. It should be remembered, however, that absolute speci-ficity of antibodies for a given molecule will rarely, if ever, be observed [34]. Crossreactivity with drug metabolites may not represent a major disadvantage if, in practice, serum concentrations of 'immunoreactive' drug correlate well with values obtained by other methods and with the clinical state of the patients stu-died. For example, such a correlation does exist in the case of digoxin; this cor-relation, however, does not necessarily apply to other drugs because digoxin is somewhat unusual in that it is not extensively degraded in man, and in that seve-ral of its major metabolites are both pharmacologically and immunologically active [14].

Antibodies to a given drug will often react with related drugs of the same class, but this crossreactivity should not constitute a major problem clinically if it can be established with certainty that the patient is receiving a given drug and has not recently received a chemically related agent [14].

If problems are encountered in obtaining antibodies of satisfactory speci-ficity for use in an immunoassay procedure, it is important to remember that diffe-rent individual animals may produce antibodies which vary greatly in specificity; one should, therefore, examine several antisera to select the one with optimal specificity. Moreover, insofar as the specificity of antihapten antibodies appears to be directed primarily against that portion of the hapten molecule furthest from the site of conjugation to the carrier, antibodies of different specificity can usually be obtained if the hapten is coupled to the carrier *via* a different func-

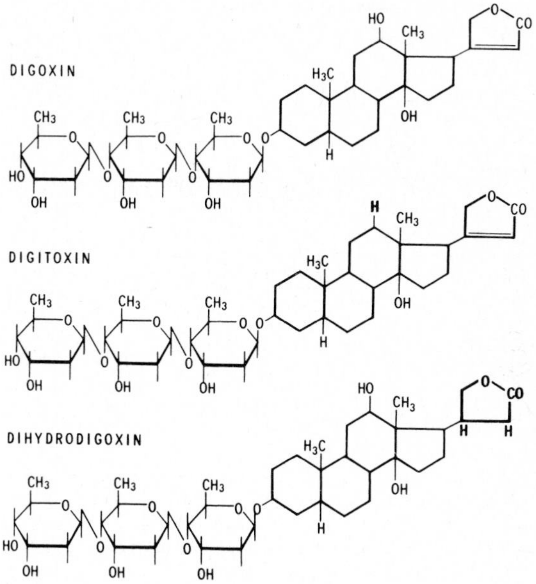

Fig. 3. Structural formulas
of digoxin, digitoxin and
dihydrodigoxin. The portions
of the digitoxin and dihydrodigoxin molecules, respectively, which differ structurally
from digoxin are shown in
bold.
Reprinted with permission from
Butler et al. [29].

DIGOXIN

DIGITOXIN

DIHYDRODIGOXIN

tional group [26, 31, 32].

Antiserum to a given
drug usually contains a
heterogeneous population of
antidrug antibodies with
different avidities or association constants. In general,
the greater the affinity of
antibody for drug, the more
sensitive will be the immunoassay which can be developed
and the simpler it will be
to make assay behaviour con-
tant and reproducible. Accordingly, the determination of
association constants is useful in the selection of antisera for use in immunoassay work; it is, however, not essential since the avidity of antibodies may be
inferred from a variety of measurements of hapten-antibody interactions [59].

Recent studies have also emphasized that dissociation constants of drug-
antibody complexes may be important when, in an immunoassay procedure, the adsorbent used to separate free from antibody-bound drug competes with antibody for
drug molecules which dissociate from antibody during the separation step [78, 79].

It should be pointed out that no two antisera to any antigen may ever be
considered to be identical either in specificity or in affinity. Even in antisera obtained at different times from a single animal, striking changes in the
affinity and specificity of antidrug antibodies have been observed with time [44].
Thus, published results regarding the specificity or affinity of antidrug antibodies should never be extrapolated to one's own antisera; furthermore, it would
seem reasonable to require commercial suppliers of drug antisera or of drug immunoassay kits to provide data concerning specificity and affinity with every sample
sold.

Antibody titre

By antibody titre is meant the greatest dilution of antibody which will produce a
given degree of binding of a stated amount of a drug [59]. The higher the titre,
the more determinations one can perform with a given volume of antiserum. Thus,
antidigoxin sera frequently can be used at dilutions theoretically great enough to
allow 200,000 digoxin determinations to be performed with 1 ml of antiserum. However, a high-titred antiserum is useless unless both specificity and affinity are
satisfactory.

Performance of immunoassays

Immunoassay methods for the measurement of drugs are based upon the ability of
drugs to inhibit the reaction between drug-specific antibodies and the correspon-

Fig. 4. Representative standard curve
for serum digoxin radioimmunoassay procedure. *In the presence of increasing
concentrations of non-radioactive digoxin
(in known reference standard solutions),
the percentage of [³H]digoxin (3ng) bound
by a constant amount of rabbit antidigoxin serum (50 μl of a 1:2500 dilution)
decreases from 59% in the absence of unlabelled digoxin to 16% in the presence
of 5 ng (mμg) of unlabelled digoxin. If,
under identical conditions, a patient's
serum reduces binding of [³H]digoxin to
29%, that serum contains 2 ng digoxin
per ml.*
Reprinted with permission from Butler
[30].

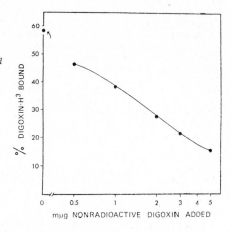

ding drug-carrier conjugate or the corresponding labelled hapten. Using principles delineated by Berson and Yalow [1-3], increasing concentrations of a
known standard solution of the drug are incubated with constant predetermined
amounts of drug-specific antibody and of drug-carrier conjugate, or of labelled
drug, under conditions of antigen excess. A standard curve (illustrated for
serum digoxin in Fig. 4) is then constructed, upon which decreasing amounts of
interaction between labelled drug and antibody can be shown to correspond with
increasing concentrations of unlabelled drug. If the biological fluid to be
assayed (a) does not interfere with the drug-antibody reaction, (b) does not
degrade the drug, and (c) does not contain substances which cross-react significantly with the drug antibody, the concentration of the drug in that biological
fluid can be determined from the degree to which it inhibits the reaction between
antibody and drug-carrier conjugate or labelled drug, when compared with a
simultaneously performed standard curve [31, 59, 66, 80].

Inhibition of complement fixation [40] or of passive haemagglutination[81]
has been used to measure drugs. However, because of their greater sensitivity,
precision, rapidity and convenience, greater experience has been obtained with
immunoassay methods which employ radioactively or physicochemically labelled
drugs or drug derivatives.

Until recently, most of the studies with labelled haptens employed radioactively labelled drugs or drug derivatives. Many methods are now available for
the separation of free, unbound radiolabelled drug from antibody-bound radioactivity in the development of RIA procedures [31, 57-60]. These include electrophoresis, gel filtration, adsorption systems (e.g. dextran-coated charcoal, membrane filtration), solvent and salt precipitation systems, solid-phase antibody
procedures and the double antibody method. Because of its convenience and rapidity, the dextran-coated charcoal method of Herbert *et al.* [61] has been widely
used in drug RIA procedures. It involves the almost instantaneous adsorption of
non-antibody-bound drug onto charcoal particles and its rapid centrifugal separation from antibody-bound radioactivity; thus, it is not useful where radiolabelled
drugs or drug derivatives are not effectively adsorbed to the charcoal or where,
with a high dissociation constant for a drug-antibody complex, results vary with
time as dissociated drug is progressively adsorbed to charcoal as a function of
the duration of the charcoal incubation step in the immunoassay procedure [79].
Because of such problems with adsorption methods, many newly developed RIA procedures have employed either the double antibody method or a solid-phase antibody
procedure. Theoretically, 'immunoradiometric' assay procedures employing radio-
iodinated antibody [82] may also be used, but extensive experience has not yet

been obtained with such procedures in the assay of drugs.

To eliminate some of the technical problems associated with the use of radiolabelled drugs in clinical laboratories or in automated equipment, physico-chemically-labelled drugs have recently been employed in the development of non-isotopic immunoassay procedures. For example, spin-labelled drugs have been used in an immunoassay procedure which takes advantage of the fact that the mobility of free radicals of spin-labelled drugs in the free, unbound state differs from that when bound to specific antibody, as measured in an electron spin resonance spectro-meter. This technique has proved useful in screening biological fluids in the detection of opiates and other drugs of abuse [83, 84]. Another, perhaps more useful, method has very recently been introduced into clinical use. It is based on the fact that antidrug antibodies will inactivate drug-enzyme conjugates in a reproducible manner which is readily quantifiable by simple spectrophotometric assays of enzymatic activity; increasing quantities of drug will reduce the degree of enzyme inactivation in a reproducible and predictable manner which can be used as the basis for a simple immunoassay procedure [69-73].

Limitations and problems

It is most convenient when an immunoassay procedure can be carried out with untrea-ted serum, plasma, or other biological fluid. In some instances, however, prior treatment or separatory procedures may be necessary to inactivate substances which degrade the drug being studied. In other cases, prior extractions or separatory procedures may be necessary to concentrate a drug, to remove it from a normal binding site on a plasma protein in the test serum, or to separate the drug from certain of its metabolites or from other structurally related compounds also capable of inhibiting the drug-antibody interaction [26, 31]. In RIA procedures, the presence of a radioisotope (administered for diagnostic or therapeutic pur-poses) in a patient's serum constitutes a potential source of error, if the pre-sence of the isotope is not known to the laboratory. In RIA procedures entailing liquid scintillation counting, chemiluminescence produced by urine and certain sera (especially from azotaemic patients) may also interfere with assay results. Neither of these sources of error in RIA, however, should cause a problem if pro-per control procedures are carried out [70, 79].

Although antibodies are stable for many years if properly stored in concen-trated form, deterioration of antisera may occur if appropriate precautions are not taken. Deterioration of radiolabelled drugs or drug derivatives may also occur with time; this is particularly true in the case of radio-iodinated deriva-tives of drugs [85]. Similarly, great care must be exercised in the preparation and storage of the drug standards used in the construction of standard immunoassay curves, because results in unknown specimens will be calculated on the basis of values obtained with these standards of pre-determined, known concentration [86].

As with all drug assay procedures, immunoassay methods will yield useful information only if it can be established, experimentally or clinically, that the drug concentrations in the specimens being assayed bear some relationship to a pharmacological effect of, or the clinical response to, that drug [87, 88]. In this latter connection, the time at which the specimen is best obtained with res-pect to the last dose of the drug is quite important and must be established before the immunoassay procedure can be used properly [14, 88].

COMPETITIVE PROTEIN BINDING ASSAYS OF DRUGS
General principles

Non-immunological competitive protein binding assays have enjoyed wide popularity in the field of hormonal assay since their introduction by Ekins in 1960 [4]. In recent years, such methods have been used with increasing frequency for the measurement of drug concentrations in serum and other biological fluids. The methods developed to date are identical in principle with RIA methods except that a serum or tissue protein with drug-binding properties is used to bind labelled drug in place of antibody [3, 4, 80]. As in RIA, a mixture of unlabelled and labelled drug is added to the binding protein. The competitive binding method, like RIA, requires separation of protein-bound from free, unbound radioactivity, followed by construction of a standard curve (similar to the RIA standard curve shown in Fig. 4) from which drug concentrations in unknown test specimens can then be determined.

Specific examples

In Table 3 are listed some drugs for which competitive protein binding assay methods have been developed. The methotrexate assay employs dihydrofolate reductase, obtained from mouse ascites tumour, as the drug-binding protein [89].Assays for cardiac glycosides employ Na^+, K^+-ATPase from guinea pig brain as the cardenolide-binding protein [90]. Assays for prednisolone [91-94] and other synthetic steroids with glucocorticoid activity [95] have employed either plasma corticosterone-binding globulin (transcortin) [91-94] or the cytosol from rat hepatoma tissue culture cells [95] as the glucocorticoid-binding reagent. Several assays for synthetic steroid drugs with progestational or other biological properties have employed tissue or serum proteins which bind progesterone. For example, assays for medrogestone [96], norethindrone [97], and danazol [98] utilize progesterone-binding globulin from pregnant guinea pig serum, while an assay for clogestone acetate employs a progesterone-binding protein obtained from rat uterus [99].

References

1. Berson, S.A. & Yalow, R.S., Adv. Biol. Med. Phys. 6 (1958) 349-430.

2. Berson, S.A. & Yalow, R.S., Harvey Lect. 62 (1966) 107-163.

3. Berson, S.A. & Yalow, R.S. in Immunobiology: Current Knowledge of Basic Concepts in Immunology and Their Clinical Applications (Good, R.A. & Fisher, D.W., eds.), Sinauer, Stamford, Connecticut (1971) pp. 287-293.

4. Ekins, R.P., Clin. Chim. Acta 5 (1960) 453-459.

5. Rothenberg, S.P., Proc. Soc. Exp. Biol. Med. 108 (1961) 45-48.

6. Murphy, B.E.P., Nature (Lond.) 201 (1964) 679-682.

7. Waxman, S., Schreiber, C. & Herbert, V., Blood 38 (1971) 219-228.

8. Butler, V.P., Jr., Metabolism 22 (1973) 1145-1153.

9. Spector, S., Ann. Rev. Pharmacol. 13 (1973) 359-370.

10. Marks, V., Morris, B.A. & Teale, J.D., Brit. Med. Bull. 30 (1974) 80-86.

11. Mulé, S.J., Sunshine, I., Braude, M. & Willette, R.E., Immunoassays for Drugs Subject to Abuse, CRC Press, Cleveland (1974).

12. Butler, V.P., Jr., J. Immunol. Meth. 7 (1975) 1-24.

13. Langone, J.J., Van Vunakis, H. & Levine, L., Acc. Chem. Res. 8 (1975) 335-342.

14. Butler, V.P., Jr., Progr. Cardiovasc. Dis. 14 (1972) 571-600.

15. Butler, V.P., Jr. & Lindenbaum, J., Amer. J. Med. 58 (1975) 460-469.

16. Smith, T.W., Amer. J. Med. 58 (1975) 470-476.

17. Koch-Weser, J., Duhme, D.W. & Greenblatt, D.J., Clin. Pharmacol. Therap. 16 (1974) 284-287.

18. Booker, H.E. & Darcey, B.A., Clin. Chem. 21 (1975) 1766-1768.

19. Lindenbaum, J., Mellow, M.H., Blacksone, M.O. & Butler, V.P., Jr., New Engl. J. Med. 285 (1971) 1344-1347.

20. Shaw, T.R.D., Howard, M.R. & Hamer, J., *Lancet 2* (1972) 303-307.

21. Wagner, J.G., Christensen, M., Sakmar, E., Blair, D., Yates, D., Willis, P.W. III, Sedman, A.J. & Stoll, R.G., *J. Amer. Med. Ass. 224* (1973) 199-204.

22. Preibisz, J.J., Butler, V.P., Jr. & Lindenbaum, J., *Ann. Int. Med. 81* (1974) 469-474.

23. Selden, R. & Smith, T.W., *Circulation 45* (1972) 1176-1182.

24. Weintraub, M., Au, W.Y.W. & Lasagna, L., *J. Amer. Med. Ass. 224* (1973) 481-485.

25. Landsteiner, K., *The Specificity of Serological Reactions,* Revised edn., Dover Publications, New York (1962) pp. 156-210.

26. Butler, V.P., Jr. & Beiser, S.M., *Adv. Immunol. 17* (1973) 255-310.

27. Butler, V.P., Jr. & Chen, J.P., *Proc. Nat. Acad. Sci. (U.S.A.) 57* (1967) 71-78.

28. Erlanger, B.F. & Beiser, S.M., *Proc. Nat. Acad. Sci. (U.S.A.) 52* (1964) 68-74.

29. Butler, V.P., Jr., Schmidt, D.H., Watson, J.F. & Gardner, J.D., *Ann. N.Y. Acad. Sci. 242* (1974) 717-730.

30. Butler, V.P., Jr., *New Engl. J. Med. 283* (1970) 1150-1156.

31. Parker, C.W., *Progr. Clin. Pathol. 4* (1972) 103-141.

32. Erlanger, B.F., *Pharmacol. Rev. 25* (1973) 271-280.

33. Beiser, S.M., Butler, V.P., Jr. & Erlanger, B.F. in *Textbook of Immunopathology,* 2nd edn. (Miescher, P.A. & Muller-Eberhard, H.J., eds.), Grune & Stratton, New York (1976) *in press.*

34. Vaughan, J.R., Jr. & Osato, R.L., *J. Amer. Chem. Soc. 74* (1952) 676-678.

35. Erlanger, B.F., Borek, F., Beiser, S.M. & Lieberman, S., *J. Biol. Chem. 228* (1957) 713-727.

36. Goodfriend, T.L., Levine, L. & Fasman, G.D., *Science 144* (1964) 1344-1346.

37. Weliky, N. & Weetall, H.H., *Immunochemistry 2* (1965) 293-322.

38. Haber, E., Page, L.B. & Jacoby, G.A., *Biochemistry 4* (1965) 693-698.

39. Anderer, F.A., *Biochim. Biophys. Acta 71* (1963) 246-248.

40. Hamburger, R.N., *Science 152* (1966) 203-205.

41. Tigelaar, R.E., Rapport, R.L. II, Inman, J.K. & Kupferberg, H.J., *Clin. Chim. Acta 43* (1973) 231-241.

42. Little, J.R. & Donahue, H. in *Methods in Immunology and Immunochemistry,* Vol. 2 (Williams, C.A. & Chase, M.W., eds.), Academic Press, New York (1968) pp. 163-174.

43. Butler, V.P., Jr., Beiser, S.M., Erlanger, B.F., Tanenbaum, S.W., Cohen, S. & Bendich, A., *Proc. Nat. Acad. Sci. (U.S.A.) 48* (1962) 1597-1602.

44. Smith, T.W., Butler, V.P., Jr., & Haber, E., *Biochemistry 9* (1970) 331-337.

45. Dumasia, M.C., Chapman, D.I., Moss, M.S. & O'Connor, C., *Biochem. J. 133* (1973) 401-404.

46. Lewis, J.E., Nelson, J.C. & Elder, H.A., *Nature New Biol. 239* (1972) 214-216.

47. Cheng, L.T., Kim, S.Y., Chung, A. & Castro, A., *FEBS Lett. 36* (1973) 339-342.

48. Chung, A., Kim, S.Y., Cheng, L.T. & Castro, A., *Experientia 29* (1973) 820-821.

49. Cook, C.E., Kepler, J.A. & Christensen, H.D., *Res. Commun. Chem. Pathol. Pharmacol. 5* (1973) 767-774.

50. Mahon, W.A., Ezer, J. & Wilson, T.W., *Antimicrob. Ag. Chemother. 3* (1973) 585-589.

51. Freund, J., Thomson, K.J., Hough, H.B., Sommer, H.E. & Pisani, T.M., *J. Immunol. 60* (1948) 383-398.

52. Jaffe, B.M., Smith, J.W., Newton, W.T. & Parker, C.W., *Science 171* (1971) 494-496.

53. Vaitukaitis, J., Robbins, J.B., Nieschlag, E. & Ross, G.T., *J. Clin. Endocrin. Metab. 33* (1971) 988-991.

54. Chase, M.W. in *Methods in Immunology and Immunochemistry,* Vol. 1 (Williams, C.A. & Chase, M.W., eds.), Academic Press, New York (1967) pp. 197-224; 237-306.

55. Hurn, B.A.L., *Brit. Med. Bull. 30* (1974) 26-28 *(see also ref.* 85 , *pp. 121-142).*

56. Eisen, H.N., *Methods Med. Res. 10* (1964) 106-114.

57. Hunter, W.M. & Ganguli, P.C. in *Radioimmunoassay Methods* (Kirkham, K.E. & Hunter, W.M., eds.), Churchill Livingstone, Edinburgh (1971) pp. 243-257.

58. Daughaday, W.H. & Jacobs, L.S. in *Principles of Competitive Protein-Binding Assays* (Odell, W.D. & Daughaday, W.H., eds.), Lippincott, Philadelphia (1971) pp. 303-324.

59. Hunter, W.M. in *Handbook of Experimental Immunology,* 2nd edn. (Weir, D.M., ed.), Blackwell, Oxford (1973) pp. 17.1—17.36.

60. Ratcliffe, J.G., *Brit. Med. Bull. 30* (1974) 32-37.

61. Herbert, V., Lau, K.-S., Gottlieb, C.W. & Bleicher, S.J., *J. Clin. Endocrin. Metab. 25* (1965) 1375-1384.

62. Haber, E., Page, L.B. & Richards, F.F., *Anal. Biochem. 12* (1965) 163-172.

63. Genuth, S., Frohman, L.A. & Lebovitz, H.E., *J. Clin. Endocrin. Metab. 25* (1965) 1043-1049.

64. Gershman, H., Powers, E., Levine, L. & Van Vunakis, H., *Prostaglandins 1* (1972) 407-423.

65. Van Vunakis, H. & Levine, L. in *Immunoassays for Drugs Subject to Abuse* (Mulé, S.J., Sunshine, I., Braude, M. & Willette, R.E., eds.), CRC Press, Cleveland (1974) pp. 23-35.

66. Yalow, R.S. & Berson, S.A., *Meth. Biochem. Anal. 12* (1964) 69-96.

67. Morgan, C.R. & Lazarow, A., *Diabetes 12* (1963) 115-126.

68. Wilzbach, K.E., *J. Amer. Chem. Soc. 79* (1957) 1013.

69. Butler, V.P., Jr., *Lancet 1* (1971) 186.

70. Engvall, E. & Perlmann, P., *Immunochemistry 8* (1971) 871-874.

71. Rubenstein, K.E., Schneider, R.S. & Ullman, E.F., *Biochem. Biophys. Res. Commun. 47* (1972) 846-851.

72. Schneider, R.S., Lindquist, P., Wong, E.T., Rubenstein, K.E. & Ullman, E.F., *Clin. Chem. 19* (1973) 82]-825.

73. Broughton, A. & Ross, D.L., *Clin. Chem. 21* (1975) 186-189.

74. Mäkelä, O., *Immunology 10* (1966) 81-86.

75. Haimovich, J. & Sela, M., *J. Immunol. 97* (1966) 338-343.

76. Andrieu, J.M., Mamas, S. & Dray, F., *Prostaglandins 6* (1974) 15-22.

77. Smith, T.W., Butler, V.P., Jr. & Haber, E., *New Engl. J. Med. 281* (1969) 1212-1216.

78. Meade, R.C. & Kleist, T.J., *J. Lab. Clin. Med. 80* (1972) 748-754.

79. Smith, T.W. & Haber, E., *Pharmacol. Rev. 25* (1973) 219-228.

80. Ekins, R.P., *Brit. Med. Bull. 30* (1974) 3-11.

81. Adler, F.L. in *Immunoassays for Drugs Subject to Abuse* (Mulé, S.J., Sunshine, I., Braude, M. & Willette, R.E., eds.), CRC Press, Cleveland (1974) pp.37-43.

82. Woodhead, J.S., Addison, G.M. & Hales, C.N., *Brit. Med. Bull. 30* (1974) 44-49.

83. Leute, R.K., Ullman, E.F., Goldstein, A. & Herzenberg, L.A., *Nature New Biol. 236* (1972) 93-94.

84. Schneider, R.S., Bastiani, R.J., Leute, R.K., Rubenstein, K.E. & Ullman, E.F. in *Immunoassays for Drugs Subject to Abuse* (Mulé, S.J., Sunshine, I., Braude, M. & Willette, R.E., eds.), CRC Press, Cleveland (1974) pp. 45-72.

85. Kirkham, K.E. & Hunter, W.M. (eds.), *Radioimmunoassay Methods,* Churchill Livingstone, Edinburgh (1971) pp. 100-104 & 189-193.

86. Bangham, D.R. & Cotes, P.M., *Brit. Med. Bull. 30* (1974) 12-17.

87. Brodie, B.B. & Reid, W.D. in *Fundamentals of Drug Metabolism and Drug Disposition* (LaDu, B.N., Mandel, H.G. & Way, E.L., eds.), Williams & Wilkins, Baltimore (1971) pp. 328-339.

88. Koch-Weser, J., *New Engl. J. Med. 287* (1972) 227-231.

89. Arons, E., Rothenberg, S.P., da Costa, M., Fischer, C. & Iqbal, M.P., *Cancer Res. 35* (1975) 2033-2038.

90. Brooker, G. & Jelliffe, R.W., *Circulation 45* (1972) 20-36.

91. Sandberg, D.H., Bacallao, C.Z. & Cleveland, W.W., *Biochem. Med. 4* (1970) 383-390.

92. English, J., Chakraborty, J. & Marks, V., *Ann. Clin. Biochem. 11* (1974) 11-14.

93. Leclercq, R. & Copinschi, G., *J. Pharmacokin. Biopharmaceut. 2* (1974) 175-187.

94. Wilson, C.G., Ssendagire, R., May, C.S. & Paterson, J.W., *Brit. J. Clin. Pharmacol. 2* (1975) 321-325.

95. Ballard, P.L., Carter, J.P., Graham, B.S. & Baxter, J.D., *J. Clin. Endocrin. Metab. 41* (1975) 290-304.

96. Jagarinec, N. & Givner, M.L., *Steroids 23* (1974) 561-578.

97. Okerholm, R.A., Keeley, F.J., Peterson, F.E., Smith, T.C. & Glazko, A.J., *Clin. Res. 21* (1973) 499.

98. Creange, J.E. & Potts, G.O., *Steroids 23* (1974) 411-420.

99. Stern, M.D. & Givner, M.L., *J. Clin. Endocrin. Metab. 40* (1975) 728-731.

Acknowledgements

The author's work is supported by grants from the United States Public Health Service (HL 10608), the New York Heart Association, the American Heart Association (72-853), and the Burroughs Wellcome Company. The author is the recipient of an Irma T. Hirschl Career Scientist Award.

ION-PAIR SOLVENT EXTRACTION AND CHROMATOGRAPHY

G-3

Göran Schill
Dept. of Analytical Pharmaceutical Chemistry,
University of Uppsala,
S-751 23 Uppsala, Sweden.

Ionized organic compounds can be extracted into organic solvents as ion pairs with
a counter-ion, and the ion pairs can in the organic phase form adducts with un-
charged complexing agents. The extent of extraction is controlled by the nature
of the organic solvent and the ion-pairing and/or the adduct-forming agent, and by
the concentration of these agents. The procedures are easy to adapt to both hydro-
philic and hydrophobic samples, but they are particularly useful for the extraction
of charged aprotic compounds and hydrophilic acids and bases.

The methods can be used in batch extractions as well as in partition chromatography
with straight and reversed phases. The selectivity depends on the binding within
the ion pairs and the complexes, as well as on the composition of the complexes.

Optical determination techniques can be used even for non-absorbing samples, if the
counter-ion has a high absorbance or fluorescence. It will then be possible to
quantify down to 0.01 n-mol of sample.

Examples are given of extractions and isolations from complex samples and biologi-
cal material: quaternary ammonium ions, amines (e.g. amitriptyline, nortriptyline,
clomipramine, alprenolol and de-alkylated and hydroxylated metabolites), carboxylic
and sulphonic acids (e.g. benzoic, mandelic and phenylacetic acid derivatives),
sulphonamides, barbiturates, glucuronides and sulphates (e.g. corticosteroid and
oestrogen metabolites). [For 'classical' solvent extraction, see the next 2 articles.-Ed.]

Drugs and metabolites are usually present in biological material in very low concentrations, and the determination will, as a rule, require methods with very high
sensitivity. In bioanalysis, the main interest is often focused on the development
of highly sensitive quantitation techniques, whilst the earlier stages of the procedure, particularly the isolation processes, follow traditional lines.

An isolation procedure that is not adapted to the actual problem can, however, have a highly disastrous influence on the result of an analytical determination. The yield can be low and also varying due to lack of control of important
conditions. An unsuitable isolation process can also decrease the sensitivity of
the quantitation step by not removing disturbing sample components.

A good isolation procedure must have *high selectivity,* i.e. give large
differences in distribution ratio between structurally closely related compounds.
However, the selectivity can be fully utilized only if the system is *highly*
flexible and offers the possibility of adjusting the distribution ratio to a
level suitable for extractive or chromatographic isolation.

CONTROL OF THE DISTRIBUTION RATIO

Liquid-liquid partition procedures can be given high flexibility if the distribution process is combined with complexation in one of the phases, usually the organic. The principle can be applied to both uncharged and charged compounds, but
only the latter case will be discussed here.

A cationic compound Q^+ can be extracted into an organic phase as an ion
pair with an anion X^-:

[Continued at foot of next p.

Table 1. Extraction constants of tetrabutylammonium ion pairs [1].
Organic phase: chloroform. *Ionic strength:* 0.1. E_{QX} *values for the sulphates are from ref.* [2].

Class	Anionic component	log E_{QX}
Inorganic	Cl^-	-0.11
	Br^-	1.29
	I^-	3.01
	ClO_4^-	3.48
Sulphonic acid	Toluene-4-sulphonic acid	2.33
	Naphthalene-2-sulphonic acid	3.45
	Anthracene-2-sulphonic acid	5.11
Sulphate	Phenylpropyl sulphate	4.20
	2-Napthyl sulphate	4.90
Phenol	Picric acid	5.91
	2,4-Dinitro-1-naphthol	6.45
Carboxylic acid	Acetic acid	-2.12
	Phenylacetic acid	0.27
	Benzoic acid	0.39
	Salicylic acid	2.42

Table 2. Extraction constants of glucuronic acid conjugates of corticosterone derivatives [2].
Organic phase: chloroform.
Counter-ion: tetrapentylammonium.

Glucuronic acid derivative of	log E_{QX}
Deoxycorticosterone	4.50
11-Deoxycortisol	3.66
11-Dehydrocorticosterone	3.17
Cortisone	2.95

Table 3. Extraction constants of cholic acid derivatives [2, 3].
Organic phase: chloroform. TBA = tetrabutylammonium, TPeA = tetrapentylammonium.

Anion	Cation	log E_{QX}
Cholate	TPeA	2.22
Glycocholate	TPeA	2.37*
Taurocholate	TPeA	3.81
Deoxycholate	TBA	2.23
Glycodeoxycholate	TBA	2.30
Taurodeoxycholate	TBA	3.90
Chenodeoxycholate	TBA	2.19
Glycochenodeoxycholate	TBA	2.35
Taurochenodeoxycholate	TBA	4.08
Dehydrocholate	TBA	2.10
Glycodehydrocholate	TBA	2.33
Taurodehydrocholate	TBA	3.97

[TEXT, continued]   * *conditional constant*

$$Q^+_{aq} + X^-_{aq} = QX_{org} \qquad \text{equilibrium constant: } E_{QX}.$$

This gives the following expression for the distribution ratio:

$$D_Q = [QX]_{org}/[Q^+]_{aq} = E_{QX} \cdot [X^-]_{aq}. \tag{1}$$

The distribution ratio of Q^+ (D_Q) is governed by the nature of the organic solvent and the counter-ion X^- (which affects the extraction constant E_{QX}) and by the concentration of X^- in the aqueous phase, i.e. by three parameters.

The distribution ratio can be varied within wide limits by the choice of counter-ion. Some examples of the influence of the anion are given in Table 1, which shows extraction constants of tetrabutyl-ammonium ion pairs with anions of widely different kinds from hydrophilic· inorganic to highly hydrophobic organic [1].

The ion-pair technique can be used for all kinds of ionizable compounds, but it offers particular advantages for substances that are impossible or difficult to extract in uncharged form, i.e. aprotic ions and highly hydrophilic acids and bases. Such compounds often appear as drugs or metabolites: quaternary ammonium ions, aminophenols, amino acids, sulphuric and glucuronic acid conjugates.

Ion-pair extraction of glucuronides of some corticosterone derivatives is illustrated in Table 2. The glucuronides are rather hydrophilic but they can be extracted as ion pairs with tetrapentylammonium. The complexation with tetrapentylammonium gives an increase with 20 alkyl carbons, and the resulting ion pair will be rather hydrophobic and easily extracted into the organic phase [2].

Cholic acids and their conjugates can be extracted into chloroform as ion pairs with tetrapentyl- or tetrabutyl-ammonium (Table 3). The cholic acids and their glycine derivatives have extraction constants of the same magnitude, while the taurine conjugates have considerably higher constants [3].

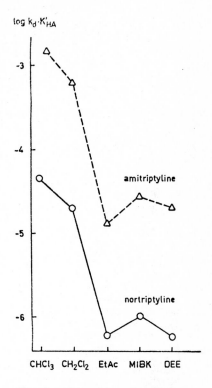

Fig. 1. Extraction of amitriptyline and nortriptyline as bases. EtAc = ethyl acetate; MIBK = methylisobutyl ketone; DEE = diethyl ether.
Figs. 1 & 2 have appeared in ref. 4 (acknowledgement: Pergamon Press).

SELECTIVITY

The ion-pair technique also opens good possibilities for varying the extraction selectivity. The extraction of a secondary amine, nortriptyline, and its *N*-methyl derivative, amitriptyline, in the traditional mode as bases is demonstrated in Fig. 1. The hydrogen-donating chloroform gives considerably higher partition coefficients (k_d) than the hydrogen-accepting solvents (ethyl acetate, methylisobutyl ketone and diethyl ether), but the selectivity (i.e. the difference between the logarithms of the partition coefficients) is essentially independent of the solvent properties.

The situation is quite different in ion-pair extraction (Fig. 2). The extraction constant changes with the nature of the organic solvent, but the selectivity (i.e. the difference between the logarithms of the extraction constants) is no longer independent of the solvent properties. Also, it is obviously dependent on the properties of the counter-ion since quite different selectivity changes are obtained when Cl^- and ClO_4^- are used as counter-ions. The highest selectivity for ammonium ions of different degree of substitution is obtained with a counter-ion of good hydrogen-accepting ability (Cl^-) and with a hydrogen-donating solvent that mainly solvates the anion component of the ion pair ($CHCl_3$, CH_2Cl_2) [4].

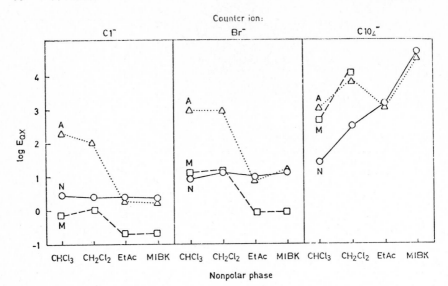

Fig. 2. Extraction of nortriptyline (N), amitriptyline (A)
and *N*-methyl-amitriptyline (M)
as ion pairs.

Table 4. Structure-extraction constant
relationships.
Organic phase: chloroform or methylene
chloride.

Structural change	$\Delta \log E$
+ CH_2 (alkyl or aryl)	+0.5
+ OH (alcoholic)	-1
+ OH (phenolic)	-2
+ NR_3 (tertiary amine)	-1
Tertiary → secondary alkyl-ammonium	-0.5
Tertiary → primary alkyl-ammonium	-1
Tertiary → quaternary alkylammonium*	-2

* *same number of alkyl carbons*

Structural changes in the
ion pair will in such systems
give rise to considerable changes
in the extraction constant. Some
examples are given in Table 4
[5, 6]. For the polar groups,
the given figures are rather
approximate.

COMPLEX FORMATION IN THE
ORGANIC PHASE

The versatility of the ion-pair
extraction procedure can be considerably increased by adding
to the organic phase an agent
S that can form complexes with
the ion pair.

$$QX_{org} + nS_{org} = (QX \cdot S_n)_{org} \qquad \text{\textit{equilibrium constant:} } k_n$$

If the ion pair QX and the complex $QX \cdot S_n$ are present in the organic phase, the
equilibrium constants, E_{QX} and k_n, can be combined into a new extraction constant
[4]. Substitution in eq (1) gives

$$D_Q = E_{QX} \cdot [X^-] \cdot (1 + k_n \cdot [S]^n_{org}) \qquad (2)$$

Four parameters will now control the extraction: the nature and the concentration
of the counter-ion X^- and the nature and the concentration of the complexing agent S.

An illustration is given in Fig. 3. Four amines with different degrees of
substitution are extracted as ion pairs with naphthalene-2-sulphonate. The organic

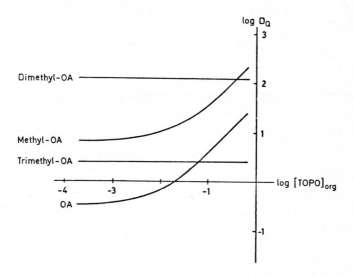

Fig. 3. Extraction of ion pairs with trioctylphosphineoxide
(TOPO) as complexing agent. *Counter-ion:* naphthalene-2-
sulphonate, 0.05 M. *Organic phase:* chloroform.
OA   = octylammonium.
Methyl-OA   = *N*-methyloctylammonium.
Dimethyl-OA = *N,N*-dimethyloctylammonium.
Trimethyl-OA = *N,N,N*-trimethyloctylammonium.

From ref. [7].
Acknowledgement
for this & other
Figs.: Acta Pharm.
                Suecica.

phase contains trioctylphosphineoxide (TOPO) as complexing agent. A logarithmic
plot of D_Q *versus* the TOPO concentration shows a large increase of the distribution ratio with the TOPO concentration for the primary and the secondary ammonium
ions, while the tertiary and the quaternary are not affected. It is apparent
that an agent like TOPO which only gives complexes with ion pairs of primary and
secondary ammonium ions can have a large influence on the extraction selectivity
[7].

ION-PAIR EXTRACTION IN PHOTOMETRY AND FLUORIMETRY

Ion-pair extraction has, for more than 30 years (but under another name), been
used for transforming ions into compounds with high absorbance, simply by extracting them with counter-ions of high molar absorptivity. Amounts down to 1 μg/ml
can be determined by such procedures.

The fluorimetric technique will by an analogous procedure enable determinations to be performed down to 10 ng/ml. As an example, Table 5 shows an assay
method for propantheline, a quaternary ammonium ion, in plasma [8]. The method
also demonstrates how the ion-pair technique can be used to overcome disturbances
from the matrix, e.g. protein-binding of the drug.

The first step is an extraction of propentheline as perchlorate. Theoretically, a distribution ratio D = 100 should be necessary, but it was found that
a counter-ion concentration corresponding to D = 10,000 was required to overcome
disturbances from the plasma. The next step is a purification. The final purification is made in the third step where a transformation into an ion pair with
the highly fluorescent anion dimethoxyanthracene-sulphonate is obtained. The
ion pair is determined fluorimetrically. The limiting concentration is 10 ng/ml
of plasma, with which a yield of about 80% is achieved.

Table 5. Determination of propantheline in plasma.
Organic phase: dichloromethane. Q = propantheline, A = amines, HX = acids,
AS = dimethoxyanthracene sulphonate.

Extraction	Sample	Reagent	pH	Extracted
1	Plasma	$HClO_4$ 0.1 M	3	$QClO_4$, $HAClO_4$, HX
2	Organic phase from 1	$NaClO_4$ 10^{-2} M	13	$QClO_4$, (A)
3	Organic phase from 2	AS $10^{-4.7}$ M	11	QAS (fluorimetric determination)

Table 6. Distribution of *N,N*-dimethylprotriptyline (MPT) [9].
Organic phase: dichloromethane. Initial concentration: 3×10^{-7} M. Fluorimetric
determination of MPT in both phases.

Glass equipment	Aqueous phase	pH	Ionic strength	Recovery, %
Acid-washed	Phosphate buffer	7.3	0.1	95 ± 4*
" "	" "	7.3	0.01	87 ± 6
Silanized	" "	7.3	0.1	74
"	" "	7.3	0.01	62 ± 4
"	Water	–	–	52 ± 1

*S.D.

The yield is somewhat low, but as a rule it is difficult to obtain quantitative recoveries at concentration levels below 10^{-7} mol/l due to adsorption onto phase boundaries, mainly the walls of glass vessels. A study made on a highly fluorescent quaternary ammonium ion in 10^{-7} M solution is shown in Table 6 to illustrate the difficulties. The recovery decreases with decreasing ionic strength, and it is also obvious that silanization of the glass will increase the losses.

In this concentration range serum can have a considerable influence on the extraction yield. Normally, serum can be expected to decrease the yield by protein binding, but the reverse has also been observed as demonstrated in Fig. 4 [9]. The increase of the distribution ratio of the quaternary ammonium ion may be due to ion-pair extraction with the anion of a weak organic acid present in the serum.

LIQUID CHROMATOGRAPHY

The ion-pair extraction principle has also found use in partition chromatography, both in straight- and in reversed-phase systems. In both cases the counter-ion is added to

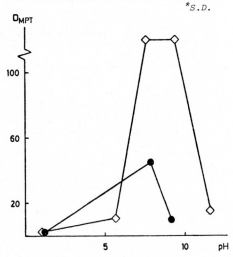

Fig. 4. Distribution of *N,N*-dimethylprotriptyline (MPT) in the presence of serum. *From ref.[9].*
Organic phase: dichloromethane.
Aqueous phase: serum + phosphate buffer: 1 + 1,● ; 1 + 7,◇.
Initial concentration of MPT: 5×10^{-8} M.

the aqueous phase.

The principles for regulation of the retention time of a cation Q^+ appear from the expression for the retention time t_R:

$$t_R = \frac{L}{v} (1 + k') \quad \text{where } L = \text{column length, } v = \text{linear speed of the mobile phase.} \tag{3}$$

In a system with a stationary aqueous phase (straight phase) the capacity factor k' is given by:

$$k' = \frac{1}{E_{QX} \cdot [X^-]} \cdot \frac{V_s}{V_m} \quad \text{where } V_s/V_m \text{ is the phase volume ratio in the column.} \tag{4}$$

The retention time t_R decreases with increasing concentration of the counter-ion X^-.

In a system with a mobile aqueous phase (reversed phase)

$$k' = E_{QX} \cdot [X^-] \cdot \frac{V_s}{V_m} \tag{5}$$

and t_R increases with the counter-ion concentration.

The versatility of the ion-pair systems makes them very useful in chromatography. It is easy to adapt the systems to different kinds of samples and to regulate k' to a suitable level. Also, they can give high selectivity: the separation factors will then be large, and comparatively few theoretical plates will be needed, which will reduce the time for the separation.

The chromatographic systems have a very good long-term stability if they are carefully thermostatted and if the mobile and the stationary phase are equilibrated with each other. The sample should, as a rule, be injected as an ion-pair with the counter-ion of the stationary phase; yet amines and acids can be injected in uncharged form if the sample concentration is much lower than the counter-ion concentration of the stationary phase.

STRAIGHT-PHASE SYSTEMS

Phase systems with high selectivity according to the above-mentioned principles will allow the separation of compounds with very small structural differences. Quinidine and dihydroquinidine can be separated with perchlorate as counter-ion and with a mixture of dichloromethane and 1-butanol (19 + 1) as mobile phase (Fig. 5 [10]). In spite of the close structural resemblance (a double bond in quinidine is hydrated in dihydroquinidine) a separation factor of 1.4 is obtained.

A similar phase system has been used for separation of isomeric aminophenols (Fig. 6 [11]). The three compounds are monohydroxy derivatives of a phenylalkyl amine, alprenolol. The separation is probably due to differences in intramolecular hydrogen bonding between the phenolic group and an oxygen in the side-chain.

Metabolism of drugs will often give rise to structural changes that give high separation factors. An example is given in Fig. 7 [12] which shows the separation of alprenolol from its main metabolites. The separation factor between the parent compound and the de-isopropyl derivative is about 5, while the 4-hydroxy derivative gives a separation factor of about 50.

Anionic metabolic products can be separated in systems with quaternary alkylammonium ions in the aqueous phase. Fig. 8 shows the separation of a number of steroidal sulphuric acid conjugates with tetrapropylammonium as counter-ion, while

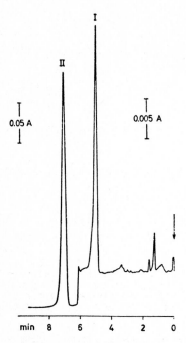

Fig. 5. Separation of dihydro-
quinidine (I) and quinidine (II)
as perchlorate ion pairs.
Support: LiChrosorb SI 100 (10 μm).
Stationary phase: HClO₄(0.2 M) +
NaClO₄(0.8 M).
Mobile phase: dichloromethane +
1-butanol (95 + 5).

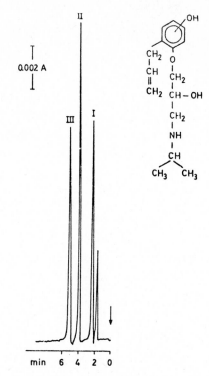

Fig. 6. Separation of positional isomer
of hydroxyalprenolol as perchlorate ion
pairs. I: 6-hydroxyalprenolol; II: 5-
hydroxyalprenolol; III: 4-hydroxyalpre-
nolol. *From ref. [11].*
Support: Partisil 10 (10 μm).
Stationary phase: HClO₄(0.2 M) + NaClO₄
(0.8 M).
Mobile phase: 1,2-dichloroethane + 1-
butanol (95 + 5).

separation of some glucuronides with
tetrapentylammonium as counter-ion
is demonstrated in Fig. 9 [13].

AMPLIFICATION OF THE DETECTOR RESPONSE

Photometric detectors are widely used in HPLC due to their high stability and sensitivity. The ion-pair principle offers unique possibilities of obtaining a high
response on this kind of detector by use of a counter-ion with high molar absorptivity at the measuring wavelength. An increase in response for cations can be obtained, for example, with picrate [14] and naphthalene-2-sulphonate [15] as counter-
ions. An example is given in Fig. 10 which shows the separation of homologous primary alkylamines with 0.1 M naphthalene-2-sulphonate as the stationary phase. The
ion pairs have a molar absorptivity of 3000, which enables <15 ng of amine to be
determined. Quaternized derivatives of protriptyline and imipramine have been used
as response-increasing counter-ions in the chromatography of anionic compounds [16].
Molar absorptivities of >10,000 can be obtained.

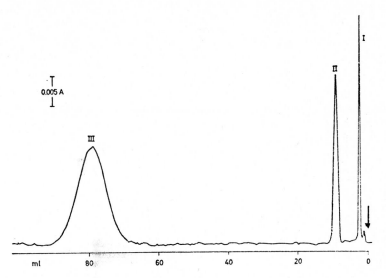

Fig. 7. Separation of alprenolol (I), de-isopropylalprenolol (II) and
4-hydroxyalprenolol (III). *From ref. [12].*
Support: cellulose (37-74 μm).
Stationary phase: $HClO_4$ (0.1 M) + $NaClO_4$ (0.9 M).
Mobile phase: cyclohexane + 1-pentanol (93 + 7).

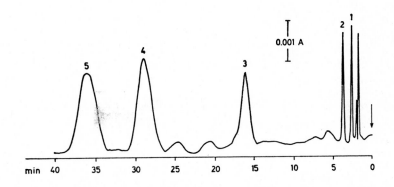

Fig. 8. Separation of steriodal sulphuric acid conjugates.
Support: Lichrospher SI 1000 (10 μm). 1: equilin-3-sulphate; 2: 17-α-
dihydroequilin-3-sulphate; 3: estradiol-3-sulphate; 4: oestriol-17-sulphate;
5: oestradiol-17-sulphate. *From ref. [13].*
Stationary phase: tetrapropylammonium (0.1 M), pH 7.0.
Mobile phase: chloroform + 1-butanol (19 + 1).

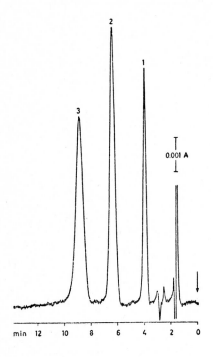

Fig. 9 *(on left)*. Separation of glucuronides. 1: 8-quinolyl glucuronic acid; 2: 2-naphthyl glucuronic acid; 3: 4-methylumbelliferyl glucuronic acid. *From ref. [13].*
Support: LiChrosphere SI 100 (10 μm).
Stationary phase: tetrapentylammonium (0.065 M).
Mobile phase: chloroform + 1-butanol (19 + 1).

Fig. 10 *(below)*. Separation of primary aliphatic amines. Pr = propylamine; Bu = butylamine; Pe = pentylamine; He = hexylamine. *From ref. [15].*
Stationary phase: naphthalene-2-sulphonate (0.1 M).
Mobile phase: chloroform + 1-pentanol (9 + 1).
Support: cellulose (37-74 μm).

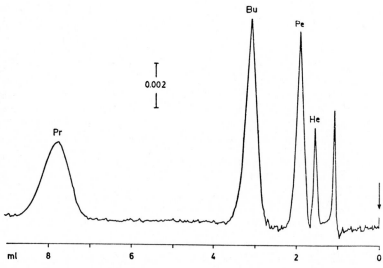

BIOLOGICAL SAMPLES

The high selectivity and good separating efficiency of the ion-pair systems make them useful for isolations even from rather impure extracts of biological samples.

An isolation of a quaternary ammonium compound from serum is demonstrated in Fig. 11 [10]. The compound is extracted with dichloromethane as the perchlorate and the organic phase is evaporated. The residue is dissolved in the mobile phase and, without further purification, injected onto a separation column with perchlorate as the stationary phase. A well-isolated sample peak is obtained.

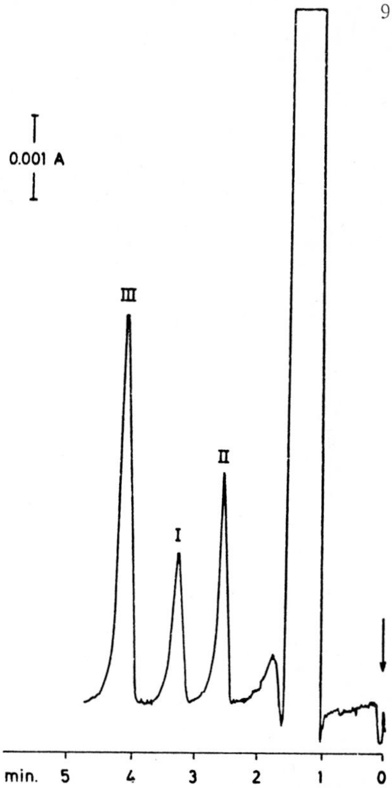

Determination of a tertiary amine, clomipramine, and its de-methyl metabolite in plasma is demonstrated in Fig. 12 [17]. The plasma is made alkaline, and the amines are extracted as bases with diethyl ether, re-extracted into 0.01 M H_2SO_4 and, after rendering the solution alkaline, finally extracted into 1,2-dichloroethane. The sample solution is injected onto a separation column with methanesulphonic acid (0.1 M) as the stationary phase. Quantitation is made by use of desipramine as internal standard.

Quantitative extraction of a hydrophilic, aprotic ion can, as a rule, be obtained only by use of a highly hydrophobic counter-ion. An example is given in Fig. 13, which demonstrates a method for determination of acetylcholine, a quaternary ammonium ion, in rat ischias nerve [18]. The extraction is made with dichloromethane and di-t-butyl-2-hydroxybenzenesulphonate as counter-ion. The chromatographic isolation is made with picrate as counter-ion in order to obtain a suitable retention and a detector response of sufficient magnitude (the picrate ion pair has a molar absorptivity of 10,000). Disturbances from the sulphonate are avoided by addition of tetrabutylammonium as displacer [19]. The acetylcholine peak is well defined and, down to a few ng, can be determined with acceptable precision by peak-area measurement.

Fig. 11. Determination of a quaternary ammonium compound in plasma.
Support: LiChrosorb SI 100 (10 μm).
I: 120 ng (corresponding to 400 ng/ml plasma).
Stationary phase: $HClO_4$ (0.2 M) + $NaClO_4$ (0.8 M).
Mobile phase: 1-butanol + dichloromethane + hexane (20 + 30 + 50).

REVERSED-PHASE SYSTEMS

The extraction from biological material is a time-consuming procedure, and there is a high demand for methods that will enable a direct injection of biological fluids. Ion-pair chromatographic systems with aqueous mobile phases are very suitable for that purpose.

The reversed-phase systems are particularly useful in the separation of hydrophilic compounds. A separation of five benzoic acid derivatives and two benzenesulphonates is demonstrated in Fig. 14 [20]. Silanized silica particles

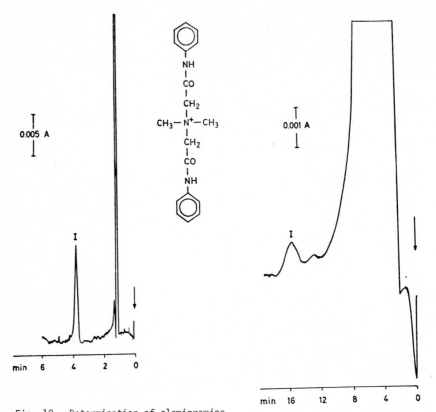

Fig. 12. Determination of clomipramine and de-methylclomipramine in plasma. I: clomipramine, 50 ng; II: de-methylclomipramine, 50 ng; III: desipramine (internal standard), 100 ng. *From ref. [17].* *Support:* Partisil 10 (10 μm). *Stationary phase:* methanesulphonic acid (0.1 M). *Mobile phase:* n-hexane + dichloromethane + 1-butanol (45 + 45 + 10).

Fig. 13. Determination of acetylcholine (I) in rat ischias nerve as picrate ion-pair. *From ref. [18].* *Support:* cellulose Munktell 410 (37-74 μm). *Stationary phase:* 0.06 M picrate, pH 6.5. *Mobile phase:* chloroform + 1-butanol (96 + 4).

are used as support, pentanol as the stationary phase and an aqueous solution of tetrabutylammonium as the mobile phase. The retardation increases with increasing hydrophobic character, and benzoic acids with hydrophilic substituents are eluted first. The positional isomers are well separated: 4-substituted compounds are more hydrophilic than 3-substituted.

The selectivity and versatility of the reversed-phase systems with pentanol as stationary phase is demonstrated in a series of separations: mandelic and phenylacetic acid derivatives in connection with catecholamine metabolism in Figs. 15 and 16, nicotinic acid derivatives in Fig. 17 [21].

Good separation has also been obtained with butyronitrile as the stationary

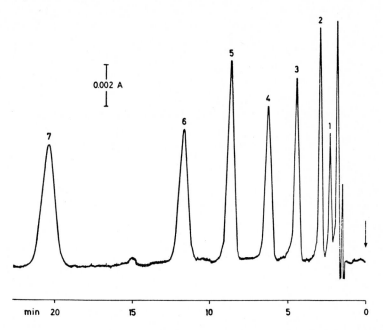

Fig. 14. Separation of benzoic acid and benzenesulphonic acid derivatives.
1: 4-aminobenzoic acid; 2: 3-aminobenzoic acid; 3: 4-hydroxybenzoic acid;
4: 3-hydroxybenzoic acid; 5: benzenesulphonic acid; 6: benzoic acid; 7:
toluene-4-sulphonic acid.
Support: LiChrosorb SI 60 silanized (10 μm).
Stationary phase: 1-pentanol.
Mobile phase: tetrabutylammonium (0.03 M), pH 7.4.

*Figs. 14 & 20 have
appeared in ref.[20]
(an Elsevier journal).*

phase. Fig. 18 shows a separation of barbiturates, while sulphonamide separations
are demonstrated in Fig. 19 [22].

The reversed-phase systems are excellent for gradient elution: the eluting
power of the mobile phase is easily increased by decreasing the concentration of
the counter-ion. An example is given in Fig. 20. The tetrabutylammonium concentration decreases from 0.1 M to zero with the first 5 ml of the mobile phase. Components of very different hydrophobic character can now be separated within a short
time, and the last peak in the chromatogram is only slightly wider than the first
[20].

The gradient technique can also be used to avoid a decrease of separating
efficiency when large-volume samples are injected [20].

Studies entailing isolations from unpurified plasma have shown that many
successive samples can be injected without inconvenient loss of separating efficiency. Further improvement of the column stability can be obtained by use of
pre-columns, back-flushing and other technical aids.

The reversed-phase systems are very simple to use and to adapt to different
kinds of samples, and it is likely that they will considerably broaden the field
of application of ion-pair partition chromatography.

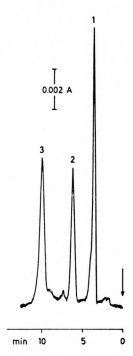

Fig. 15. Separation of hydrophilic carboxylic acids. 1: 4-hydroxy-3-methoxymandelic acid; 2: 4-hydroxy-3-methoxyphenylacetic acid; 3: mandelic acid. *From ref. [21].*
Support: LiChrosorb SI 60 silanized (10 μm).
Stationary phase: 1-pentanol.
Mobile phase: tetrabutylammonium (0.1 M), pH 7.4.

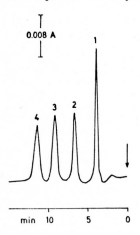

Fig. 16. Separation of phenylacetic acid derivatives. 1: 4-hydroxy-3-methoxyphenyl-acetic acid; 2: 3,4-dimethoxyphenylacetic acid; 3: 3,4,5-trimethoxyphenylacetic acid; 4: 4-methoxyphenylacetic acid. *From ref. [21].*
Support: LiChrosorb SI 60, silanized (10 μm).
Stationary phase: 1-pentanol.
Mobile phase: tetrabutylammonium (0.03 M), pH 7.4.

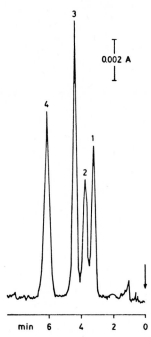

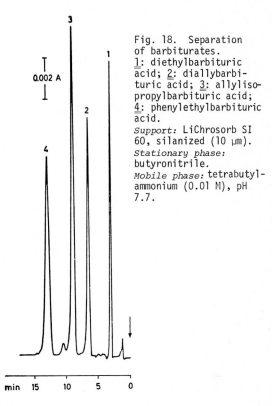

Fig. 18. Separation
of barbiturates.
1: diethylbarbituric
acid; 2: diallybarbi-
turic acid; 3: allyliso-
propylbarbituric acid;
4: phenylethylbarbituric
acid.
Support: LiChrosorb SI
60, silanized (10 μm).
Stationary phase:
butyronitrile.
Mobile phase: tetrabutylammonium (0.01 M), pH
7.7.

Fig. 17. Separation of
nicotinic acid derivatives.
1: nicotinic acid; 2:
isonicotinic acid; 3:
3-hydroxymethyl-5-fluoro-
pyridine; 4: 5-fluoroni-
cotinic acid. *From ref. [21].*
Support: LiChrosorb SI 60,
silanized (10 μm).
Stationary phase: 1-pentanol.
Mobile phase: tetrabutylammonium (0.03 M), pH 7.4.

Fig. 19 *(on right).* Separation
of sulphonamides. 1: 2-sulpha-
nilamidopyrimidine; 2: 3-
methoxy-2-sulphanilamidopyra-
zine; 3: 4-methyl-2-sulphanila-
midopyrimidine; 4: 5-methyl-
3-sulphanilamidoisoxazole;
5: 2,4-dimethyl-6-sulphanila-
midopyrimidine.
Support: LiChrosorb SI 60,
silanized (10 μm).
Stationary phase: butyronitrile.
Mobile phase: tetrabutylammonium
(0.01 M), pH 7.9.

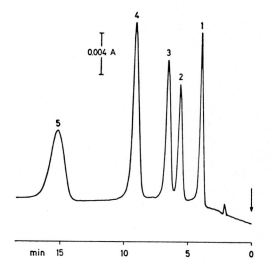

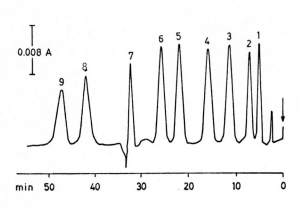

Fig. 20. Reversed-phase, ion-pair partition chromatography with gradient elution. 1: 4-aminobenzoic acid; 2: 3-aminobenzoic acid; 3: 4-hydroxybenzoic acid; 4: 3-hydroxybenzoic acid; 5: benzenesulphonic acid; 6: benzoic acid; 7: toluene-4-sulphonic acid; 8: 2,4-dimethylbenzenesulphonic acid; 9: 2-hydroxybenzoic acid. *Support:* LiChrosorb SI 60, silanized (30 μm). *Stationary phase:* 1-pentanol. *Mobile phase:* phosphate buffer pH 7.4 with a linear tetrabutylammonium gradient from 0.1 M to zero in the first 5 ml.

References

1. Schill, G., in *Ion Exchange and Solvent Extraction,* Vol. 6 (Marinsky, J.A. & Marcus, Y., eds.), Marcel Dekker, New York (1974) pp. 1-57.

2. Fransson, B. & Schill, G., *Acta Pharm. Suecica 12* (1975) 107-118.

3. Fransson, B. & Schill, G., *Acta Pharm. Suecica 12* (1975) 417-424.

4. Modin, R. & Schill, G., *Talanta 22* (1975) 1017-1022.

5. Gustavii, K., *Acta Pharm. Suecica 4* (1967) 233-246.

6. Persson, B.A., *Acta Pharm. Suecica 5* (1968) 335-342.

7. Schröder-Nielsen, M., *Acta Pharm. Suecica, in press.*

8. Westerlund, D. & Karset, K.H., *Anal. Chim. Acta 67* (1973) 99-106.

9. Westerlund, D. & Theodorsen, A., *Acta Pharm. Suecica 12* (1975) 127-148.

10. Persson, B.A., *personal communication.*

11. Borg, K.O., Gabrielsson, M. & Jönsson, T.E., *Proc. International Solvent Extr. Conf. ISEC 1974,* Vol. III, Soc. Chem. Ind., London (1974) pp. 2173-2181.

12. Borg, K.O., Gabrielsson, M. & Jönsson, T.E., *Acta Pharm. Suecica 11* (1974) 313-324.

13. Fransson, B., *Acta Pharm. Suecica, in press.*

14. Eksborg, S. & Schill, G., *Anal. Chem. 45* (1973) 2092-2100.

15. Eksborg, S., *Acta Pharm. Suecica 12* (1975) 19-36.

16. Lagerström, P.O. & Theodorsen, A., *Acta Pharm. Suecica 12* (1975) 429-434.

17. Lagerström, P.O., Carlsson, I. & Persson, B.A., *Acta Pharm. Suecica, in press.*

18. Ulin, B., Gustavii, K. & Persson, B.A., *J. Pharm. Pharmacol., in press.*

19. Eksborg, S. & Schill, G., *Acta Pharm. Suecica 12* (1975) 1-8.

20. Wahlund, K.G., *J. Chromatog. 115* (1975) 411.

21. Wahlund, K.G., *J. Chromatog., in press.*

22. Johansson, M. & Wahlund, K.G., *to be published.*

G-NC

Handling of conjugates, and study of metabolites[*]

Remark by L.E. Martin: Not all glucuronides are hydrolyzed by β-glucuronidase. Moreover, alkyl sulphate esters are not hydrolyzed by arylsulphatase. *Remark by* R.A. Chalmers: With the anion-exchange method described below (Art. S-6), acidic conjugates including β-glucuronides and glycine conjugates are quantitatively extracted, although an alternative GC system would be required, e.g. a 1% loaded column compared to the 10% loading used for low molecular mass organic acids. In this way it is possible to study directly intact conjugates which may also be identified by direct MS including the high-resolution approach (cf. the trichloroethanol β-glucuronide example in Art. S-6).

Comment by A.W. Forrey: The argument that glucuronides and other conjugates could usefully be isolated intact, in the study of drug metabolites, is a good one. Selected individual families of conjugates can then be subjected to appropriate work-up procedures. We are using this approach in the study of [35S]frusemide in resistant patients. *Viewpoint put forward by* C.R. Jones: It is arguable whether we should indeed concentrate upon identifying the conjugates rather than aglycones. A single aglycone can give rise to several conjugates, and therefore the task of identifying the aglycones may well be simpler and cheaper. Additionally, the aglycone is much more likely to be responsible for any toxic or therapeutic effects than is the conjugate. Perhaps we should be aiming at the purification of the hydrolytic enzymes in order to reduce side-reactions.

Comment by D.A. Cowan (*following remarks by* D.B. Faber): We believe that it is essential to determine the physico-chemical properties of chemically synthesized compounds which can then be shown to be identical with the metabolites of a particular drug. Although it is a chicken-and-egg situation, we feel it best to decide on the possible identity of metabolites and synthesize these compounds. Then we can determine whether an observed process is occurring metabolically or chemically.

Strategy of method development

Approach advocated by G. Schill.— One should start by determining relevant physico-chemical data, particularly distribution coefficient (uncharged compound), acid dissociation constants, extraction constants (ion-pair equilibria; equation 2 in Art. G-3) and molar absorptivity. These constants give highly concentrated information about the analytically significant properties of the compound. 'Trial-and-error' will in most cases take considerably longer than will the construction of a theoretically based method as the outcome of measuring constants etc. The 'constants determination technique' has, moreover, the advantage of giving a basis for the modifications of the preliminary technique that are usually necessary.

Should the initial emphasis be on sample preparation or on detection ?[*]

The balance of opinion was in favour of the latter, in a discussion opened by S.S. Brown. D.B. Faber: I prefer firstly to investigate detection possibilities in relation to the sensitivity required, and then to develop a simple sample preparation procedure which avoids chemical changes and keeps the original profile from the moment of sampling (e.g. in connection with the total fate of a drug, with toxicological analyses and therapy control); thirdly, the complexity of drug treatment and interactions calls for improvement of both separation and detection techniques. J.J. de Ridder: A detection technique is a pre-requisite for developing sample preparation procedures; otherwise one is working blind. Either, for low-level determinations, one develops a detection technique and then sample preparation, or the latter can come first where the compound is available in radio-labelled form so that one can continuously follow the progress of sample preparation trials.

---

[*] *from a 'Panel Discussion' which actually concluded the Techniques Forum; relevant to E. Reid's contribution (Art. G-1) which opens this Section.*

[Subject-matter relating to Art. G-1 continues on pp. 105-106.- ED.]

Immunoassays/Protein-binding assays (Art. G-2, by V.P. Butler)

Question by A.P.A. Woolley.— In view of the longer half-life of ^{14}C as compared with ^{125}I and ^{3}H, what do you see as the role of ^{14}C in RIA ? *Reply by* V.P.Butler.— When one states that ^{14}C has a long half-life (5730 years), one is stating that relatively few atoms of ^{14}C will disintegrate per second or minute. The shorter half-lives of ^{3}H (12.26 years) and of ^{125}I (60.2 days) indicate that many more atoms of these radioisotopes will disintegrate per unit time than will atoms of ^{14}C. According to my calculations, a gram-atom of ^{3}H will undergo 467 times more disintegrations per unit time, and a gram-atom of ^{125}I 35,000 times more disintegrations, than will a gram-atom of ^{14}C. Thus, one can achieve much higher specific activities (disintegrations per unit time per unit mass) with ^{3}H- or ^{125}I-labelling than one can with ^{14}C-labelling.[*] High specific activities or radiolabelled compounds are required for optimal sensitivity of RIA methods, as well as for conservation of antisera stocks. Therefore, I doubt whether ^{14}C-labelled compounds will be used extensively in RIA or competitive protein binding assay studies.

Question by L.S. Jackson.— Is any information available on techniques for precipitation by second antibody in the presence of dextran-ammonium sulphate, for instance, to make this a more suitable technique for RIA drug screening methods ? The aim would be to utilize the specificity of the second antibody in immunoassays. *Reply by* V.P. Butler.— I am not familiar with the use of either of these reagents to accelerate precipitate formation by second antibody when a double-antibody method is used. Thus I can only speculate as to their possible effects. Dextran, of course, has been used to promote the precipitation of antigen-antibody complexes, so it might be useful in this regard. Some single-antibody immunoassay methods employ ammonium sulphate to precipitate antigen-antibody or hapten-antibody complexes. These ammonium sulphate methods are somewhat less specific and less reproducible than the double-antibody method; thus, whilst it is likely that ammonium sulphate would accelerate precipitation of soluble complexes containing the first and second antibodies, its use might have other non-specific effects on non-antibody-bound tracer which might detract from the specificity and reproducibility of double-antibody RIA methods. *RIA & drugs.-* Landon, J. & Moffat, A.C., *Analyst 101* (1976) 225-243.-*ED.*

Ion-pair[†] methods (Art. G-3, by G. Schill)

Answer to D. Dell: Normal coating techniques are used for deposition of stationary phases such as perchloric acid and sodium perchlorate on silica. *Question by* A. Bye.— What is the relative importance of particle size of columns as compared with the ion-pairing properties of the compound ? *Reply.—* The situation is complex, but small particles add extra effects outside ion-pairing.

Question by R.E. Majors.— In the normal phase method (i.e. aqueous stationary phase, relatively non-polar mobile phase), use of a fairly polar solvent in the mobile phase might bring about dissociation of the ion pair. What effect would this have on the chromatography, especially peak shape ? *Reply.—* Such dissociation of the ion pair must be avoided. Otherwise, a severe leading or trailing edge peak will result, depending on whether the normal or reverse phase mode is being used. Dissociation can be avoided by including another counter-ion in the mobile phase (i.e. saturating it with a counter-ion). For example, consider the equilibrium:

$$QX_{aq} \rightleftharpoons Q^{+}_{org} + \overset{\downarrow}{X}^{-}_{org} \cdot \qquad HA^{+}_{org} + X^{-}_{org}$$

One must add a counter-ion (e.g. X^{-}_{org}) to the mobile phase to shift the equilibrium to the left and avoid dissociation.

EDITORIAL FOOTNOTES:
[*]*This point has a bearing on comments made in Art. G-1 concerning ^{14}C (as compared with ^{3}H) specific activity as a possible constraint in radioderivatization or recovery assessment.* [†] *Deplorable synonym registered by a company (Waters): "paired ion".*

SEPARATION OF DRUGS FROM BODY FLUIDS: (1) LOW-VOLUME EXTRACTION, AND (2) PROBLEMS ASSOCIATED WITH PLASMA PROTEIN

D.B. Campbell
Servier Laboratories
Greenford, Middx. UB6 7PW, U.K.

(1) Extraction procedures

Extraction procedures have, in the past, been designed to remove drugs from biological fluids with the goal of achieving the highest possible recovery with minimum contamination. (A useful review of the field has recently appeared [1].) This has been achieved with an apparent disregard of time and effort involved, and often little attempt has been made to rationalize each step in terms of effort, efficiency and precision.

    Methods are, in general, longer and more complex than are required, and once reported in the literature they are handed down from one laboratory to another with ever-increasing embellishments. Procedural dictums have been unquestioningly accepted, one example being the recommendation that for drug extraction the organic solvent to aqueous phase ratio should be 10 : 1 [2]. The technique now described uses an organic-to-aqueous phase ratio of only 1 : 50, and has achieved the same extraction capability for all but one of the drugs studied.

Table 1. Recoveries of drugs from urine with a low volume of chloroform. *The values in ITALICS were obtained with radiolabelled drugs, and assume 100 µl of chloroform for quantitation purposes.*

Drug	% recovery ±S.D.
Amphetamine	78 ±5
Fenfluramine*	90 ±4
"	*93 ±1*
Gliclazide ('1702')	*72 ±4*
Indapamide ('1520')	*0 ±5*
Methadone	83 ±3
Methylamphetamine	80 ±5
Norfenfluramine	85 ±5
Pethidine	99 ±1
Piribedil ('495')	*93 ±1*

* Conventional extraction with diethyl ether gave 92% recovery (on basis of all the solvent)

Methods, and procedure for urine

Of the 9 drugs investigated, two (indapamide and gliclazide) were acidic, and the others as listed in Table 1 were basic. All had partition coefficients between chloroform and water, pH 7.4, of >15, except for indapamide. Except when ^{14}C-labelled drugs were used (as indicated in Table 1), estimation was by GC methods [3]. To urine (5 ml, pH-adjusted) in a tapered tube was added 100 µl of chloroform containing a suitable internal standard. After vortex-mixing for 30 sec (even 5 sec gave 90% extraction for fenfluramine) and centrifugation, an aliquot of the organic phase was injected directly into the GC apparatus.

Results and comments

Recoveries and reproducibility are as good as by existing methods (Table 1), except for the especially water-soluble compound indapamide. With no evaporation step the total time for extraction is only 2 min — a 10-20 fold decrease over that in previous methods. Moreover, unpurified solvent can be used, and the overlying aqueous layer prevents evaporation. With such short mixing times, no contaminating material enters the solvent, and thus the GC traces are very clean. When drug solutions in 5 ml of chloroform in untreated 30 ml glass tubes were shaken for 10 min to check for adsorption onto glass, this was found to be low, although significant for piribedil and fenfluramine (3.5%) and for 2 acidic drugs (2%). Evaporation to dryness caused losses (14-48%) of all the drugs.

    A variation of this procedure is applicable to plasma: 50 µl is extracted with 50 µl of solvent with internal standard in a 1 ml Dreyer tube. For 14 hypnotics that have been investigated, recoveries have varied from 43% for barbitone to 100% for glutethimide [4]. This micro-technique has wide application for all drugs with plasma concentrations >1 µg/ml; an appropriate pH is used for each.

(2) Protein-binding problems

Many drugs are bound to plasma or tissue protein, and it is sometimes necessary to break down the drug/protein complex and remove contaminants prior to extraction. Numerous protein-precipitation procedures have been used to achieve this dissociation, but often without prior knowledge of recoveries or of the stability of the drug under the conditions used.

Stevens & Bunker [5] have investigated recoveries of some 36 basic compounds from whole blood, employing various protein-precipitation procedures as used in forensic toxicology. Tungstic acid [6], ammonium sulphate [7], aluminium chloride [8], hydrochloric acid [9], trichloroacetic acid and perchloric acid were investigated. Their results (Table 2) show that only with perchloric acid were all the tested compounds extracted: for the 12 tested, the extractability was >10% (but better than 50% in only one instance). Only half of the compounds were extracted better than 10% using tungstic acid or ammonium sulphate, compared with four-fifths using aluminium chloride, 5 M HCl, trichloroacetic or perchloric acid. Although 5 M HCl gave higher recoveries, cocaine, colchicine, aphenadrine and phenazone could not be recovered in any yield. Only colchicine was lost completely using aluminium chloride. Low recoveries were shown to arise from both drug precipitation and degradation.

Table 2. Extraction of basic compounds from whole blood with different protein-precipitation procedures [5].

| | Distribution of cpds. | | |
PRECIPITANT	Up to 80%	Up to only 50%	Up to only 10%
Tests on a wide range of compounds*			
Tungstic acid	2	18	33
Ammonium sulphate	2	18	26
Aluminium chloride	5	29	35
5 M HCl at 80°	13	30	32
Tests on only 12 of the compounds			
Trichloroacetic acid	2	8	10
Perchloric acid	1	11	12

* Antazoline   Strychnine   Tryptamine
Chloroquine   Thiorida-   Pethidine
Dextropro-   zine   Codeine
  poxyphene   Trifluo-   Morphine
Imipramine   perazine   Phenazone
Orphenadrine   Papaverine   Mescaline
Quinine   Methaqua-   Methylam-
Amitriptyl-   lone   phetamine
 line   Cocaine   Tranyl-
Chlorprom-   Nicotine   cypromine
 azine   Mepyramine   Amphetamine
Methadone   Caffeine   Ephedrine
Opipramol   Colchicine
Paraquat   Tyramine
Perphenazine   Lignocaine

For the majority of drugs in fresh, clean samples, protein precipitation is unnecessary; but in forensic samples when blood and tissue samples have decomposed, precipitation may be required, and the aluminium chloride method is recommended as being the 'safest'.

1. Reid, E., Analyst 101 (1976) 1-18.
2. Jackson, J.V., Isolation and Identification of Drugs (Clarke, E.G.C., ed.), Pharmaceutical Press, London (1969) p. 16.
3. Ramsey, J. & Campbell, D.B., J. Chromatog. 63 (1971) 303-308.
4. Flanagan, R., personal communication.   5. Stevens, H.M. & Bunker, V.W. (1976),
6. Valor, P., Ind. Eng. Chem. (Anal. edn.) 8 (1946) 456.   [to be published.
7. Nicholls, L.C., Toxicology in the Scientific Investigation of Crime, Butterworth, London (1956) p. 348.
8. Stevens, H.M., J. Forens. Sci. Soc. 7 (1967) 184-193.
9. Dubost, P. & Pascal, S. Ann. Pharm. Franc. 11 (1953) 615-619.

Comments and questions (with replies by D.B. Campbell) on the foregoing (pp. 105-106)

(1) (J.S. Cridland)-Possible variation: use a less dense solvent than the aqueous phase, the risk of adsorptive losses being minimized by silylation of tubes - which leads to a reversal of the meniscus of the aqueous phase. Queries.-Why use chloroform? Was the alcohol washed out before use (could account for chloroform losses into urine phase)? (J.E. Fairbrother). Do prolonged extractions worsen contamination? (C.R. Jones). — Unwashed chloroform was used since it separates into tapered part of the tube & the vol. can be seen. Precision & recoveries are unaffected by 'losses' of chloroform into urine. Contamination is not a problem with extraction times <30 sec; >30 sec leads to emulsions. (2) Fresh plasma samples protein-bind drug &/or marker more than old samples (D.A. Cowan). Protein binding could be worse with anionic drugs than with the cations (amines) tested; best to extract without prior precipitation (G. Schill).—Latter agreed by D.B. Campbell, where samples 'clean'; acid drugs generally bind more strongly than bases.

Section on Sample preparation

SOLVENT EXTRACTION

S-1

C.R. Jones
Dept. of Drug Metabolism,
Wellcome Research Laboratories,
Beckenham, Kent, BR3 3BS, U.K.

Each laboratory has its own techniques for developing suitable methods for solvent extraction of compounds present in biological fluids at the µg or ng level. Because of the large number of possible solvents and conditions it is desirable to adopt a logical approach to the selection. The thoroughness of the 'clean-up' needed will depend upon the subsequent analysis, e.g. a GC method may require only a simple primary extraction.

Some biological samples are best extracted in solid form, e.g. freeze-dried, perhaps by a sequence of solvents chosen in order of increasing polarity.

Liquid-liquid extraction is more familiar, but requires a careful choice of solvent, the properties of which can be compared before use so as to enable a shortlist of suitable candidates to be compiled. Other factors which are important include: method and duration of mixing, presence of inorganic salts, volume ratios, presence of a second solvent, solubilities, etc. These are discussed with reference to problems which have arisen and their subsequent solutions.

Insofar as the Forum which has led to this book was aimed at the practicalities of drug assay, the emphasis of this article will be on practical considerations.

The aim of solvent extraction is to separate the wanted compound from the unwanted background. It can reasonably be regarded as the one technique with which we all get involved, and although we exploit the same few underlying principles I am sure that we all have our own favourite methods. So it seems best that I explain the approach which we use in our unit at Wellcome when developing an extraction method for drug assay, and include examples from various sources to serve as a focus. I shall confine myself mainly to those cases where there are a large number of samples containing a single component for measurement or identification.

The early origins of solvent extraction are lost in the past, and certainly it was used extensively in the last century; but its use to separate trace substances from biological samples was put on a rational basis by Brodie and his co-workers in a series of papers in the 1940's [1]. We will, then, consider the approaches which we use now and which are based upon those principles.

LIQUID-SOLID EXTRACTION METHODS

Before dealing with liquid-liquid methods it is worth considering some aspects of liquid-solid extraction. Extraction of solid samples is often particularly suitable for highly polar compounds which would otherwise tend to remain in the aqueous phase; it may also be useful for those amphoteric compounds which cannot be easily extracted from water at any pH. A convenient aspect of this technique is that polar solvents miscible with water can be used. Solid biological samples most frequently encountered are:-
(a) freeze-dried — e.g. tissues;
(b) dehydrated — e.g. addition of anhydrous sodium sulphate to whole blood;
(c) coated onto a finely divided solid support.

When urine is to be freeze-dried it is convenient to add a quantity of a cellulose filtering aid so that a fine dried powder results. Similarly if an alcoholic extract of faeces is rotary-evaporated, the resulting thick brown 'varnish'

Table 1. Typical
eluotropic series
for extracting
solid samples

n-hexane	
carbon tetrachloride	
di-isopropyl ether	
toluene	*increasing polarity*
chloroform	
1,2-dichloro-ethane	
acetone	
ethyl acetate	
ethanol	
methanol	
water	

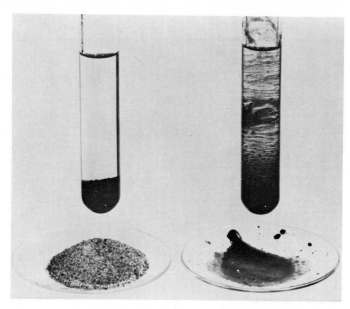

Fig. 1. Processing of faeces extracts *(see text)*.
Bottom left: Beads coated with the alcohol-extracted
material. *Bottom right:* Material isolated without beads.
Above: Appearance after shaking with chloroform.

around the inside of the flask is very difficult to deal with. If, however, suffi-cient glass ballotini beads are added before rotary evaporation, each bead is sepa-rately coated and thus a convenient finely divided sample results which can be poured like liquid and after extraction does not require centrifugation. Fig. 1 shows a heap of such coated beads which have been poured through a fine funnel onto a watch-glass alongside a second watch-glass containing the normal dried faeces ex-tract. Also shown are the tubes containing these samples after shaking with chloro-form.

Once the solid samples have been obtained, the next consideration is the choice of solvent, and when developing a method it is useful to work down a list of solvents of increasing polarity. Table 1 shows a list based upon a typical eluo-tropic series as published in most chromatography books. The preferred solvent is usually the least polar one which will efficiently extract the required substance. This will often follow a solvent of lower polarity which has removed some inter-fering constituents.

LIQUID-LIQUID EXTRACTION METHODS

These procedures depend upon the intended subsequent steps.

(a) If the extraction is to be followed by another separation such as GC, TLC or HPLC then it may suffice for the 'clean-up' to be only marginal. Such a simple one-step procedure has been described as a preamble to GC [2]. De Angelis *et al.* [3] used a typically uncomplicated extraction of diaminopyrimidines before quanti-tation by TLC.

(b) If the final measurement is highly specific, such as a colorimetric or a fluo-rescence assay, then again a simple extraction will often suffice. Tetracyclines, for example, can be directly extracted from plasma into amyl acetate, and measured after the addition of a fluorogenic reagent [4].

(c) If the extract is to be subjected to a final direct non-specific measurement, a more elaborate and exacting procedure is required which may involve transfer into and out of organic solvents, with aqueous washes included too. This is the type with which most of us are concerned at various times.

Optimization

Whatever method is chosen, success depends upon optimizing the conditions. It is well worth approaching this systematically, the first task being to choose the solvent.

Choice of solvent

The properties of the ideal solvent, in my view, are listed below and are examined in turn. Other workers may well have different ideas.

1) Cheap or easily recoverable.

2) Non-toxic and not highly flammable.

I doubt whether anyone will quarrel with these, but at times we all have to compromise and hence, for example, diethyl ether is often used despite the danger of fire.

3) Immiscible with water.

When a solvent is partly miscible with water the expected volume changes of the two phases can be partly avoided by presaturating the solvent with water. However this will not avoid the transfer of polar solutes along with the water dissolved in the solvent. Butanol, by dissolving about 20% water (w/w), is particularly bad in this respect, hence the high background of contaminants with this solvent.

4) Of convenient specific gravity.

What is considered convenient depends upon the order of operations. If the required phase has an inconvenient specific gravity it can sometimes be adjusted by the addition of appropriate inert solvent so as to make it float or sink in water, e.g. hexane or carbon tetrachloride.

5) Of suitable volatility.

Subsequent evaporation will require a high volatility, but it should be noted that considerable volume losses of a volatile upper phase can occur during even a short centrifugation if the tubes are not capped.

6) Of high chemical stability and inertness.

Although these properties are obviously important they are sometimes overlooked. For instance, shaking ethyl acetate with mineral acid can cause some hydrolysis to produce ethanol and acetic acid, both of which tend to increase the miscibility of the phases. Ketones although usually satisfactory can be rather reactive so that acetone is not suitable for use with some amines.

7) Transparent to UV and non-quenching for liquid scintillation counting.

Whether these are important considerations depends entirely upon the final method of measurement.

8) Not prone to form an emulsion.

It is not possible to predict whether an emulsion is likely, but a good rule-of-thumb is that if a solvent is ideal in all other respects it is bound to form an emulsion! Emulsions are the enemy of efficient extraction because of the large surface area of interface which they present. They are better avoided rather than broken up later, so a long, gentle agitation is to be preferred to a short, vigorous one. If it is necessary to break an emulsion it can be done by spinning hard, touching with a glass rod, passing through filter paper, repeatedly freezing and thawing, and so on. But it is likely that there will be significant losses at the fragments of emulsion which remain.

9) Dissolves the un-ionized but not the ionized form of the compound.

Selective extraction by means of different pH values depends upon this property of the solvent. Solvents can be conveniently assessed by setting up tubes containing the required substance dissolved in water at pH values above and below its pK_a. Each is then shaken with solvents as shown in Fig. 2. A good choice would be one in which there was a large difference between the concentrations in the same solvent at high and low pH.

This simple assessment will usually quickly lead to a suitable choice and avoid the dangers of too theoretical an approach. For example, one recommended method for extracting the basic drug pyrimethamine from urine included a pre-wash with chloroform of urine acidified with HCl, the chloroform washings then being discarded. Unfortunately pyrimethamine hydrochloride is soluble in chloroform, which ensured that almost all the drug was thrown away with the washings.

I have short-listed some organic solvents in Table 2, in rough order of increasing polarity. It is convenient when assessing solvents to examine about five covering the range of this list, and when the results are known a narrower selection can then be made, so that the least polar solvent which will efficiently extract the desired constituent can be chosen. This list does not take into account the selectivity of solvents, which will vary with the nature of the solute and which is usually not predictable. Sometimes a suitable extraction is achieved by a mixture of two solvents, but this must be determined by trial and error.

Mixing

This is often done too vigorously and for too long a time. It can conveniently be achieved with a minimum of emulsion formation by making use of a mechanical tube roller or by gentle end-over-end mixing as illustrated in Fig. 3. The illustrated 'tumble-mixer' has been in continual use for about five years and substantially similar equipment is now offered commercially.

A suitable duration of mixing is usually determined by plotting the measured transfer into solvent against time, which follows a simple exponential. A compromise between what is ideal and what is practicable can then be chosen. It is possible, however, to be too careful. We had a compound which was extracted from alkaline plasma into solvent then back into aqueous acid. A 10-min mixing was acceptable for the first transfer, but 20 min was used. The overall recovery was then found to be disappointing. It eventually transpired that plasma protein was slowly transferring along with the drug, so that protein binding retarded the final extraction. Fig. 4 illustrates the dependence of the last transfer upon the duration of mixing for the first.

Salting-out

Sometimes the presence of a high concentration of inorganic salts aids the transfer from aqueous to solvent phase, but sometimes it actually hinders it. This must be tried in practice.

The presence of high concentrations of electrolyte can also affect the miscibility of solvents. For example, if sufficient anhydrous sodium carbonate is added to 10% (v/v) ethanol, the latter will separate from the water and can be removed for analysis.

Partition coefficients

Measurements of partition coefficients can be of great value, but they can also be misleading especially where there is a degree of miscibility of the phases. Thus when an amidinourea was back-extracted from di-isopropyl ether containing 10% (v/v) *n*-butanol into an equal volume of dilute acid, it was found that the concentration in the aqueous phase was only about 8 times that of the other phase. Yet when the volume ratio was 20 : 1 the ratio of concentrations was found to favour the acid by a factor of 50.

Presence of a second solvent

This is commonly recommended usually in the form of an alcohol, especially to reduce the likelihood of adsorption to glass or to protein. In the example quoted above, the working range of concentrations was increased very substantially by adding butanol to the ether.

Solubility

It is worth determining the solubility of the compound in the organic solvent and in the final aqueous phase, so as to determine whether the system will deal with an adequate range of concentrations. For instance it is no use using sulphuric acid for the final back-extraction if the sulphate is not sufficiently soluble. However, simple solubility experiments are only a guide. Sometimes the pH for optimal solubility does not coincide with that for optimal transfer, which again must be determined by trial and error.

Adsorption onto glass

This is more likely from non-polar solvents, being much more noticeable at very low concentrations.

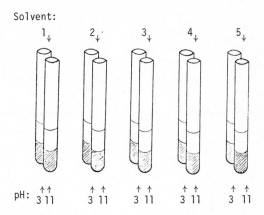

Fig. 2. Assessment of solvents for extraction at low and high pH.

Table 2. Short-list of solvents for liquid-liquid extraction. *The listing is in approximate order of increasing polarity.*

	UV cut-off, nm	b.p., °C	Price ratio	Remarks
n-hexane	210	69	6.3	low flash-point
cyclohexane	210	81	1.7	
carbon tetrachloride	265	77	1.5	toxic
benzene	280	80	1.0	toxic
toluene	285	111	1.1	
diisopropyl ether	220	68	(1.0)	low flash-point; peroxides
diethyl ether	220	35	1.7	low flash-point; peroxides
amyl acetate	285	149	2.2	
chloroform	245	61	2.0	
1,2-dichloro-ethane	230	83	1.7	toxic
methylisobutyl ketone	330	116	2.0	
ethyl acetate	260	77	2.0	
n-butanol	215	118	2.2	dissolves too much water

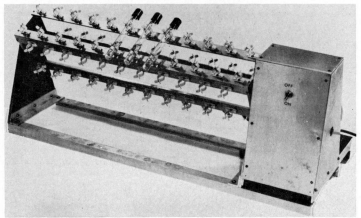

Fig. 3.
Mechanical
'tumbler-mixer'.

Below:
Fig. 4.
Efficiency of
back-extraction
of basic drug from
organic solvent
into 0.1 N HCl
after an initial
extraction from
plasma into the
solvent.

Probably many of the instances
quoted for loss through adsorption on glass are in fact due
to losses of a different sort,
but undoubtedly it can occur.
As mentioned above, the addition
of small amounts of polar solvents, especially alcohols, can
help, and so can silanization
of glassware; but these measures
are not always effective.   If
radio-labelled compounds are
being measured then addition
of 'cold' carrier is the preferred method.

VALIDATION OF THE METHOD

When these various factors have
been optimized the extraction
method must be shown to possess:

a) adequate sensitivity and suitable working range of concentrations;
b) low background interference;
c) adequate specificity;
d) adequate reproducibility.

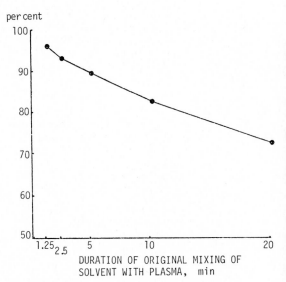

per cent

DURATION OF ORIGINAL MIXING OF
SOLVENT WITH PLASMA, min

    In practice if the recovery is less than about 75% the reproducibility is
unlikely to be suitable, but this depends upon the reasons for the losses. If they
are due to adsorption, evaporation or inadequate mixing, etc., the recovery will
be variable. If it is due, for example, to poor partition, it may be acceptably
constant. In any event an internal standard is desirable, if available.

CONCLUDING COMMENTS

This presentation is inevitably a somewhat sketchy and inadequate coverage of this
vast subject. I have not dealt with special techniques which have instead been
covered by other contributors, including sample preparation for GC and HPLC *(see
especially* Arts.G-1&S-5) and ion-pair extraction (Art.G-3), but I have tried to
indicate what kind of approach is practicable when one is faced with developing a
suitable solvent-extraction method.

References

1. Brodie, B.B., Udenfriend, S. & Baer, J.E., *J. Biol. Chem. 168* (1947) 299-309.

2. Ramsey, J. & Campbell, D.B., *J.Chromatog. 63* (1971) 303-308 *(see also* this Volume, Art. G-NC).

3. De Angelis, R.L., Simmons, W.S. & Nichol, C.A., *J.Chromatog. 106* (1975) 41-49.

4. Lever, M., *Biochem. Med. 6* (1972) 216-222.

Useful sources of information

Weissberger, A., Proskauer, E.S., Riddick, J.A. & Toops, E.E., eds., *Organic Solvents,* Vol. 7 of *Techniques of Organic Chemistry,* 2nd edn. Interscience, New York (1955).

Brodie, B.B., *Basic Principles in the Development of Methods of Drug Assay,* in *Handbook of Experimental Pharmacology,* 1st edn., Vol. 28, part 2 (Eichler, O., series ed.), Springer-Verlag, Berlin (1971).

Titus, E.O., *Isolation Procedures - Liquid Extraction and Isolation Techniques* in *Fundamentals of Drug Metabolism and Drug Disposition,* 1st edn. (La Du, B.N., Mandel, H.G. & Way, E.L., eds.), Williams and Wilkins, Baltimore (1971) pp. 419-436.

SOLVENT EXTRACTION AS APPLIED TO FLUPHENAZINE AND ITS METABOLITES

S-2

R. Whelpton and S.H. Curry
Department of Pharmacology and Therapeutics
The London Hospital Medical College
Turner Street, London, E1 2AD, U.K.

A number of attempts have been made to assay fluphenazine and its metabolites in biological samples collected following the administration of therapeutic doses in man [1-6]; but progress has been severely limited by:
1) difficulties in separation of pharmacologically interesting compounds;
2) the small quantities involved;
3) low sensitivity of available detection systems.

We have approached this problem by selective solvent extraction of fluphenazine and its metabolites from biological samples collected after doses of ^{14}C-labelled samples of the drug.

When compounds are extracted from solutions of controlled pH into suitable solvents, or mixtures of solvents, typical sigmoidal curves are obtained [7]. This approach facilitates the separation of fluphenazine, fluphenazine sulphoxide and 7-hydroxy-fluphenazine from each other. Fluphenazine is extracted into heptane such that it is 50% extracted from pH 5.6 buffer and is totally extracted (>99%) from solutions with pH 9.0 or greater. 7-Hydroxyfluphenazine is only partly extracted into hep-tane, reaching a maximum value (~10%) between pH 8 and pH 10, and for practical purposes, fluphenazine sulphoxide may be considered not to be extracted into hep-tane. All three compounds may be extracted into toluene and are 50% extracted at the following pH values: FPZ, 3.7; FPZSO, 7.7; 7-OH FPZ, 6.0 and 11.6. This approach not only enables the compounds of interest to be separated prior to quanti-tative analysis but also serves as a useful qualitative check on the materials in a particular extract.

This paper is intended to demonstrate how the concept of pH-dependent partition ratios, originally used in drug analysis by Brodie *et al.* in 1947 [8], can be applied to the identification and quantification of fluphenazine and some of its metabolites following administration of radioactively labelled fluphenazine to man.

Fortunately for the investigator, the metabolism of drug molecules generally leads to the production of metabolites which are more polar than the parent com-pound, and this change of polarity may be utilized in such a way as to allow the separation of that parent compound from its metabolites. Fig. 1 shows the molecu-lar formulae of fluphenazine and some of the metabolites possible. The pathways include sulphoxidation, *N*-oxidation and ring hydroxylation. Conjugation can occur at either the phenolic or the alcoholic hydroxyl groups. We shall confine our dis-cussion to those compounds for which we have reference material, namely, fluphena-zine, 7-hydroxyfluphenazine and fluphenazine sulphoxide.

EXTRACTION

When a dilute solution of an ionizable solute is shaken with an immiscible organic solvent, the solute will be distributed between the two phases, the ratio of the concentration in each phase being a function of:

[Continued overleaf, foot of p.

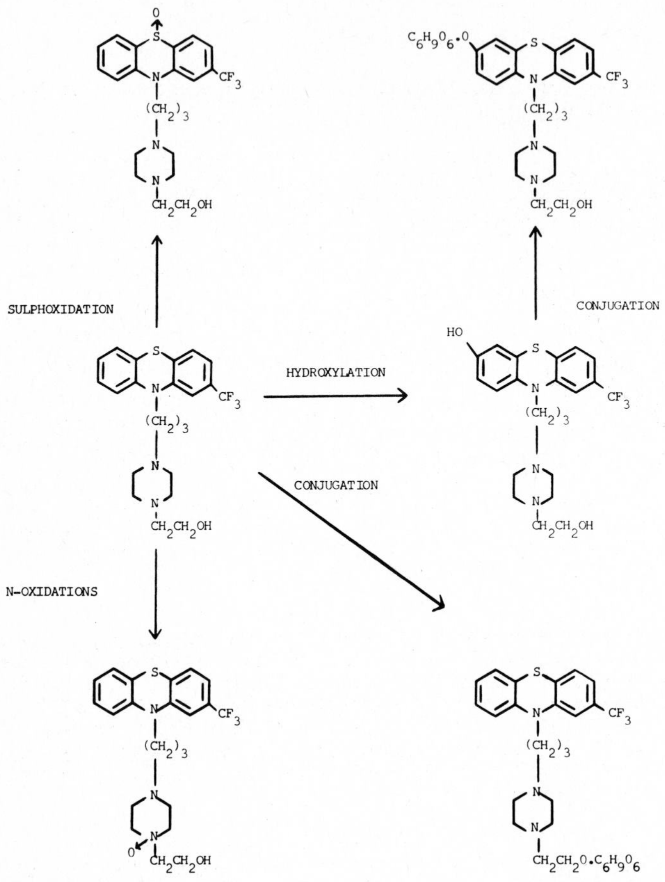

Fig. 1. Biotrans-
formation of flu-
phenazine.

a) the partition coefficient of the neutral species;
b) the pKa of the solute;
c) the pH of the aqueous phase.
By adjusting the pH of the aqueous phase the degree to which the solute is extracted into one phase or the other can be varied. For the solute A:

$$\begin{array}{ll}
\text{SOLVENT} & A \\
\text{-----------} & \big\updownarrow\text{(1)}\text{-----------------} \\
\text{AQUEOUS} & A \rightleftharpoons AH^+ \\
& \text{(2)}
\end{array}$$

equilibrium (1) is the partitioning of the uncharged form. Equilibrium (2) is pH-
dependent and the degree of ionization is given by the Henderson-Hasselbalch equation. Leo *et al.* [9] have suggested that the term partition coefficient should be
reserved for the distribution of the unionized species while the experimental data
uncorrected for ionization, dimerization, etc., should be referred to as the 'partition ratio'. Van der Kleijn [10] chooses the terms 'true partition coefficient'

(TPC) and 'apparent partition coefficient' (APC) and relates the two:

$$TPC = APC\ (1 + 10^{pK_a - pH})$$

when the solute is a base. Note that for a particular solvent the value of TPC is a constant and is independent of pH.

One way of presenting pH partition data is to plot log APC against pH and to use the resulting straight line to obtain the value of TPC. When the numerical value of the pH of the buffer is the same as the pK_a of the solute then the solute is 50% ionized and the APC determined at this pH is half of the value of the TPC, i.e.:

$$2 \times APC_{(pH = pK_a)} = TPC.$$

When using pH partitioning to extract compounds from aqueous media it is more convenient to plot the percentage of compound in the organic phase against the pH of the aqueous phase. Sigmoidal curves of the type seen in Fig. 2 *(upper graph)* arise from this type of plot. Solutions of controlled pH were shaken with equal volumes of heptane containing fluphenazine (D) or one of its esters (A-C). As the pH of the aqueous phase increased so the proportion of material in the heptane increased from almost zero to virtually 100%. Lower pH values than those needed to extract fluphenazine would allow the extraction of the more lipophilic fluphenazine esters. Manipulation of pH enables the therapeutically important decanoate and enanthate esters to be separated from fluphenazine.

Fluphenazine sulphoxide and 7-hydroxyfluphenazine do not extract into heptane from solutions with pH values greater than 13. These compounds will extract into toluene (Fig. 2, *lower graph)*. Fluphenazine extracts into toluene at slightly lower pH values than it does into heptane. 7-Hydroxyfluphenazine produces a 'bell-shape' curve because ionization of the phenolic hydroxyl group results in it not being extracted at high pH values. The extraction of fluphenazine sulphoxide leads to a 'stepped' curve which suggests the presence of either two compounds or two ionizable groups. TLC of the aqueous and organic layers at each pH has confirmed the presence of only one compound.

By utilizing the data of Fig. 2 these compounds can be systematically separated prior to radioactive measurement. The solution under test is adjusted to pH 14 and extracted with heptane. If fluphenazine enanthate or decanoate has been administered then the heptane is washed with buffer of pH 3 to separate the esters from fluphenazine. Fluphenazine sulphoxide is extracted into toluene before the pH is readjusted to pH 9. A further toluene extraction removes the 7-hydroxyfluphenazine.

When the compounds were added to blank urine and then extracted, the recovery of material from urine was not significantly different from that obtained from solutions in water. However, when fluphenazine was added to plasma the amount recovered was in the order of 50-60% of that added. Amyl or hexyl alcohols added to the heptane increased the recovery of fluphenazine, but this also changed the partition ratios and hence the specificity of the extraction. Instead, a known amount of non-radioactive fluphenazine was added to each plasma sample before extraction, and the concentration of fluphenazine in the heptane extract was obtained by measuring the UV absorption before the heptane was transferred to scintillation vials. Thus the concentration in each sample could be corrected for the reduced recovery from plasma.

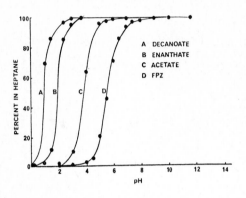

Fig. 2. *Upper part.* - Partition characteristics of fluphenazine, fluphenazine acetate, fluphenazine enanthate and fluphenazine decanoate, between heptane and buffer solutions of various pH values.
Lower part. - Partition characteristics of fluphenazine, 7-hydroxyfluphenazine and fluphenazine sulphoxide, distributed between toluene and buffer solutions of various pH values.

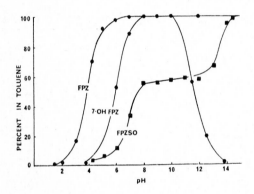

SPECIFICITY

Not only do techniques entailing pH partition provide a method of separating a drug from its more polar metabolites but, since the pH partition is characteristic of a particular compound, it may be used to confirm that that compound has been extracted. The solvent containing the extracted compound is 'back-washed' with buffers of different pH values to obtain the partition characteristics of the solute. These are compared with the partition of an authentic sample. The heptane extract of a faecal sample obtained following an intramuscular dose of ^{14}C-fluphenazine hydrochloride was washed with buffer solutions. Fig. 3 *(upper graph)* shows the results *(broken line)* from this backwashing compared with the extraction of an authentic sample of fluphenazine *(solid line)*. The same approach has been applied to the toluene extract which is expected to contain 7-hydroxyfluphenazine (Fig. 3, *lower graph*). The agreement between extracted radioactivity and non-radioactive authentic 7-hydroxyfluphenazine is good. Further confirmation of the specificity of the method was obtained by subjecting the individual extracts to TLC analysis (Fig. 4). The heptane extract contains only fluphenazine and the toluene extract from pH 9 solution contains only 7-hydroxyfluphenazine. The extract from pH 14 solution shows the presence of a small amount of fluphenazine sulphoxide and a little fluphenazine which has been carried over from the previous extraction.

For pharmacokinetic calculations the most important extraction is probably that which extracts unmetabolized fluphenazine from plasma. The heptane extract

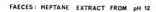

FAECES: HEPTANE EXTRACT FROM pH 12

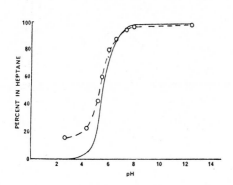

Fig. 3. *Upper part*. - Partition characteristics of radioactivity extracted into heptane from faecal homogenate at pH 12, (o---o) compared with standard reference fluphenazine *(solid line)*.
Lower part. - Partition characteristics of radioactivity extracted into toluene from faecal homogenate at pH 9 *(broken line)*, after removal of fluphenazine and fluphenazine sulphoxide, compared with standard reference 7-hydroxyfluphenazine.

FAECES : TOLUENE EXTRACT FROM pH 9

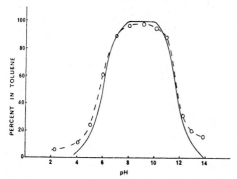

from plasma was treated in the same way as described for the faecal extracts. Because the heptane-extractable radioactivity from plasma is much less than that from faeces it was not possible to use more than three pH values for back-washing. The percentage in the heptane was determined via the UV absorption of the cold internal standard and then by counting the radioactivity. The residues after aliquots had been removed for counting were pooled and used for TLC. Fig. 5 and Table 1 confirm that the specificity of the method when applied to plasma allows the measurement of fluphenazine independently of its metabolites.

Table 1. Partitioning, related to pH, of heptane-extractable radioactivity from plasma

pH	Heptane-extracted, % UV	Radioactive
5.20	20	13
5.52	36	39
6.08	53	56

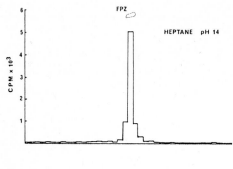

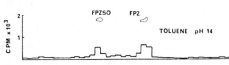

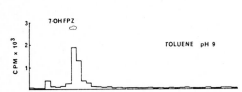

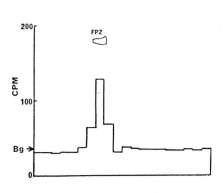

Fig. 5. TLC of heptane-extractable radioactivity from plasma, showing a single peak, well resolved from the background level, corresponding to fluphenazine.

Fig. 4. TLC of radioactivity obtained following extraction with heptane, and then toluene, of a faecal homogenate adjusted to pH 14, and then further extraction with toluene after readjusting to pH 9.

References

1. Smulevitch, A.B., Minsker, E.L., Mazayera, N.A., Volkava, R.P. & Lukanina, S.K., *Comprehensive Psychiatry 14* (1973) 227-233.

2. McIssac, W. Paper presented to *CINP Triannual Meeting* (1971), quoted in ref.3.

3. Schreiber, E.C. & Grozier, M.L., *Therapie 28* (1973) 441-449.

4. Larsen, N.-E. & Naestoft, J. *Med. Lab. Tech. 30* (1973) 129-132.

5. Kelsey, M.I., Kesiner, A. & Moscatelli, E.A. *J.Chromatog. 75* (1973) 294.

6. Forrest, F.M., Forrest, I.S. & Mason, A.S. *Amer. J. Psychiatry 118* (1961) 300-307.

7. Curry, S.H. *Anal. Chem. 40* (1968) 1251-1255.

8. Brodie, B.B., Udefriend, S., Baer, J.E., Dill, W., Chenkin, T., Downing, G., Taggert, J.V. & Josephson, E.S., *J. Biol. Chem. 168* (1947) 299-329.

9. Leo, A., Hansch, C. & Elkins, D., *Chem. Rev. 71* (1971) 525.

10. Van der Kleijn, E., *Arch. Int. Pharmacodyn. 179* (1969) 225-250.

THE QUANTITATIVE FREEZE-DRYING OF ORGANIC COMPOUNDS OF LOW RELATIVE MOLECULAR MASS

S-3

R.A. Chalmers
Division of Inherited Metabolic Diseases,
Medical Research Council Clinical Research Centre,
Harrow, HA1 3UJ, U.K.

The use of extraction procedures that present the metabolites of interest in aqueous media often necessitates the reduction of the extract to dryness before derivative formation and/or further analysis. Many organic compounds are steam-volatile or are thermally and chemically labile, resulting in high losses or artefact formation then rotary evaporation is used. Freeze-drying then becomes the preferred method; when compounds of low relative molecular mass are studied, considerable losses still occur due to volatilization during the conventional freeze-drying process. These losses have been related to the latent heats of vaporization or sublimation of the compounds concerned and to the variation of their vaporization or sublimation pressures with temperature. As reliable data on latent heats are seldom available, a method has been developed for their calculation from molecular group contributions. The thermochemical data derived from the use of both calculated and experimentally-determined latent heats have enabled the selection of the optimum freeze-drying conditions for organic acidic metabolites, and full recoveries of the acids studied have been obtained. The thermochemical data obtained may also be of use in the estimation of the relative volatilities of compounds under study by GC and other techniques.

The problems of extracting organic acids from physiological fluids have been discussed in an accompanying article [1]. The method of choice for these compounds (anion-exchange chromatography) presents the extracted acids as a dilute aqueous solution. When GC or other analytical methods are to be used for the further separation and study of the metabolites, this dilute aqueous solution must be reduced to dryness prior to the preparation of suitable derivatives. Many of the organic acids and other compounds of interest in metabolic studies are steam-volatile or chemically or thermally unstable, and drying processes such as rotary or flash evaporation cannot be used. Freeze-drying (lyophilization) becomes the preferred method. However, losses are still encountered in the freeze-drying of low molecular weight organic compounds. This article is concerned with the selection of optimum drying conditions for such compounds, with the minimum of exploratory experiments. Whilst the methods used will be exemplified by low molecular weight organic acids, the principles apply generally to other classes of organic compounds.

THEORETICAL BASIS OF THE METHOD

During conventional freeze-drying, the sample is frozen as a shell and then placed under vacuum to remove the water and other volatiles by sublimation, thereby minimizing sample losses due to steam volatilization and thermal or chemical decomposition. The sample remains cold throughout the drying process while water (ice) remains in the flask, due to heat being taken up from the sample and the surrounding air to provide the sublimation energy required. During this stage, little loss of the low molecular weight compounds occurs; but when all the water has been removed, the sample warms up to room temperature while remaining under vacuum, and volatilization of the sample commences. Table 1, *upper part (the lower part is considered later)*, illustrates the increased losses that occur when an aqueous solution of some representative organic acids is freeze-dried under conventional conditions for varying times. The longer the time under vacuum after reduction to dryness, the greater the

Table 1. Recoveries of organic acids after freeze-drying.
The values are expressed as per cent. The acids were determined as TMS
derivatives by GC, as in an accompanying paper [1].

	Glycollic	Oxalic	Glyoxylic	Glyoxylic ethoxime	Succinic	Fumaric	L-Malic	Citric
Effect of time under vacuum, without optimization of conditions (SEE TEXT)								
7 h*	79.6	80.3	41.9	-	109.5	99.7	73.3	77.5
15 h	57.7	43.3	42.1	-	111.1	100.7	72.1	72.7
19 h	54.7	44.3	45.6	-	106.1	98.7	78.2	81.0
31 h	39.1	34.4	39.7	-	103.3	96.1	68.5	74.9
Recoveries with theoretically selected conditions (0.5 torr, -10°; SEE LATER IN TEXT)								
7 h*	96.8	108.7	35.7	-	111.1	102.2	81.1	96.1
17 h	95.6	110.9	30.1	84.1	113.1	101.0	79.3	92.8

* *just dry*

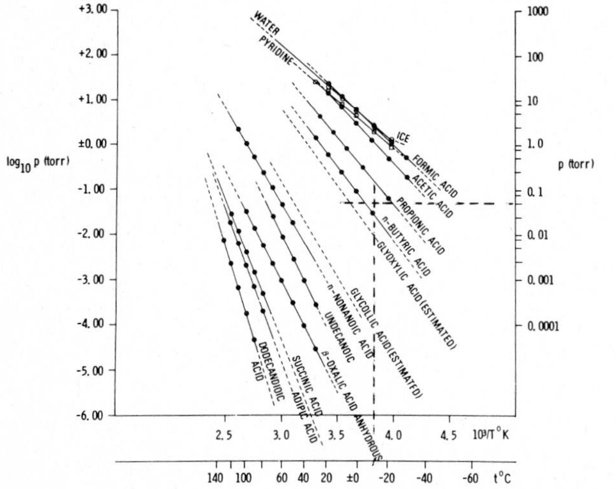

Fig. 1. Pressure-
temperature diagrams
for aliphatic carbox-
ylic acids, water and
pyridine.
The optimum freeze-
drying conditions of
0.5 torr and -10° are
indicated by the
broken vertical and
horizontal lines.

losses of the lower molecular weight acids. Most freeze-drying is carried out overnight, and thus the 15-19 h figures are most representative of normal results.

The losses observed are due to the vaporization or sublimation of the acids
under the conditions used, and are thus related to the variation of the vaporization
and sublimation pressures of the acids with temperature and to their latent heats of
vaporization or sublimation. Consideration of these factors allows the determination
of the volatility of the acids and the selection of the optimum conditions for freeze-
drying with minimal losses.

The Clapeyron-Clausius equation applies: $\dfrac{d(\ln p)}{dT} = \dfrac{\Delta H}{RT^2}$

where p is the pressure, T is the temperature in degrees Kelvin, ΔH is the compound's
latent heat of vaporization (ΔH_V) or sublimation (ΔH_S), and R is the gas constant.

ΔH is temperature-independent over short temperature ranges (of about 50-100°), particularly for solid crystalline materials. Assuming that the vapour behaves ideally, the equation provides a reasonably good fit of vapour and sublimation pressure data, even for the carboxylic acids which are known to have very imperfect vapours [2].

On integrating and taking common logarithms, the equation becomes

$$\log_{10}p = A - \Delta H/2.303RT$$

where A is a constant, and thus $\log_{10}p$ may be plotted against $1/T$ to give a straight line with a slope of $- \Delta H/2.303\ R$.

CALCULATION OF LATENT HEATS OF VAPORIZATION

The use of this equation requires knowledge of the latent heats of vaporization or sublimation of the compounds concerned. Little reliable experimental data are available, particularly for oxygen-containing organic compounds of interest in metabolic studies, and a method has been developed for the calculation of these latent heats from molecular group contributions. The latter have been calculated in turn by consideration of homologous series of compounds that contain the groups of interest and for which reliable experimental data exist [2, 3]. Some values are shown in Table 2. It has been assumed for the purposes of these calculations that the contributions of C—C bonds in which both carbon atoms are sp³ hybridized are zero [3, 4].

Using this data it has been possible to calculate the latent heats of vaporization of a range of organic acids for comparison with experimental data (Table 3), both as used in the original calculations and as obtained subsequently from the literature. Agreement between calculated and experimental data for ΔH_v is reasonably good, whereas discrepancies occur between calculated ΔH_v and experimental ΔH_s values. These discrepancies are due to crystal lattice geometry factors which are in turn related to the melting point of the compound [3, 5]. This is most clearly seen by comparison of the values for ΔH_v and ΔH_s for undecanoic acid, and for maleic and fumaric acids (*cis* and *trans* butenedioic acids respectively). Calculated values of ΔH_v for some acids and other organic compounds for which experimental data are not available are also included in Table 3. More extensive data are given elsewhere [3, 6].

SELECTION OF OPTIMUM FREEZE-DRYING CONDITIONS AND THEIR VALIDATION

Using the calculated and experimentally determined latent heats, graphs have been constructed of pressure against temperature for a range of the acids of interest, and for water, acetic acid and pyridine (Fig. 1), which are the constituents of the buffer used in the extraction of organic acids from physiological fluids [1]. Comparison of the lines obtained has enabled the optimum freeze-drying conditions of - 10° and 0.5 torr to be selected (Fig. 1). Under these conditions, relatively rapid volatilization of the buffer constituents should occur, while retaining most of the acids of interest in the residue. The most volatile oxo acids, pyruvic and glyoxylic acids, are stabilized prior to freeze-drying as their ethoximes [1], and only the short-chain fatty acids are lost during the freeze-drying process. These short chain C_2—C_5 acids and other volatile organic compounds may be determined by alternative procedures [6]. Table 1, *lower part,* shows the recoveries obtained from aqueous pyridinium acetate buffer of a range of acids when dried under the theoretically selected conditions.

CONCLUSIONS

It has been possible therefore to select the optimum freeze-drying conditions for organic acids of low relative molecular mass with a minimum of experimental work. The methods used are applicable to other classes of organic compounds, and are generally helpful

Table 2. Molecular group contributions to latent heats of vaporization of organic compounds.
Values represent k-cal per g formula weight at 25°C [3].

Group	ΔH_v
C—C	0
C=C	1.07
C≡C	3.04
C—H *primary*	0.45
C—H *secondary*	0.60
C—H *tertiary*	0.65
C—CO$_2$H	11.0
C—OH	7.42
C—CHO	4.73
C—CO—C	3.99
C—O—C	1.38

in the calculation of the relative volatilities of a wide range of organic compounds including aromatic compounds and esters, with useful applications to a variety of other techniques including GC [6].

Table 3. Calculated and determined latent heats of vaporization (ΔH_v) and sublimation (ΔH_s) of some organic acids.
Values represent k-cal per g formula weight [3].
Values for additional acids and some other low molecular weight aliphatic compounds are given elsewhere [3, 6].

	Melting point,°C	ΔH_v calculated	ΔH_v determined	ΔH_s determined
Formic	8	11.65	11.0	-
Acetic	17	12.3	12.5	-
Propionic	-20	13.5	13.7	-
n-Butyric	-8	14.7	15.2	-
Glyoxylic	98*	15.7	-	-
Pyruvic	14	16.3	-	-
Glycollic	80	19.6	-	-
Lactic	25	20.4	-	-
n-Nonanoic	15	20.7	19.7	-
Oxalic (β form)	101†	22.0	-	22.3
n-Undecanoic	28	23.3	23.4	29.0
Maleic	130	24.4	-	26.3
Fumaric	286	24.4	-	32.5
Succinic	184	24.4	-	28.1
L-Malic	100	31.3	-	-
Citric	153	42.8	-	-

*monohydrate   †dihydrate

References

1. Chalmers, R.A., this volume (1975) pp. 135-140.

2. Cox, J.D. & Pilcher, G., *Thermochemistry of Organic and Organometallic Compounds,* Academic Press, London & New York (1970).

3. Chalmers, R.A. & Watts, R.W.E., *Analyst, Lond.* 97 (1972) 224-232.

4. Laidler, K.J., *Can. J. Chem.* 34 (1956) 626-648.

5. Bondi, A., *J. Chem. Engng. Data 8* (1963) 371-377.

6. Chalmers, R.A., Bickle, S. & Watts, R.W.E., *Clin. Chim. Acta 52* (1974) 31-41.

SAMPLE PREPARATION BY CHEMICAL MASKING

S-4

J. Chamberlain
Hoechst Pharmaceutical Research Laboratories,
Milton Keynes, Bucks. MK7 7AJ, U.K.

The goal of sample preparation in analytical work is to present the sample to an analytical end-point in such a way that only the compound under investigation is detected. The most obvious way to do this is by the physical removal of all other substances. Another extreme approach is to have a specific end-point and use a relatively crude sample. Usually one combines the two approaches, and the major effort in analytical development tends to be in the removal of substances which interfere with that particular end-point. This paper gives several examples of a different general approach where interfering compounds are not removed, but a series of chemical reactions are applied to prepare the sample for measurement of a specific substance. These include pH changes or chemical reduction to provide a 'blank' from the sample, chemical oxidation to provide more specific derivatives for EC detection in GC, masking of alcohols to provide more specific enol hepta-fluorbutyrates for EC detection in GC, and masking of primary amines for measure-ment of secondary amines by isotope derivative assay.

This volume has arisen from a Techniques Forum titled 'Assay of Drugs and other Trace Substances in Biological Fluids', and although various types of analytical instrumentation are discussed, the underlying theme is sample preparation. Undoubtedly, sample preparation depends on the type of instrumentation used and the goal of sample preparation can be simply stated to be, "to present the sample to an analytical end-point in such a way that only the compound under investigation is detected". The two extreme ways of achieving this goal are:
a) to remove all substances not to be measured and apply a non-specific end-point, e.g. removal of water to determine dry-weight;
b) use a crude sample and a highly specific end-point, e.g. a geiger counter to detect radioactivity.

Better examples of both extremes can be taken from the history of steroid hormone assays. In the mid-1960's, GC was used extensively. In most cases, the relatively non-specific flame-ionization detector was used as the end-point and, in addition to the separating power of the GC column, two successive TLC systems were often used. Van der Molen and Groen [1] in a method describing the assay of several steroids in single blood samples stated that they generally tried to purify their samples to such an extent that the compound under investigation appeared as an isolated peak on the GC trace. Exley's flow chart shows that the assay for plasma testosterone required two TLC systems and a paper chromatographic system [2]. Even so, the relatively specific electron-capture detector (ECD) was used as the end-point, although here it was the sensitivity rather than the specificity of this detector that was required.

If such elaborate purifications were necessary for the determination of plasma testosterone in 1966 (and indeed they were), it must have been difficult to envisage a method at the other extreme - no purification but very specific detection.

Such a technique began to be realized with the introduction of competitive protein binding into the steroid field in 1967, mainly by Beverley Murphy [3]. Radioimmunoassay (which is essentially the sampe type of method) could be made even more specific, and Chen, Zorn, Hallberg and Wieland [4] described an antibody which could be used to measure testosterone in extracted but unchromatographed plasma.

Usually, one uses a combination of the two extremes. That is, the major effort in the development of an analytical method is in the removal of substances which interfere with a particular end-point. If the end-point is GC, then the contaminants which will be the problem are those with similar retentivity to the compound being measured; if the end-point is colorimetric then the effort is directed at removing compounds which absorb in the same region as the compound being measured.

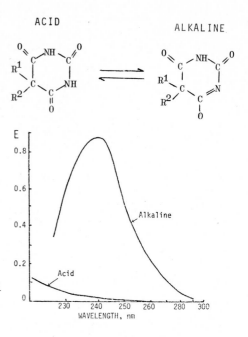

Fig. 1.   Effect of pH on the UV-absorption spectrum of barbiturates.

EXAMPLES OF 'CHEMICAL MASKING'

This paper describes selected examples where the accent is not on removing interfering materials, but on manipulating the sample in such a way that these materials are not detected. For want of a better expression, I have called this chemical masking. The main advantage of this type of method should be to combine the cheapness of reagents and instruments, where non-specific detection is used, with minimal losses of sample in the specific detection methods, where fewer transfers are usually involved.

One of the simplest examples of chemical masking is the effect of changing the pH of a solution. Barbiturates have a characteristic absorption at 240 nm in alkaline solution which disappears in acid solution (Fig. 1). In fact, this was originally used in the assay of barbiturates where the acidified extract is used as the control for measurements at pH 10 [5]. Thus, in the context of using pH changes as a chemical masking agent, acidification could be used to eliminate the interference of barbiturates in assays requiring UV-absorption measurements. Similarly, where phenols are potentially interfering with UV-absorption measurements, the interference can be partly masked by a change in pH, which shifts the position of the absorption rather than eliminates it completely.

In much the same way that acidification was used to produce a 'control' sample for barbiturates, reduction with sodium borohydride has been used to produce a 'control' sample for 3-oxo-Δ^4 steroids. A typical 3-oxo-Δ^4 steroid, such as progesterone, absorbs at 240 nm. Reduction of the oxo group was found to completely eliminate this absorption (Fig. 2), and a method for specific determination of progesterone was suggested. The procedure could also be used to eliminate absorption by conjugated ketones in other UV assays.

When one considers GC with ECD, it is usual to think in terms of halogenated compounds which are themselves electron-capturing, e.g. DDT, aldrin, dieldrin, etc., or of making halogenated derivatives, e.g. chloroacetates, heptafluorobutyrates, pentafluoro phenylhydrazones. The disadvantage of the latter approach is the difficulty in removing excess reagents or other derivatized components of a mixture. What is not often appreciated is that some structures can be electron-capturing without being halogenated. If such a structure can be produced by a simple chemical transformation, it can offer advantages over the derivatization

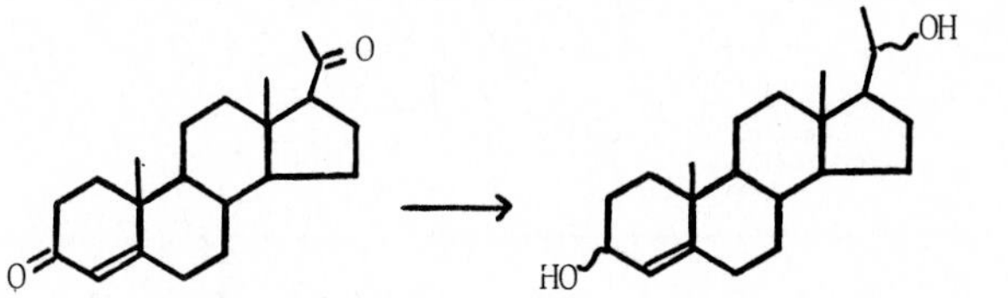

Fig. 2. Reduction of a UV-absorbing group (in progesterone) to a non-UV-absorbing group.

procedures. A good example is in the determination of 6-oxygenated corticosteroids by oxidation of a crude urine extract with chromium trioxide [6]. The product, androst-4-ene-3, 6,11,17-tetrone (Fig. 3), is stable to GC and has strong electron-capturing properties by virtue of the 3,6,-dioxo-Δ^4 group. In this analysis, the oxidation step itself is instrumental in providing a 'clean' extract by changing the GC characteristics of biological contaminants.

A method which we developed using several masking procedures was for the assay of urinary aldosterone. The advent of radio-immunoassay made this method obsolete before it was used in clinical samples [V.T. James, Art. T-1, *this Vol.*]; however, I now present it for academic interest.

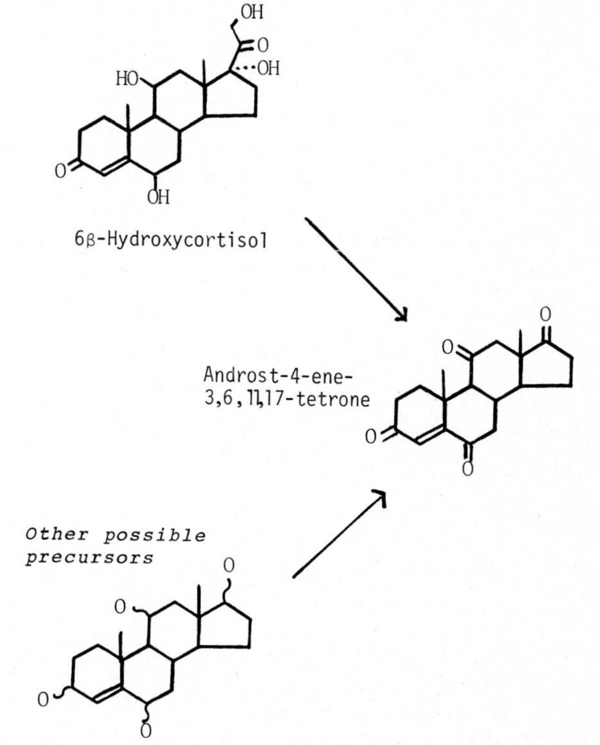

6β-Hydroxycortisol

Androst-4-ene-3,6,11,17-tetrone

Other possible precursors

Fig. 3. Oxidation of 6β-hydroxycortisol to a strongly electron-capturing, chromatographically stable compound.

Aldosterone (I, Fig. 4) is a very labile compound and not at all amenable to GC, even as a silyl derivative. Because of the levels involved, a sensitive endpoint was required, and because of its similarity to other urinary steroids, multiple chromatographic purifications would be needed, as already described for testosterone. A simple, rapid and specific assay for urinary aldosterone did not look promising. As a first step, oxidation converted aldosterone to a stable product, the γ-lactone (II). The γ-lactone did not have a high enough affinity for thermal electrons, so it was necessary to form a derivative. A promising derivative was the enol heptafluorobutyrate (III).

Theoretically, there should be no primary or secondary alcohols in the mixture to form interfering heptafluorobutyrates, as the initial oxidation will have converted these into acids or ketones. However, we found that chromium trioxide did not convert aldosterone to the γ-lactone in high yield; accordingly, the milder

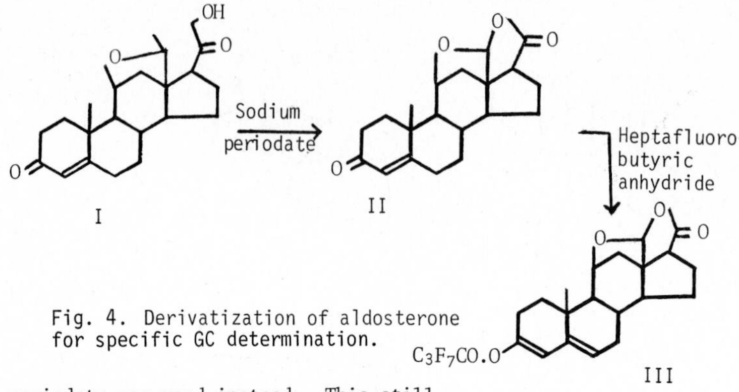

Fig. 4. Derivatization of aldosterone
for specific GC determination.

reagent sodium periodate was used instead. This still
left the problem of the hydroxy compounds. The problem
was effectively solved by blocking these groups with
acetic anhydride, which under the right conditions does
not acylate enols. It is useful to review the sequence
(Fig. 4) and see how the method has become quite specific for aldosterone with very few transfer procedures
and no chromatography other than GC.

Acidified urine is extracted with diethyl ether.
The periodate oxidation converts 20-oxo-21-hydroxy steroids to 17-carboxylic acids;
these are removed with an alkaline wash along with phenols. 20-Oxo-17,21-dihydroxy
steroids are converted to 17-oxo steroids. Aldosterone is oxidized to a 17-carboxy-
lic acid; but as this forms a γ-lactone, this is not removed in the alkaline wash.
Acetylation prevents remaining hydroxy steroids from forming the heptafluorobutyrate; hence in the final GC the isolated peak obtained is due not to extensive purification, but to the application of masking techniques.

Another technique which normally requires extensive purification procedures
is the method of analysis known as isotope derivative assay. In this technique, a
functional group is reacted with a labelled reagent, the product is purified and
the amount of radio-label incorporated enables the amount of material originally
present to be assessed. For example, primary and secondary amines can be determined by acetylation with tritiated acetic anhydride and the tritium content of the
purified N-acetyl derivative measured. This technique was used by Hammer and Brodie
(Fig. 5) to determine desipramine in plasma following therapeutic doses of the drug
[7]. However, the method would be expected to be less specific for the measurement
of a drug which gave rise to primary amines as metabolites. Overø [8] suggested a
modified method where the primary amine was blocked by the addition of salicylic
aldehyde, presumably to form a Schiff's base effectively masking the amine (Fig. 6).
Overø suggested the modification for the analysis of Lu 5-003, which is metabolized
to the primary amine. Analysis of rat blood following oral dosing of Lu 5-003 was
shown to give higher values than would be expected if the modification was used.
Overø suggested that salicylic aldehyde should be added routinely in all isotope
derivative assays where the possibility of the presence of primary amines could
lead to falsely high values.

What I have tried to illustrate in this article is more of a philosophical
approach to sample preparation. When faced with interfering factors in an assay,
as well as thinking in terms of how to remove these factors, we should also consider whether we can 'hide' them.

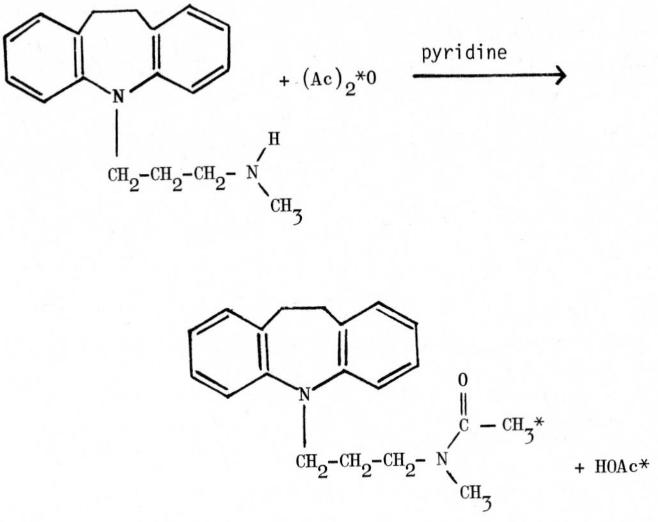
+ (Ac)2*O
pyridine
H
CH2-CH2-CH2- N
CH3
N
O
C — CH3*
+ HOAc*

Fig. 5. Isotope derivative assay for desipramine.

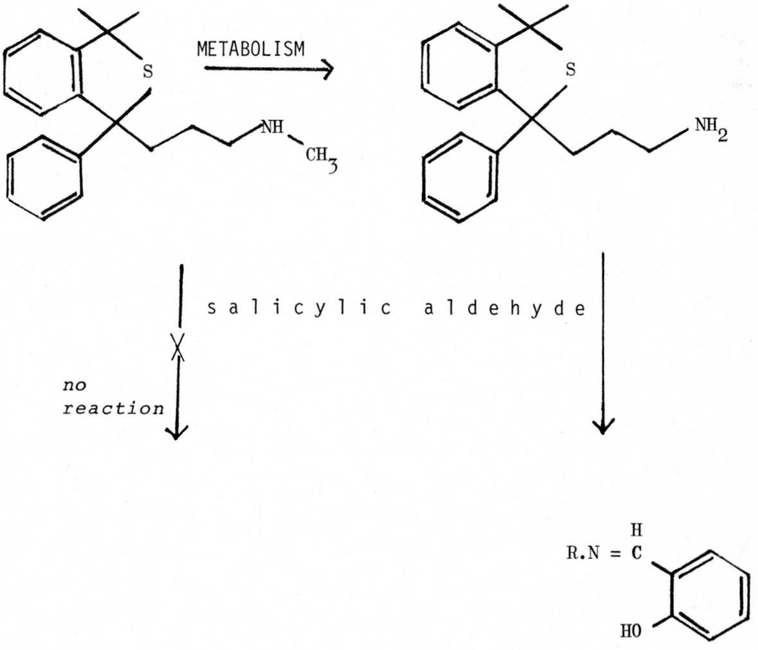
METABOLISM
S
NH
CH3
NH2
salicylic aldehyde
no reaction
H
R.N = C
HO

Fig. 6. Protection of primary amine in the isotope derivative assay for Lu 5-003. *The latter without its* $-NH_2$ *group is denoted* R.

References

1. Van der Molen, H.J. & Groen, D. in *Gas Liquid Chromatography of Steroids* (J.K. Grant, ed.), University Press, Cambridge (1967) pp. 155-177.

2. Exley, D., *Biochem. J. 107* (1968) 285-292.

3. Murphy, B.P., *J. Clin. Endocrin. 27* (1967) 973-990.

4. Chen, J.C., Zorn, E.M., Hallberg, M.C. & Wieland, R.G., *Clin. Chem. 17* (1971) 581-584.

5. Walker, J.T., Fisher, R.S. & McHugh, J.J., *Amer. J. Clin. Path. 18* (1948) 451-461.

6. Chamberlain, J., *Clin. Chim. Acta 34* (1971) 269-271.

7. Hammer, W.M. & Brodie, B.B., *J. Pharmacol. Exp. Ther. 157* (1967) 503-508.

8. Overø, K.F., *Acta Pharmacol. et Toxicol. 31* (1972) 433-440.

S-5

SAMPLE PREPARATION IN HPLC

Dennis Dell
Hoechst Pharmaceutical Research Limited,
Walton Manor, Walton,
Milton Keynes, Bucks. MK7 7AJ, U.K.

HPLC packing materials, and packed columns particularly, are considerably more expensive than GC packing materials and columns and are, therefore, less expendable. As for GC, deposition at the top of the column of lipids and/or protein from plasma samples causes a gradual deterioration of peak shape and overall column efficiency. Protein is best removed before a plasma sample is injected, and in any case a precolumn is desirable. Urine samples may be ultrafiltered and passed through XAD-2 before analysis.

For the majority of drug assays, the problems of sample preparation for HPLC are very similar to those which confront the gas chromatographer. Plasma proteins and inorganic salts do not present a problem because most drugs can be extracted from aqueous solution by an organic solvent at the appropriate pH. However, one of the theoretical advantages of HPLC over GC is that drugs can be assayed by direct injection of biological fluids. This is particularly important for compounds which are too water-soluble to allow extraction by conventional means (e.g. penicillins, cephalosporins, and drug conjugates).

If this advantage is to be realized in practice, then the presence of relatively large amounts of proteins, lipids, salts, etc., in biological fluids must be considered and, in fact, these are normally removed from the sample before chromatography.

This text is essentially a review of techniques in current use. Some of the procedures are in use in the author's laboratory and others were obtained from the literature and from unpublished personal communications.

PREPARATION METHODS FOR PLASMA AND SERUM SAMPLES

Removal of proteins by precipitation

Precipitation methods are widely used. Addition of the appropriate reagent to the plasma or serum denatures the protein, which is precipitated and can be removed by centrifugation. The use of acidic reagents such as trichloroacetic acid [1-3], perchloric acid [4], and tungstic acid [5] has been described. If the compound being analyzed is unstable at low pH, then ethanol or methanol is a suitable alternative. Ethanol will precipitate protein from plasma provided that not less than two vol. ethanol to one vol. plasma are added.

Removal of proteins by ultrafiltration

Ultrafiltration is a technique which is well established for the sterilization of, and the removal of macromolecules from, biological fluids. This technique has not yet found widespread acceptance for protein removal in drug analysis. The main reason for this is that the filtration rate for plasma through membranes which retain compounds with a relative molecular mass greater than 1000 is slow (1 ml/h at 60 psig). When large numbers of samples have to be analyzed, the slowness makes this method of sample preparation impracticable. There is a membrane available which retains molecules above 25,000. This membrane retains 90% of the plasma globulins and albumins and would possibly allow a higher filtration rate than the 1000 relative molecular mass membrane, and give an ultrafiltrate which is suitable for HPLC analysis [6]. An ultrafiltrate of plasma obtained in this way would, of course, only give a measure of unbound, rather than total, drug.

For the analysis of oxypurines, Pfadenhauer [7] removed most of the protein in plasma by ultrafiltration through a membrane filter which removed proteins of relative molecular mass greater than 50,000.

The use of pre-columns

The use of pre-columns for protein removal has also been reported. For the analysis of frusemide by direct injection of plasma, Forrey and co-workers [8] used a pre-column which contained the same material as the main separation column (pellicular cation-exchange). The mobile phase was phosphate buffer at pH 2.5 and, under these conditions, protein accumulated on the pre-column, which had to be replaced whenever the back-pressure in the column began to build up.

In the above-mentioned analysis of oxypurines, Pfadenhauer injected plasma ultrafiltrate onto a pre-column containing the same adsorbent as the main separation column (25-35 μm silica). The pre-column effectively trapped the residual protein and other constituents precipitated by the mobile phase (diethyl ether, n-propanol, and 5% acetic acid).

The removal of lipids

In adsorption chromatography, methylene chloride or diethyl ether will elute neutral lipids and methylene chloride/methanol or methanol will elute phospholipids. However, these eluted lipids will not normally interfere if a UV detector is being used because of the very low molar absorption of these compounds.

Retention of lipids on reverse-phase columns leading to a deterioration in column efficiency has been reported [9, 10]. Salmon [10] has found that purging the column with chloroform following every hundred injections of ether-extracted plasma removes accumulated lipids. Removal of neutral lipids by selective solvent extraction can be accomplished if the drug itself is not extracted from the aqueous phase into ether or methylene chloride. For example, Bayne [11] extracted acetazolamide from acidified plasma with ethyl acetate. The solvent was evaporated and the residue dissolved in pH 2 glycine buffer. The yellow pigments and lipids were extracted with methylene chloride and the purified drug was extracted from the aqueous phase with ethyl acetate.

Use of activated charcoal

For the determination of anticonvulsants in serum, Adams and Vandemark [12] added charcoal to diluted serum containing an internal standard. The mixture was agitated, centrifuged, and the aqueous phase discarded. The charcoal was then mixed with an organic solvent to dissolve the drugs. This procedure is an alternative to liquid/liquid extraction and depends for its success on the compounds of interest being:
i) readily adsorbed onto charcoal from the plasma sample, and
ii) efficiently extracted from the charcoal by the organic solvent.
The use of dextran-coated charcoal, as in RIA methods, may be expected to provide a milder adsorbing reagent.

PREPARATION METHODS FOR URINE SAMPLES

Whereas the problems associated with preparation of plasma samples for HPLC are mainly concerned with the removal of protein and lipids, the problems associated with urine are mainly those of sample concentration and removal of inorganic salts or small molecular weight components which may have similar chromatographic properties to the compounds being assayed. The separation of these latter compounds is usually approached by variation of the chromatographic conditions, the consideration of which is outside the scope of this paper.

    We have found that a reverse-phase column which has deteriorated as a result
of repeated injections of undiluted urine may be regenerated by purging with methanol or dimethylformamide (Fig. 1).

    Before injecting urine, suspended solids may be removed by centrifugation or
by filtering the urine through a 0.4 μm 'Millipore' membrane. Another procedure
involves passing urine through the Amberlite resin XAD-2; inorganic salts are not
retained and the organic components may be eluted with methanol. Thus, desalting
and concentration are accomplished in one step. For the analysis of porphyrins in
urine, Jackson [13] adsorbed the urine sample onto talc and eluted the porphyrins
with a mixture of ethanol and Tris buffer.

CONCLUSION

For those drugs which cannot readily be extracted from biological fluids it is evident that a sufficiently 'clean' sample for HPLC analysis can be obtained provided
attention is paid to the removal of endogenous constituents.

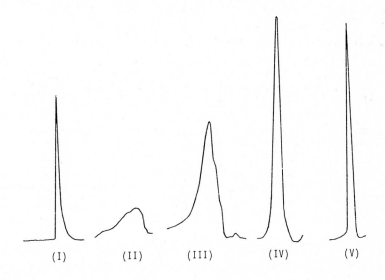

Fig.1. Regeneration of a μBondapak C_{18} column after loss of efficiency following
injections of unfiltered urine.
(I) represents the peak shape of a cephalosporin antibiotic injected as an aqueous
solution onto a C_{18} reverse-phase column. The mobile phase was a mixture of
methanol and 1% acetic acid. Urine had not been injected onto the column at this
stage.
Unfiltered urine (containing precipitated inorganic phosphates) from a volunteer
who had received a dose of this cephalosporin was injected; the first five 10 μl
injections gave the normal peak shape (I). The sixth injection gave peak shape
(II), indicating a sudden deterioration in column efficiency. Washing the column
successively with aqueous methanol (III), chloroform (IV), and warm dimethylformamide (V) gave peak shapes as shown.
The purging of the column was performed with 25 column volumes of each solvent,
and the clean-up process was monitored by injecting an aqueous solution of this
compound after each solvent treatment. The gradual improvement in peak shape can
be observed (III-V), although the column could not be used for quantitative work
until it had been further purged with the mobile phase used for the analysis.

References

1. Brown, P.R. & Parkes, R.E., *Anal. Chem. 45* (1973) 948-951.
2. Bighley, L.D., Wurster, D.E., Cruden-Loeb, D. & Smith, R.V., *J. Chromatog. 110* (1975) 375-380.
3. Brown, P.R., Parkes, R.E. & Herod, J., *Clin. Chem. 19* (1973) 919-922.
4. Solem, E., Agarwal, D.P. & Goedde, H.W., *Clin. Chim. Acta 59* (1975) 203-207.
5. Ings, R.M.J., McFadzean, J.A. & Ormerod, W.E., *Xenobiotica 5* (1975) 223-235.
6. *Molecular Filtration, AR 801* (Technical Bulletin), Millipore Corporation, Bedford, Mass. (1974).
7. Pfadenhauer, E.A., *J. Chromatog. 81* (1973) 85-91.
8. Blair, A.D., Forrey, A.W., Meijsen, T. B. & Cutler, R.E., *J. Pharm. Sci. 64* (1975) 1334-1338.
9. Cosgrove, M. (I.C.I. Pharmaceuticals Ltd., Alderley Park, U.K.), *personal communication.*
10. Salmon, J.R., *this volume,* Art. T-7 [T. Cowen & J.R. Salmon].
11. Bayne, W.F., Rogers, G. & Crisologo, N., *J. Pharm. Sci. 64* (1975) 402-404.
12. Adams, R.F. & Vandemark, F.L., *Clin. Chem. 22* (1976) 25-31.
13. Evans, N., Jackson, A.H., Matlin, S.A. & Towill, R., in *The Application of High Pressure Liquid Chromatography to Clinical Chemistry* (Dixon, P.F., Gray, C.H., Lim, C.K. & Stoll, M.S., eds.), Academic Press, London (1976) *in press.*

S-6 ANION EXCHANGERS FOR QUANTITATIVELY EXTRACTING
ORGANIC ACIDS FROM URINE AND OTHER FLUIDS

R.A. Chalmers
Division of Inherited Metabolic Diseases,
Medical Research Council Clinical Research Centre,
Harrow, HA1 3UJ, U.K.

Successful determination of organic constituents of biological fluids depends on the efficiency of the extraction procedure used. The complex variety of metabolites in urine and other fluids necessitates their fractionation into subgroups for further analysis. Conventional methods use solvents for extraction and fractionation; but these techniques are particularly unsuited to the extraction of organic acids due to their unfavourable partition coefficients between aqueous solution and organic solvents. Ion-exchange techniques for extraction and fractionation are preferable, in that good quantitation is essential for meaningful metabolic studies such as the clinical evaluation of a drug and its metabolites.

A comparative study of some anion-exchange materials has shown that some of the more labile acidic metabolites decompose on polystyrene-based resins and the more polar compounds are often incompletely eluted. DEAE-Sephadex has proved particularly suitable for the extraction of organic acids from urine and other biological fluids. All anionic compounds with pKa values below about 5.5, including anionic drugs and metabolites and conjugates with glycine and glucuronic acid, are extracted. The urine or other protein-free biological fluid is applied directly to the column. Neutral and basic compounds are removed by water washing and may be further fractionated by ion-exchange procedures. The acids are eluted with aqueous pyridinium acetate buffer and, after quantitative freeze-drying, are suitable for analysis by GC or other chromatographic methods. Particular groups, such as the more hydrophobic aromatic acids, may be accentuated by further selective extraction of the freeze-dried residue.

Despite the increased sensitivity and selectivity of modern identification techniques, some of which are discussed elsewhere in this Volume, the successful determination of any organic constituents of biological fluids and tissues is still very dependent on the efficiency of the extraction process used. The study of intermediary metabolism, including the metabolism of drugs, has often been hampered by the need for a suitable method for the isolation of the metabolites of interest from the biological material. Even with the introduction of modern separation techniques such as electrophoresis, GC and HPLC, there remain the problems of the quantitative and selective aspects of the necessary initial extraction process.

The complexity of the metabolites present in most physiological fluids, particularly urine, demands their fractionation into sub-groups prior to further separation, quantitation and identification. These metabolites may be most simply and conveniently classified as acidic, basic, and neutral (and amphoteric) compounds, this classification providing the basis for any extraction system. This paper is specifically concerned with the first of these groups of compounds. Besides the wide range of naturally-occurring organic acids, many drugs and other administered compounds are themselves anionic in nature, and others that are themselves neutral or basic are metabolized to anionic species. In meaningful metabolic studies, all of these metabolites need to be identified and quantitated, and thus the study of the acidic metabolites is important.

These acidic metabolites are polar, their polarity often being enhanced by the presence of other oxygen- or sulphur-containing functional groups; they are thus generally very hydrophilic, making their extraction difficult in practice. Provided, however, that they can be quantitatively extracted and separated from the other non-acidic compounds, it is possible to overcome other analytical problems not to be considered here, viz. the concentration of the extract [1], separation of the individual metabolites, quantitation and identification. The most widely used analytical methods for organic acids are GC and on-line GC-MS, after conversion into volatile and stable derivatives such as the trimethylsilyl (TMS) esters of carboxylic acid groups, TMS ethers of hydroxyl groups, and o-ethyloximes (ethoximes) of carbonyl groups, as used in the work described in this paper. Details of these methods and derivatives are given elsewhere [2, 3], free acids or weak salts being required for trimethylsilylation; the acidic metabolites are extracted as a group for derivative preparation and GC.

EXTRACTION METHODS

Extraction methods that have been used for acidic metabolites include solvent extraction, adsorption onto non-functional materials, partition chromatography, and anion-exchange chromatography. This paper is primarily concerned with the latter method but the reasons for the selection of anion-exchange extraction need some comment and explanation.

Most organic acids have unfavourable partition coefficients between aqueous media and organic solvents such as diethyl ether, ethyl and methyl acetates, and acetonitrile. Solvent extraction has been shown to be generally unsuitable for comprehensive extraction and quantitative studies on organic acids, even with the use of continuous liquid-liquid extractions from hot acidified solutions over 24-h periods. In addition, solvent extraction, even under the most suitable conditions of concentration and pH, is non-specific: varying proportions of all of the soluble metabolites are extracted into the solvents used, often more efficiently than the organic acids. Thus, qualitative work can be difficult even with the aid of MS. Many hydrophilic acids are not extracted at all, and important metabolites may completely escape detection [3, 4].

Non-functional adsorbents such as alumina, XAD-2 and Sephadex are similarly non-specific and at best only semi-quantitative for small hydrophilic molecules.[*] In this laboratory, XAD-2 and Sephadex (G-10 or G-25) have proved unsuitable for the extraction of organic acids from aqueous solutions. Partition chromatography with silicic acid (silica gel) columns presents similar problems and, due to the occurrence of partial fractionation, is not suitable as an extraction method. Attempts to analyze organic acids in physiological fluids directly, utilizing the fractionation on these columns [e.g. 5, 6, 7, 8] have been limited by the poor resolution and by the problems encountered in detecting molecules that have little UV absorbance and therefore call for indicator or oxidation procedures, necessarily insensitive.

ANION-EXCHANGE EXTRACTION METHODS

There is a wide range of anion exchangers available for use, with a variety of functional groups attached to different supporting materials, including polystyrene and other polyaromatic resins, cellulose, agarose and dextran. Most early work on the extraction of organic acids from biological materials was done using Dowex 1, a strongly-basic resin with quaternary ammonium groups on a polystyrene-divinylbenzene lattice, with the resin in the acetate, formate, or chloride forms and with the corresponding aqueous acid used as eluant. Dowex 2, a slightly less basic resin, has also been used, in the formate form with formic acid elution. However, recoveries from Dowex 1 [9, 10, 11] or Dowex 2 [12] are often low and non-reproducible, with decomposition of some of the more chemically-labile acids occurring on the strongly basic resins [10, and author's observations].

*EDITOR'S NOTE: Articles G-1 & T-2 (amongst others) are relevant: alumina does have a predilection for molecules with vicinal hydroxyl groups.

In addition to these resins, Biorex 9, a strongly basic resin with pyridinium functional groups, has also been used in these laboratories. Very similar results to those with the other Dowex resins were obtained, with the acids being fractionated to some extent, and eluted roughly in order of their pK_a values. Acids of lower pK_a values were very difficult to remove from the resins without the use of strong mineral acid eluants.

In order to minimize the fractionation and in an attempt to improve recoveries, weakly basic anion exchangers such as Dowex 3 × 4A, with polyamine functional groups on a polystyrene-divinylbenzene lattice, were also studied. Fractionation and incomplete elution still occurred however, and the latter in particular appears to be a feature of these polyaromatic resins.

The best results in these laboratories have been achieved using the weakly basic dextran-derived A25 DEAE (diethylaminoethyl)-Sephadex with pH 7 pyridinium acetate buffer elution, based on the method used by Jaakonmaki *et al.* [13] to extract a glucosiduronic acid from rat urine. Although a slight degree of fractionation may occur, the organic acids are completely eluted quantitatively as a group. The method is thus most suitable for the extraction of the organic acids for further analysis by GC. The quantitative aspects of the method have been studied in detail [3], and the general procedure that has been developed is described below.

General anion-exchange procedure using DEAE-Sephadex

The overall procedure used in these laboratories is summarized in Fig. 1. An aliquot of urine (neutralized to pH 7; generally equivalent to 3 mg of creatinine) or other protein-free physiological fluid is applied to the resin column (45 × 7 mm), which has been pre-washed with water and 0.5 M aqueous pyridinium acetate buffer. The column is washed with 2 aliquots of water, the washings containing the neutral and basic metabolites. These may be further separated by cation-exchange chromatography and analyzed in detail [14]. The acidic metabolites are eluted from the column with 15 ml of 1.5 M aqueous pyridinium acetate buffer into a flask containing *o*-ethoxylamine hydrochloride (to stabilize the oxo acids as their ethoximes). The pyridinium counter-ion is essential in the elution step since acetic acid alone is insufficiently acidic to elute most naturally occurring acids. The eluate is freeze-dried under controlled conditions [1], and the acids are finally analyzed by GC and/or GC-MS as their TMS derivatives.

Quantitative recoveries of a representative range of physiologically important organic acids have been obtained both from aqueous solutions and from urine [3]. The method allows the extraction of all anionic compounds with pK_a values below about 5.5, including glucuronides and other conjugated species, and has been applied to other protein-free physiological fluids such as deproteinized blood plasma, amniotic fluid, and cerebrospinal fluid.

APPLICATIONS

Fig. 2 illustrates a typical chromatogram of acidic metabolites extracted from the urine of a normal subject. The metabolites include the inorganic anions sulphate and phosphate, and hippuric, citric and uric acids. Of particular interest is the series of aldonic and deoxyaldonic acids which were, except for the tetronic acids [15], first discovered in urine in these laboratories using the methods described above [4, 14]. They include 4-, 3-, and 2- deoxytetronic acids, and tetronic acids erythronic acid and threonic acid, 2-deoxypentonic acid, pentonic acids, deoxyhexonic acid and the hexonic acids such as gluconic acid. All of these compounds are polyhydroxy monocarboxylic acids and are not extracted by solvents such as diethyl ether, ethyl acetate and methyl acetate [4].

The use of similar methods, based on those described above, has recently been described by Thompson & Markey [16], but these workers attempted to remove inorganic

ANALYTICAL METHODS FOR ORGANIC ACIDS

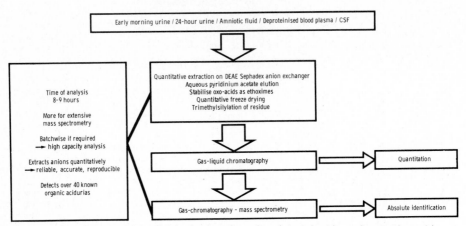

Fig. 1. Summary of analytical procedure for determination of organic acids in physiological fluids. *On-line GC-MS (BOTTOM, CENTRE) is an alternative to conventional GC, not a sequel to it.*

sulphate and phosphate by precipitation as their barium salts. This procedure has the effect of precipitating and co-precipitating most of the organic acids as well, particularly the higher molecular weight aldonic acids and those acids with multiple carboxylic acid groups, and cannot be recommended. Sulphate and phosphate obscure little of the chromatograms obtained using non-polar stationary phases such as OV1, SE30, and OV 101, and their removal is generally unnecessary except for specialized applications [A.M. Lawson, R.A. Chalmers & R.W.E. Watts, unpublished].

The presence of the acids as a group in the freeze-dried eluate allows the use of different procedures to fractionate or study them further, with the know-ledge that all the compounds present are acidic in nature. For example, the aro-matic acid and other hydrophobic acid components of the extract may be further accentuated by solvent extraction of the freeze-dried and stabilized DEAE -Sephadex extract. Fig. 3 illustrates the organic acid component of an extract of urine from a normal subject that is accentuated by this procedure, after reconstitution of the dried residue in 2 ml of water, acidification to pH 1, sodium chloride satu-ration and solvent extraction with ether and ethyl acetate. The solvents were re-moved with a stream of nitrogen and the residue trimethylsilylated with the same quantity of reagent as used for the sample shown in Fig. 2. As can be seen, the hydrophobic and aromatic acids are more readily observed whereas the hydrophilic aliphatic and polyhydroxyacids are not extracted. The aromatic acids present at very low levels may be further accentuated by use of less reagent in the trimethyl-silation stage [A.M. Lawson, R.A. Chalmers & R.W.E. Watts, unpublished].

The possible applications of these techniques are numerous, both in the study of natural metabolites and those of administered compounds such as drugs and parenteral nutrients. Many pharmaceutical preparations are themselves anionic or are metabolized by oxidation, deamination and oxidation, or by conjugation with glucuronic acid and amino acids such as glycine or glutamine to anionic species that are then observed in the acidic fraction. This may be illustrated by the simple example of chloral hydrate. This drug and other hypnotics of the trichloro-methyl group (such as trichloroethanol hydrogen sodium phosphate [trichlorofos sodium], and trichlorobutanol [chloretone]), are used extensively for the sedation of paediatric and other patients. Chloral hydrate is metabolized *in vivo* to its active form, trichloroethanol, which is itself metabolized by oxidation to

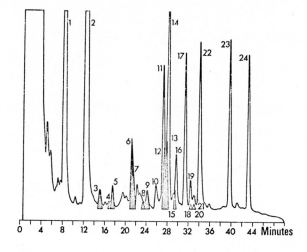

Fig. 2. Gas chromatogram of urinary acidic metabolites extracted from the urine of a normal subject using DEAE-Sephadex. In Figs. 2-4 the metabolites were separated as their ethoxime and trimethylsilyl (TMS) derivatives on 10% OV101 on HP Chromosorb W, 80-100 mesh, by temperature programming from 110° to 285° at 4°/min, with a 5 min initial isothermal delay.

Peak identifications:
1) sulphate; 2) phosphate; 3) 4-deoxytetronic acid; 4) 3-deoxytetronic acid; 5) 2-deoxytetronic acid; 6) erythronic acid; 7) threonic acid; 8) a deoxypentonic acid; 9) 2-deoxypentonic acid; 10) *cis*-aconitic acid; 11) hippuric acid; 12) & 13) pentonic acids; 14) citric acid; 15) deoxyhexonic acid; 16) glucono-1,5-lactone; 17) undecandioic acid *(serving as acidic internal standard)*; 18) a hexonic acid; 19) glucuronic acid; 20) gluconic acid; 21) glucaric acid; 22) uric acid; 23) *n*-tetracosane *(internal standard)*; 24) *n*-hexacosane *(internal standard)*.
The aldonic and deoxyaldonic acids are shaded in order to make their relative positions more apparent.

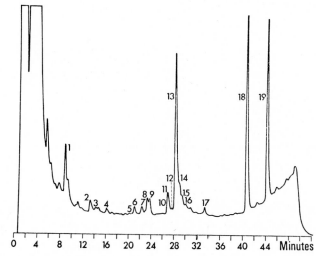

Fig. 3. Gas chromatogram of hydrophobic urinary acidic metabolites extracted from the urine of a normal subject by: DEAE-Sephadex extraction, quantitative freeze-drying; reconstitution of the residue in 2 ml water, acidification and sodium chloride saturation followed by re-extraction with ether (× 3) and ethyl acetate (× 3). For separation conditions, see Legend to Fig. 2.
Peak identifications: 1) cresol; 2) phosphate; 3) succinic acid; 4) 4-deoxytetronic acid; 5) adipic acid; 6) 3-methyladipic acid; 7) 2-hydroxyglutaric acid; 8) 3-hydroxy-3-methyl-glutaric acid; 9) 4-hydroxyphenylacetic acid; 10) vanillic acid; 11) homovanillic acid; 12) 4-hydroxymandelic acid; 13) hippuric acid; 14) citric acid; 15) *m*-hydroxy-phenylhydracrylic acid; 16) vanilmandelic acid; 17) unidentified aromatic acid; 18) *n*-tetracosane *(internal standard)*; 19) *n*-hexacesane *(internal standard)*.

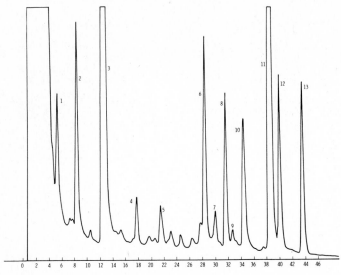

Fig. 4. Gas chroma-
togram of urinary
acidic metabolites
extracted using
DEAE-Sephadex from
the urine of a child
receiving chloral
hydrate. For sepa-
ration conditions,
see Legend to Fig.2.

*Peak identifications
of interest:*
1) trichloroacetic
acid and 11) tri-
chloroethanol-β-
glucuronide (uro-
chloralic acid).

trichloroacetic acid and conjugated with glucuronic acid to give urochloralic acid
(trichloroethanol-β-glucuronide). Both of these metabolites may be extracted and
determined by the procedure described in this paper, and Fig. 4 illustrates a typical chromatogram of urinary acidic metabolites from a child receiving chloral
hydrate, from which the excreted levels of trichloroacetic acid and of trichloroethanol-β-glucuronide may be determined.

References
1. Chalmers, R.A., this Volume, pp. 121-124.
2. Chalmers, R.A. & Watts, R.W.E., *Analyst, Lond. 97* (1972) 951-957.
3. Chalmers, R.A. & Watts, R.W.E., *Analyst, Lond. 97* (1972) 958-967.
4. Chalmers, R.A. & Lawson, A.M., *Chem. Brit. 11* (1975) 290-295.
5. Marvel, C.S. & Rands, R.D., *J. Amer. Chem. Soc. 72* (1950) 2642-2646.
6. Barness, L.A., Morrow, G., Nocho, R.E. & Maresca, R.A., *Clin. Chem. 16* (1970)
   20-23.
7. Rosevear, J.W., Pfaff, K.J. & Moffitt, E.A., *Clin. Chem. 17* (1971) 721-730.
8. Kesner, L. & Muntwyler, E., *Meths. in Enzymology 13* (1969) 415
9. Busch, H., Hurlbert, R.B. & Potter, V.R., *J. Biol. Chem. 196* (1952) 717-727.
10. Von Korff, R.W., *Meths. in Enzymology 13* (1969) 425-430.
11. Kuksis, A. & Prioreschi, P., *Anal. Biochem. 19* (1967) 468-480.
12. Zaura, D.S. & Metcoff, J., *Anal. Chem. 41* (1969) 1781-1787.
13. Jaakonmaki, P.I., Knox, K.L., Horning, E.C. & Horning, M.G., *Eur. J. Pharmacol.
    14* (1967) 63-70.
14. Lawson, A.M., Chalmers, R.A., Purkiss, P., Mitchell, F.L. & Watts, R.W.E.,
    Adv. Mass Spec. 6 (1974) 235-243 *[Proc. 6th Internat. Mass Spect. Symp.]*
15. Horning, E.C. & Horning, M.G., *Clin. Chem. 17* (1971) 802-809.
16. Thompson, J.A. & Markey, S.P., *Anal. Chem. 47* (1975) 1313-1321.

S-NC   NOTES AND COMMENTS RELATING TO SAMPLE PREPARATION

HEXANE/ACETONITRILE PARTITION SYSTEMS APPLIED TO ASSAY OF CORTICOSTEROID OINTMENTS

J.E. Fairbrother
Squibb International Development Lab., Moreton, Merseyside, L46 1OW, U.K.

Hexane/acetonitrile partition systems are useful for the preparation and 'clean-up' of samples of corticosteroid ointments prior to colorimetric, GC or HPLC assay, as will now be described. Squibb have marketed topical preparations containing triamcinolone acetonide for many years.
In early 1969 we were involved in the development of a number of ointment formulations containing triamcinolone acetonide and several related compounds. The ointments in general were formulated using either of two ointment bases, viz. 'PLASTIBASE' (polyethylene and liquid paraffin) or 'PPG' (propylene glycol and white soft paraffin).

Since the early 1960's triamcinolone acetonide, in common with most other corticosteroids, had been assayed in formulations after a sample 'clean-up' step using two colour reactions, as shown. The Nydrazid procedure involves the formation of a hydrazone between the 3-oxo group of the steroid

SAMPLE in methanol

    ADD Isonicotinic acid hydrazide in methanolic HCl

    INCUBATE 45 min at 55°

λ_{max} 405 nm   NYDRAZID REACTION

SAMPLE in ethanol

    ADD Blue Tetrazolium in ethanol

    ADD Tetramethylammonium hydroxide in ethanol

    KEEP 70 min in the dark

    ADD 1 M HCl in ethanol

λ_{max} 525 nm   BLUE TETRAZOLIUM REACTION

and the hydrazide grouping of the reagent. Thus, it can be used only to monitor changes in the steroid A ring. The Blue Tetrazolium procedure involves an oxidation-reduction reaction between the C_{17} side chain of the steroid and the blue tetrazolium reagent in alkaline solution to form a coloured formazan. Both the C_{20}-oxo and the C_{21}-oxy groups are needed for this reaction.

The extraction of the steroid from the ointment base and the removal of substances interfering in these two colour reactions was at the start of our work in 1969 generally performed using a Florisil partition chromatographic procedure. When samples of PPG ointments containing 0.025% SQ 15,112 and

COLUMN PARTITION CHROMATOGRAPHIC PROCEDURE

1. Dissolve in chloroform.
2. Partition with water (PG removed).
3. Run through Florisil column.
4. Wash column with 10% acetone in chloroform.
5. Elute with 2% water in acetone.
6. Evaporate acetone and take up in ethanol.
7. Nydrazid and Blue Tetrazolium reactions.

SQ 15,377 were examined using this procedure, poor recoveries were obtained. Some of the white soft paraffin came through the 'clean-up' procedure and retained residual quantities of acetone which interfered in the Nydrazid reaction. SQ 15,377 is esterified in the C_{21}-oxy group, making it unsuitable for determination by blue tetrazolium. Attempts to extract the ointment by boiling with hot alcohol gave unsatisfactory results and, in the case of SQ 15,377, caused a transesterification reaction to occur.

Acetonitrile had been used in the past to extract triamcinolone from a tablet formulation, and was found to be a good solvent for these other steroids. It was thought that a partition system might be devised between acetonitrile and a non-polar solvent capable of holding back the petrolatum fraction. It was found that partition of a hexane solution of the ointment with three successive aliquots of acetonitrile gave quantitative separation of the steroid from petrolatum. The observed partition coefficients between hexane and acetonitrile were 1.0×10^{-4} for triamcinolone acetonide and SQ 15,112, and 8.5×10^{-4} for SQ 15,377.

Assay procedures were then developed for these ointments, the acetonitrile extracts being evaporated to dryness and the residue taken up in chloroform to perform the Nydrazid reaction. For the Blue Tetrazolium reaction a preliminary partition between water and chloroform was required to remove the propylene glycol which interferes in the colour reaction.

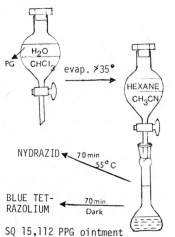

Fig. 1. SQ 15,112 PPG ointment colorimetric procedures.

Acknowledgement: J. Fay, S. Shand and J. Sutton, Squibb private communication (April 1969).

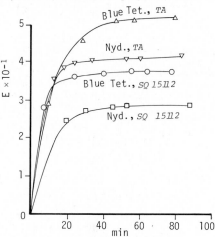

Fig. 2. Blue Tetrazolium & Nydrazid colour development in acetonitrile. The chosen λ values were 525 and 415 nm respectively, and two steroids were used.

The evaporation of the acetonitrile extracts was a lengthy business and traces of acetonitrile caused variability in the colour reactions. The direct development of the Nydrazid and Blue Tetrazolium colours was attempted on the acetonitrile extracts. This was found to be quite satisfactory after a few minor procedural changes including a slight upward shift in the λ_{max} values (Figs. 1 & 2). This separation technique using hexane-acetonitrile partition was now extended to other uses and was used as a 'clean-up' procedure prior to assay of the extracted steroid by quantitative TLC or GC (Fig. 3).

Workers in the University of Dallas had been working along similar lines, and late in 1970 Graham *et al.* [1] published a procedure which used an *n*-heptane-acetonitrile partition system to 'clean up' corticosteroid creams and ointments to enable the Nydrazid and Blue Tetrazolium reactions to be performed (Fig. 4). The procedure involved the application of an acetonitrile-*n*-heptane mixed solvent solution of the ointment to a column containing 'Celite' with an equal weight of adsorbed acetonitrile. The column was washed with *n*-heptane to remove interfering excipient materials and certain steroid degradation products, and the steroid was then eluted with chloroform. The chloroform eluate obtained in this procedure contains a significant proportion of acetonitrile, and the authors had to evaporate to dryness and take up the residue in ethanol before the colorimetric reactions could be performed.

In a later paper Graham *et al.* [2] use the procedure to separate corticosteroids from ointments containing chloroiodooxine, and for this purpose found cyclohexane-acetonitrile better than *n*-heptane-acetonitrile.

More recently we have been faced with the same problem again in the development of assay procedures for a new corticosteroid, halcinonide. Halcinonide was formulated in an ointment containing PEG 400, PEG 1500, PEG 6000 distearate and Tween 65 as excipients. The hexane-acetonitrile partition procedure again proved [3] most useful, and was used as the basic 'clean-up' procedure prior to quantitative TLC or HPLC (Fig. 5).

Thus it can clearly be seen that the hexane-acetonitrile partition system is a

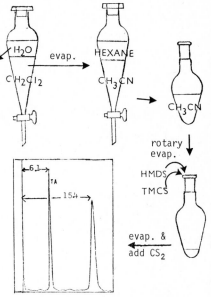

Fig. 3. SQ 15,112 PPG ointment assayed by GC procedure, with FID. HMDS and TMCS respectively denote hexamethyldisilazane and trimethyl-chlorosilane. *Acknowledgement: J.R. Salmon, Squibb private communication (July 1969).*

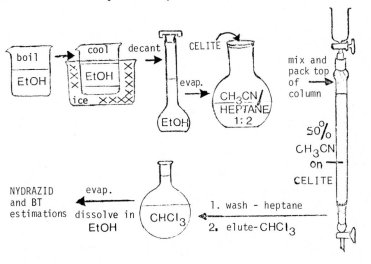

Fig. 4. Procedure of Graham *et al.* [1].

most versatile 'clean-up' tool of proven
merit. It could usefully be considered
for application outside of the corticosteroid assay field.

References

1. Graham, R.E., Williams, P.A. &
    Kenner, C.T., *J. Pharm. Sci. 59* (1970)
    1472-1476.

2. Graham, R.E., Kenner, C.T. & Biehl,
    E.R., *J. Pharm. Sci. 64* (1975) 1013-
    1017.

3. Petrie, G.A. & Nagy, D.J., *Squibb
    private communications* (Oct. 1974
    and May 1975).

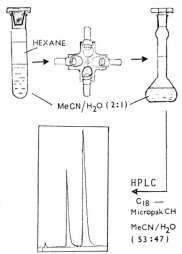

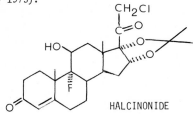

HALCINONIDE

Fig. 5. Halcinonide ointment
assayed by HPLC procedure.

APPROACHES TO SOLVENT EXTRACTION (C.R. Jones, Art. S-1)

Remark by D. Dell.— In the extraction of basified plasma with chloroform, a difficult emulsion may arise if the plasma is put into the tube
first, but no emulsion if the chloroform is put in first. *Question by*
D.B. Campbell.— Do drugs, especially amines, interact with chloroform,
with or without the presence of HCl ? *Reply by* C.R. Jones.— Amines can
interact with chloroform when heated with it in the presence of alkali,
but I am not aware of any reports of interactions occurring at room temperature during the usual relatively brief spans of solvent extractions.
However, it is advisable not to use solvents which have been standing
around for long periods especially in sunlight.

   Remarks by B. Scales.— The use of solvent mixtures can be very
beneficial in that it is often possible to select a mixture which, although not completely extracting the compound, does give minimal extraction of interfering materials and thereby a useful optimization. But
the use of simple mixtures can give rise to unexplained effects. Thus,
an acidic drug, e.g. atromid, which is quite unextractable at pH 0.5
(3 M HCl) from plasma into *n*-heptane can be completely extracted if 1%
methanol is added to the heptane. Presumably the methanol resides in
the aqueous phase but releases phosphatides to form ion-pairs with the
organic acid, which then transfers to the heptane phase. This possibility may explain the observation that a basic triphenylethylene (noval-
dex) requires 60-90 min extraction at an alkaline pH for a 95% transfer
from water to benzene, but that the extraction is complete in 3-5 min
from diluted plasma at the same pH: ion-pair formation or some type of
complex formation with phosphatides in plasma can enhance the speed of
extraction.

Remark by B.J. Millard.— We have found that losses as high as 90% may occur in the process of evaporating solutions down from, say, 2 ml to 50 μl under a stream of nitrogen in centrifuge tubes. This is a process which most analysts use at some stage, and steps should be taken to reduce these losses. One method that has been suggested is a gently heated collar placed around the tube some distance above the surface of the liquid *(cf. Scheme 2 in Art. G-1 - ED.)*.

SOLVENT EXTRACTION AS APPLIED TO FLUPHENAZINE & ITS METABOLITES (R. Whelpton & S.H. Curry, Art. S-2)

Replies by R. Whelpton *to questions*.— The extraction of fluphenazine esters is *not* pH-dependent; it depends on the lipophilicity of the esters *(answering* D. Dell). Do any special considerations apply in the choice of buffers for measuring partition coefficients over the pH range 2-14 ? (A. Bye).— Different synthetic buffers have been used to cover the range, and no problems encountered. Did you measure any blood levels of FPZ in humans using the radioactive extraction method ? (R.G.Muusze). — This work is now in progress. Fluphenazine is known to be present in the plasma following oral and injected doses. After i.m. administration of fluphenazine hydrochloride (25 mg) the peak concentration at 2 h is ∿10 ng/ml. The half-life is ∿15 h. Concentrations following oral doses and long-acting injections are lower.

Purification of solvents - *Notes contributed by A.D.R. Harrison & E. Reid*

Important though it is to use solvents of assured purity in many assay operations, budgeting constraints may preclude the purchase of ultra-pure solvents, and in any case a repeatedly used solvent may become wet or even chemically modified. A trace of moisture *per se* will obviously be inoccuous if the solvent is to be used merely for extracting an aqueous solution, but could be disastrous in preparing a drug derivative for GC-ECD assay *(see Note on this topic in Section E-NC1)*. Since the context in which the solvent will be used determines what impurities matter and have to be removed, it would be absurd to stipulate that solvents should be of immaculate purity in all respects. Elsewhere in this book there are examples (indexed under *Solvents*) of known troubles and remedies; but such information is rather scattered. By way of persuading 'old hands' in other laboratories to set down their working practices on paper, a short annotation has now been compiled.

The following examples of purification are from a description of a GC assay [1]. n-*Propanol* of 'p.a.' grade was dried by refluxing with CaH2 [expensive !] and re-distilling, the middle fraction being taken. *Acetic anhydride* and *ethyl acetate* were dried over anhydrous CaSO4 and re-distilled. *Pyridine* was refluxed with KOH pellets, distilled, and stored over KOH pellets. (Also, the nitrogen for GC, bought with 80 ppm of water, was dried by passage through a 4A molecular sieve.)

Fused CaCl2, prior to distillation, is appropriate for drying *ether* (several 24-h treatments), *dichloromethane,* and *chloroform* (but HCl may have to be washed out before use). At the outset, ether is washed with freshly made satd. FeSO4 solution (20 ml/1 of ether) and then with water; in the final distillation, it should *not* be taken to dryness, in case a trace of peroxide persists. Whilst it is traditional to store over sodium wire, a sufficient precaution with solvents such as ether may be division of the product into small portions, kept stoppered in the dark and each sufficient for only one or two experiments.

Such treatments, traditional in chemical laboratories, have been collated in a handbook which also gives physical properties of solvents with, however, little attention to UV absorption [2]. *Acetonitrile* purification has been studied [3], and two elaborate methods described with steps such as permanganate treatment; but it is uncertain what impurities matter from the point of view of HPLC assays: any acrylonitrile that may be present could interfere because of its high absorbance in the 280 nm region. Treatment with suitable alumina(s) offers a simple approach to purifying small volumes of certain solvents, e.g. peroxide-containing hydrocarbons and ethers, and to dehydrating various solvents. This approach has been set down in company literature (particularly Woelm; authors of relevant papers include G. Hesse and G. Wohlleben) together with examples of the use of alumina, in bulk or as a chromatographic thin layer, in the assay of trace organic compounds. An example of the use of aluminas in solvent purification for drug assay is the clean-up of *n*-heptane, with an aqueous H_2SO_4 wash before use [4]. To dry a wet solvent, a traditional dehydrating agent may be advantageous initially, to reduce the column size (and cost) of a subsequent alumina step.

1. Coulter, J.R. & Hahn, C.S., *J. Chromatog.* 36 (1968) 42-49.

2. Riddick, J.A. & Bunger, W.B., *Organic Solvents (Techniques of Chemistry, Vol. 2),* 3rd edn., Wiley-Interscience, New York (1970), 1041 pp.

3. Walter, M. & Ramaley, L., *Anal. Chem.* 45 (1973) 165-166.

4. Dill, W.A. & Glazko, A.J., *Clin. Chem.* 18 (1972) 675-676.

(1) FREEZE-DRYING, (2) ANION-EXCHANGERS, in sample preparation (R.A. Chalmers, Arts. S-3 & S-6)

(1) *Answers to* J. Chamberlain.- *Concerning* how the parameters for individual bonds were obtained (for ΔH_v, calc): the molecular group contributions were calculated from the experimental data then available [ref.2, Art. S-3] for several compounds each containing the group of interest, and the average group contribution to ΔH_v was then calculated [see text of the Article, & refs. 2, 3]. *Question:* May 'calc.' values have been based on the very experimental data with which they are compared, = circular argument? - The group contributions are calculated from a variety of compounds including hydrocarbons, alcohols, ethers, aldehydes, and (only for the carboxyl group contribution) carboxylic acids. Only some of the experimental values for organic acids in Table 3, as taken from the literature, were used for establishing the carboxyl contribution; but a reasonable check on the reliability of the ΔH_v estimates comes from the use of compounds lacking carboxyl groups to derive other molecular group contributions.

Answers to D.A. Cowan.— The methods used by authors (cf. [1] in Art. S-3) whose values were now used to calculate molecular group contributions included calorimetry (Wadsö and flow techniques) and the Knudsen effusion technique. *Concerning* the high m.p. of glyoxylic acid (90°) and its relatively low enthalpy change.— The m.p. shown is for the monohydrate, in which water is present as water of constitution (cf. chloral hydrate) to form what could be called dihydroxyacetic acid. This has an estimated ΔH_v of 26.5 kcal/g compared to the free aldehyde/acid value of 15.7. However, the losses observed here during freeze-drying indicate that the water is relatively easily removed under the conditions used and that the acid is present in the later stages in the free aldo form. Table 1 shows that ethoxime formation improved recovery.

(2) *Answer to* A.W. Forrey.— For volatile C_2-C_6 acids in urine, a different method is employed: the acids are released from their salts by shaking urine with AG Dowex 50W × 12 (H^+) and then the supernatant is analyzed directly by GC on Chromosorb 105 [1].

1. Chalmers, R.A., Bickle, S. & Watts, R.W.E., *Clin. Chim. Acta* 52 (1974) 31-34.

'CHEMICAL MASKING' in sample preparation (J. Chamberlain, Art. S-4)

Comment by J. Godbillon.— In determining secondary amines by radioderivatization (acetylation with [³H]acetic anhydride), a TLC purification after derivatization allows the acetyl derivatives of primary and secondary amines to be separated and contamination due to the reagent to be eliminated; this obviates protection of the primary amines before acetylation and gives better specificity in the technique.

SAMPLE PREPARATION FOR HPLC (D. Dell, Art. S-5) - *cf.* (1) above

Answer to L.S. Jackson.— I have not come across any reference to the extraction of a freeze-dried tissue homogenate (cf. extraction of freeze-dried plasma by methanol). Recently, however, R.P.W. Scott told me of an interesting technique used at Hofmann

La Roche (New Jersey). A tissue homogenate slurried with celite is freeze-dried, and the dried matrix deposited at the top of the HPLC column and eluted. Presumably the mobile phase is chosen so as to elute the compound(s) of interest, leaving behind on the celite as much as possible of the endogenous material.

   Suggestion by C.R. Jones: Might precipitated protein be removed from blocked-up columns by pumping on some proteolytic enzyme ? *Reply.-* Perhaps; but we hope to avoid the problem in future by always using a pre-column. *Editorial note.-* The use of 5% dimethyl sulphoxide has been suggested (Waters leaflet) to clean up columns.

VARIOUS SOLID-PHASE APPROACHES TO SAMPLE PREPARATION

Editorial note: Art. G-1 mentions some approaches which did feature in the Techniques Forum but which, notwithstanding their importance, have NOT appeared in Section 'S' as contributed articles. These approaches, on which some observations now follow, include: CATION-EXCHANGERS; XAD-2, CHARCOAL (adsorbents — another example being ALUMINA); LIPOPHILIC 'SEPHADEX'.

Queries and remarks on XAD-2 ('Amberlite' non-ionic resin): Is there good recovery and reproducibility, particularly with ng/ml concentrations ? (D.B. Campbell; D.L. Phillips). — For metadrenalines, good recoveries at low concentrations cannot be relied on (Art. T-2), and for other compounds the literature points to differences in recovery but lacks information on very low concentrations (E. Reid). Concerning points of technique such as flow rates *(question by J.D. Baty)*, there is helpful literature [e.g. 1]; gentle pumping during loading is permissible.

   Query by E.L. Crampton (who commented on the usefulness of XAD-2 in the routine assay of ibuprofen in serum, urine and synovial fluid): might the temperature dependence of the desorption process furnish a means of achieving some selectivity in extraction ? — In connection with tetracyclines, G.V. Samsonov reported the kinetics of the temperature effect with resins very similar to XAD-2 (J.E. Fairbrother).

Remark on charcoal by B. Scales.— Many years ago we used charcoal-celite mixtures for the adsorption of ferrocenes and metabolites (hydroxy derivatives and mono- and bis-glucuronides) from urine. An excellent clean-up and recovery was obtained by washing with water and 30% methanol in water, and eluting with 35-40% methanol in water. *Remark by* C.R. Jones.— XAD-2 tends to have replaced charcoal for drug adsorption because of the much lower adsorptive capacity of the former, which ensures that the adsorbed material is more easily released. However, there is evidence (K. Grob, *ref. 16 in Art. G-1) that* most workers use far too much charcoal. *Note by* E. Reid.— In Art. T-2 it is shown that metadrenalines in pure solution need less charcoal than urinary metadrenalines.

Editorial note.— A recent paper [2] on steroid oestrogens shows the usefulness of lipophilic (LH) Sephadex, which when followed by TLC enabled the radiochemical purity of the compounds to be established in isotope dilution studies. Various references to sample preparation procedures such as feature in the present Section are to be found in a review [3], and throughout the present book (including Art. T-2).

1. Kullberg, M.P. & Gorodetzky, C.W., *Clin. Chem.* 20 (1974) 177-183.

2. Lisboa, B.P. & Strassner, M., *J. Chromatog.* 111 (1975) 159-164.

3. Reid, E., *Analyst 101* (1976) 1-18.

Section on Tactical illustrations

Analytical case history

T-1   DETERMINATION OF ALDOSTERONE IN BIOLOGICAL FLUIDS

.V.H.T. James   and   G.A. Wilson
Department of Chemical Pathology
St. Mary's Hospital Medical School
London W2 1PG, U.K.

Requirement	*Assay sensitive to ∿20 ng/l, for plasma and urine.*
Chemistry & metabolism	*Steroid with ketol side-chain. Derivatives available for colorimetry or fluorimetry, but sensitivity poor. The hormone is unconjugated in plasma but largely conjugated with glucuronic acid in urine.*
End-step	*Radioimmunoassay.*
Sample preparation	*Hydrolysis, in case of urine. Then solvent extraction and column chromatography.*
Comments & alternatives	*Sensitivity ∿5 pg per assay tube; assay adequate for most purposes. Some drug interference. Initial radio-tracer spiking enables recoveries to be assessed. Part-automation is feasible.*
	Other published radioimmunoassays differ in the antiserum and in the method of separating the bound and free fractions in the radioimmunoassay. Some authors have employed an isotope dilution approach.

The quantitative determination of aldosterone in biological fluids presents the steroid biochemist with a challenging analytical problem. Aldosterone is a hormone of considerable biological and clinical importance, but is a chemically labile molecule and is present in relatively low concentration in fluids such as blood and urine. In blood plasma, however, aldosterone levels in a healthy subject are between 40 and 100 ng per litre, and so the prime requirement for any analytical procedure is an end-point with a very high degree of sensitivity.

There are relatively few techniques which can achieve this level of sensitivity in practice, and most of the work in this field has involved the use of the isotope dilution method or, more recently, of radioimmunoassay. These methods will now be discussed, and particular emphasis will be given to radioimmunoassay (an approach discussed by Butler - *this vol., Art.G-2*) and to the reasons which direct the choice of the various analytical steps employed.

ISOTOPE DERIVATIVE ASSAY

The first successful attempt to measure aldosterone in peripheral plasma evolved from the application of the isotope dilution derivative principle, taking advantage of the availability of high specific activity radio-labelled reagents and steroid tracers. The main advantage which this technique offers is high sensitivity, enabling amounts in the picogram range to be measured; it also has the virtue of versatility since it can be applied in principle to any compound which can be derivatized with a suitable radio-labelled reagent. On the other hand, there are disadvantages which are not to be dismissed lightly. An appropriate labelled tracer is required, and the reagents are expensive and need careful preparation to avoid problems with non-specific interference. It is a very demanding assay technically and requires first-class laboratory facilities and considerable chemical expertise. Because of the long purification procedure, productivity is low:

twenty estimations per week is about the maximum which one worker can achieve.
There is also a radiation hazard and a requirement for high quality isotope counting equipment. In spite of all these serious problems, several groups of investigators have been successful in setting up assay methods for plasma aldosterone
using the double isotope technique [1-3].

Most workers have employed [^{3}H-]acetic anhydride as reagent since this is
available commercially at high (100 Ci/mol) specific activity. The major problem
which has to be overcome is the rigorous purification of the radio-labelled derivative to remove extraneous tritium. This is achieved only after multiple chromatographic steps. In our experience, it is essential to employ freshly redistilled
reagent. The high specific activity of the anhydride encourages self-decomposition
and these products are extremely difficult to remove subsequently. Micro-distilla-
tion is carried out under vacuum several times immediately before use, and this
effectively lowers the non-specific blank value. Acetylation can be carried out
'wet', with a catalyst (pyridine); but our preference, again so as to minimize
blanks, is to carry out this stage in the vapour phase [4]. This is effective in
reducing substantially the amount of extraneous radioactivity which has to be removed. The plasma extract is applied directly to small paper strips which are exposed to [^{3}H-]acetic anhydride vapour in a small glass vessel. After reaction,
the vapour is removed by freezing and the paper strips eluted for subsequent
chromatography.

The selection of chromatographic procedures is somewhat empirical, since
the precise nature of the interfering substances is unknown. Nevertheless, systems
used for separating closely related steroids can be successfully employed. It is
also necessary to incorporate a stage in which chemical manipulation of the steroid
is carried out, so as to markedly alter the polarity of the derivative and thus
enhance the possibility of separating related substances. This stage may be
additional esterification, partial hydrolysis or oxidation (e.g. conversion of
aldosterone to the lactone), and all these methods have been employed. By repeated
chromatography (and most investigators employ up to six or more stages), it is
possible to achieve satisfactory purification of the derivative and to reduce the
'blank' to an acceptably low level, e.g. to the equivalent of 10 ng/l or less.
Applied to human plasma, the method can achieve a precision of ± 10% (C.V.) at
normal aldosterone levels [3]. However, apart from the disadvantages mentioned
above, a further serious difficulty is the relative insensitivity of the technique:
for reliable analyses, the sample has to be 20 ml, a volume unacceptably large
for clinical or repetitive analyses. The advent of radioimmunoassays has rendered
double isotope assays in the steroid field completely redundant, and in the rest
of this paper consideration will be given to the radioimmunoassay of aldosterone.

RADIOIMMUNOASSAY

The non-specific nature of the isotope derivative assay end-point necessitated a
very substantial degree of sample preparation to avoid the problem of non-specific
interference. The anticipated virtue of radioimmunoassay is the high specificity
of the end-point, permitting considerable simplification of the purification stages.
Applied to certain peptide hormones, immunoassays have achieved the ultimate in
simplification, and direct assay can be performed on the serum or urine sample
directly. So far, however, this has only rarely been achieved for steroids, and
initial purification is still required. Several authors have presented methods
for aldosterone radioimmunoassay, adopting various methods for purification.

Plasma aldosterone

Most authors have adopted an initial extraction stage, using an organic solvent.
The solvent needs to be sufficiently polar to achieve a high extraction yield, but
as non-polar as possible to minimize the extraction of extraneous and unwanted
material from plasma. It should also have a relatively low boiling point, to

facilitate removal. The solvents preferred by most authors are dichloromethane or chloroform.

The choice of purification stages is fairly wide, and it appears that several satisfactory alternatives exist. The first successful radioimmunoassay was published by Mayes *et al.* [5], who employed a silica gel column followed by paper chromatography and another silica gel column. Ito *et al.* [6] compared paper chromatography with Sephadex LH-20 and found both satisfactory, and Bayard *et al.* [7] used a single paper-chromatographic step. As an alternative to chromatographic purification, Martin & Nugent [8] used adsorption onto Fullers earth as an initial step, followed by elution, and then employed an antibody to aldosterone as a further purification stage. Varsano-Aharon & Ulick [9] adopted a similar principle, using charcoal adsorption, and Gomez-Sanchez *et al.* [10] used an antibody to aldosterone for purification. These techniques depend upon the principle that the endogenous plasma proteins bind competing steroids and retain them, whilst unbound steroids including aldosterone are selectively removed.

More recently, two methods have been published in which no chromatographic stage is employed, and the plasma extract is subjected directly to radioimmunoassay [11, 12].

The requirements for different degrees of sample purification appear to be related to the specificity of the antiserum available. One group considers that the major interfering compound in the assay is cortisol [13], and they concluded that if cortisol is removed satisfactorily, other interference is minimal. Their data are compatible with this suggestion but do not prove it. Furthermore, it is very clear that antisera are highly characteristic reagents and the same antigen produces a variety of antibodies with differing specificity. Nevertheless, it may be significant that the simplest methods have employed antibodies raised against the 3-oxime rather than the 18,21-disuccinate of aldosterone, and theoretically one would choose the former antigen for optimum specificity. It is also important to remember that the method selected for separating bound and unbound steroid can influence the specificity of the antiserum; comparisons have to be made with this in mind.

In our laboratory, we have used the double isotope assay for many years [3], subsequently changing to radioimmunoassay by the method of Mayes & Nugent [5]. The results using this latter method were compared with those from the immunoassay and have given satisfactory agreement. In subsequent work to simplify and improve the assay we have adopted the Mayes & Nugent assay as a reference method.

In our opinion, solvent extraction of the plasma sample is a simpler process than the adsorption techniques, which require thorough subsequent extraction to recover the aldosterone. In common with other investigators we have preferred dichloromethane as an extraction solvent for the reasons mentioned earlier. The solvent is distilled, and immediately prior to use is washed with water. Failure to do this engenders the risk of destroying the aldosterone, probably by phosgene which rapidly forms in chlorinated solvents like dichloromethane and chloroform.

Although most authors have employed one or more purification stages, the reports from two groups [11, 12] suggest that with appropriate antisera this purification may be unnecessary. In our hands, this has not proved to be so. Fig. 1 illustrates the comparison of the results from the reference method and the method described by McKenzie & Clements [11], using an antiserum generously donated by Dr. McKenzie. It is clear from the figure that the simplified method produces markedly lower results than the reference method, implying interference with binding, or with separation of the bound and unbound fractions which is made with charcoal in this method. Inspection of the extracts showed the presence of lipid-like material which was considered to be a likely source of interference. On this

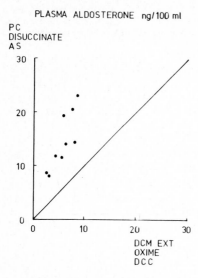

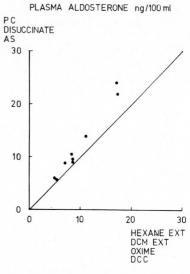

Fig. 1. Correlation between results of the 'reference method' (*see text*) for plasma aldosterone, using paper chromatography (PC), disuccinate anti-serum and ammonium sulphate separation (AS), and the method using direct extraction (DCM *denotes* dichloromethane) with oxime antiserum and dextran-coated charcoal (DCC).

Fig. 2. Correlation between results of the 'reference method' for plasma aldosterone and the method used in Fig. 1, but incorporating a pre-extraction of the plasma with hexane. *Abbreviations for Figs. 2 and 3 are as in Fig. 1 legend.*

Fig. 3. Correlation between results of the 'reference method' for plasma aldosterone and the method used in Fig. 1, but incorporating a purification stage involving column chromatography (CC).

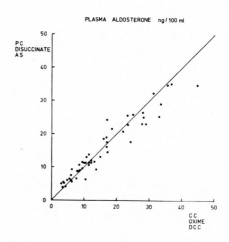

Scheme 1. Simplified radioimmunoassay for plasma aldosterone.

To 36,000 d.p.m. [^{3}H-]aldosterone (50 Ci/m-mol; hence 90 pg) is added 1.0 ml of plasma. *The same amount of labelled aldosterone is also added to a counting vial as a recovery standard.*

Extracted with 12 ml dichloromethane *(water-washed and dried over anhydrous sodium sulphate before use).*

Extract poured through filter paper onto 7 x 40 mm silica gel column - *the column having been washed before use with 2 x 5 ml hot methanol; 2 x 5 ml cold methanol; 2 x 5 ml methanol: dichloromethane (1:1); 3 x 5 ml dichloromethane.*

Column washed with 1 x 5 ml dichloromethane, then 1 x 5 ml dichloromethane: methanol (100:2).

Aldosterone eluted with 1 x 6 ml dichloromethane:methanol (100:9).

From eluate, 1.0 ml taken for recovery count, and 2 x 1.0 ml for radioimmuno-assay.

STANDARDS prepared containing 0, 10, 20, 30, 50, 70, 100 pg aldosterone per tube and an amount of [^{3}H-]aldosterone equivalent to the average recovery count per tube.

Any sample with a recovery 5% less than or greater than the standard c.p.m. tube is discarded.

To all tubes, 0.1 ml 5% propylene glycol in methanol is added. Solvent is evaporated *in vacuo* at 40°.

To all tubes is added 0.25 ml 1/16000 antibody dilution (in borate buffer containing 2% methanol and 0.1% human γ-globulin).

Tubes mixed and incubated overnight at 4°.

To all tubes is added 0.25 ml 4 mg/ml 'Norit A' charcoal in borate buffer containing 0.05% dextran 'C'. Tubes mixed and centrifuged at 4°.

From supernatant, 0.3 ml is transferred to 4.5 ml 'Instagel' scintillator and counted.

Values for $\frac{B}{B_O}$ are plotted against pg aldosterone per tube, where B = c.p.m. in assay tube and B_O = c.p.m. in zero tube.

Picogram value for sample is read from standard curve.

Concentration (ng/100 ml plasma) = pg × $\frac{RECOVERY, STANDARD}{RECOVERY, SAMPLE}$ × $\frac{1}{10}$.

---

assumption, one pre-extraction of the plasma with hexane was carried out, and the plasma was then extracted with dichloromethane and submitted to immunoassay. Fig.2 illustrates that the inclusion of this stage produces satisfactory results. As an alternative means of removing the presumed lipid-like interfering material, the dichloromethane extract of plasma was passed through a silica gel column. The method is shown in detail in Scheme 1. Fig. 3 shows a comparison of the results using this method and the reference method; the correlation is very satisfactory. Thus, although in our hands the simple method without chromatography was not satisfactory, acceptable results were obtained by use of a hexane pre-wash or of a simple column step.

These investigations were made using the antiserum against the 3-oxime-conjugate and dextran-coated charcoal (DCC) as a separatory technique. The extent to which the specificity of the method depends on these factors was investigated by using a different antiserum and also by using ammonium sulphate (AS) for separation. Using the antiserum against the 18,21-disuccinate provided by the National Institute of Arthritis, Metabolism and Digestive Diseases, Bethesda, neither DCC nor AS gave satisfactory results; in both cases, the results obtained were higher than were found by the reference method. As stated above, DCC used in conjunction with the 3-oxime antiserum was satisfactory, but AS was not. It is unwise to draw too many conclusions from these limited data, but it is clear that the antibody specificity is a limiting factor in the choice of a purification procedure and that the 3-oxime conjugate antisera may be more specific than those from the disuccinate conjugate. The separation technique for bound and unbound steroid is also important, since it conditions antiserum specificity.

In our experience adsorption of steroid onto glass reaction tubes can be a major technical problem in methods involving evaporation of extract or eluate in the reaction tube prior to radioimmunoassay. This is particularly true in the case of deoxycorticosterone and androstenedione, but it also occurs with aldosterone.

Adsorption onto glass can be variable, and result in unacceptable precision. Furthermore, if losses go unnoticed, then accuracy is affected as a result of discrepancy between the apparent recovery and the actual steroid available for radioimmunoassay in the reaction tube.

The use of propylene glycol (PG) added (as 0.1 ml of 5% PG in methanol) to the extract or eluate prior to evaporation has proved successful in preventing adsorption. Even *in vacuo* at 40°, with a boiling range of 186-188° propylene glycol does not completely evaporate from the reaction tube but leaves a thin film of liquid in which the steroid remains dissolved. Propylene glycol is readily soluble in the borate buffer system, and in our experience the presence of small amounts of PG has no apparent effect on the assay system, except to ensure constant recovery of counts into the borate buffer after evaporation of extract or eluate. Using this technique, and employing glass tubes, recoveries of aldosterone added to plasma have ranged from 94% to 100%. We have had less satisfactory results using polystyrene assay tubes.

The addition of 2% methanol to the borate buffer is made to facilitate the solubilization of steroid in the antibody mixture. The presence of γ-globulin and/or bovine serum albumin (BSA) also aids solubility in addition to providing a stable environment for the antibody. γ-Globulin also has a prime function as a co-precipitant in the AS separation stage. The amount of antibody alone is very small (1→16000 dilution), and inclusion of γ-globulin increases the mass of protein available for precipitation, making separation of bound and free steroid more satisfactory when using medium-speed centrifuges such as are available in most laboratories. The concentration of co-precipitant is important; if there is too little, separation of bound and unbound fractions may be impaired. If too much is present, some steroid may be bound non-specifically to globulin, leading to spurious results.

Some comment is also necessary on setting up standard curves. In practice it is expedient to use unextracted (or direct) standards; but before doing so, it is essential to show that standards taken through the method (extracted standards) produce identical results. In our experience, this may not be true.

In our investigation of simplified methods, standards were extracted from 5% BSA in borate buffer (cf. [11]). These standards produced a calibration curve which was less steep than for the direct standards. Since the recovery of the standards is adequate, this divergence is probably due to interference with the binding of the aldosterone by the antibody. This might be unimportant if similar interference occurred with plasma extracts; however, this is not so, and results obtained using extracted standards are lower than those obtained by the reference method. The hexane pre-extraction stage, or column chromatography, removed this interference; extracted or direct standards then produced similar results.

URINARY ALDOSTERONE

Various methods have been used for the determination of aldosterone in urine[*], but radioimmunoassay is now the method of choice. Although there is a small amount of free aldosterone in urine, almost all is present as the 18-glucuronoside. These facts dictate the necessity for a pre-extraction of the urine to remove free aldosterone and possibly other interfering compounds (including steroids) and then for hydrolysis to release the conjugated aldosterone. Pre-extraction is carried out with water-washed dichloromethane, and hydrolysis is effected by keeping the urine at pH 1 for 24 h at 37°. Although enzyme hydrolysis with β-glucuronidase will also release some aldosterone, it also hydrolyses other steroids, including tetrahydro-aldosterone, leading to interference with the immunoassay, whereas pH 1 hydrolysis appears to be more selective. In our laboratory, we have treated the hydrolysed urine in exactly the same way as for plasma in the assay of Mayes *et al.* [5], and again adopted this as the reference assay. In experiments designed to simplify this procedure, we have examined the two types of antisera available and the two separation techniques (DCC and AS) as described above.

Following hydrolysis, the urine is extracted with dichloromethane. This is then evaporated, and the extract submitted to immunoassay. Using the 3-oxime antiserum and DCC, a satisfactory correlation with the reference method was obtained (Fig. 4). Although our experience is limited, it appears that AS is also satisfactory with this antiserum (Fig. 5). Using the disuccinate antiserum, only DCC was suitable since AS produced an unsatisfactory correlation (Fig. 6).

Thus, in contrast to plasma, adequate specificity could be achieved with urine in the simple assay using either the succinate or the oxime antiserum; but it is important to note that the method of separation employed in the immunoassay stage is crucial, and conditions the specificity of the antiserum. The final method chosen for urinary aldosterone is shown in Scheme 2.

CONCLUSIONS

Reliable measurement of aldosterone, both in plasma and in urine, can be made using the immunoassay technique. The method has sufficient sensitivity to permit the use of 1.0 ml of plasma and microlitre volumes of urine. The choice of technique is conditioned to a very considerable extent by the reagent (antiserum) which is available, and the ability of some investigators to achieve considerable simplification probably relates entirely to the high specificity of their antiserum. Since antisera, even those raised against the same conjugate but in different animals, possess different characteristics of specificity, it is essential to select an analytical technique which is appropriate to the antiserum which is available. There can be no guarantee that any two antisera are identical in this respect, and prior checking is essential. It is also important to realize that the specificity of an antiserum must be considered in relation to the separation technique employed in the immunoassay stage, and it cannot be assumed that changing this will not impair the specificity of the method.

Thus, by choosing carefully the reagent and separation technique, it is possible to effect considerable simplification of the methodology, at least for plasma and urine from healthy human subjects. It does not follow that these methods can be applied to pathological sera or urines, or to other species, and the possibility of drug interference is always present.

---

[*] *See the article by J. Chamberlain earlier in this Volume. - Editor.*

URINE ALDOSTERONE µg/24 hrs

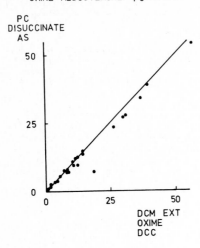

URINE ALDOSTERONE µg/24hrs

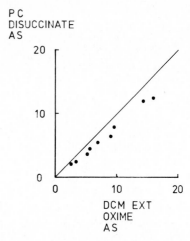

URINE ALDOSTERONE µg/24 hrs

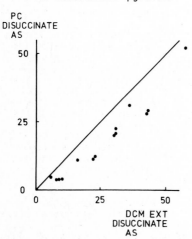

Above, left
Fig. 4. Correlation between results of the 'reference method' for urinary aldosterone, using paper chromatography (PC), disuccinate antiserum and ammonium sulphate separation (AS), and the method described in the text employing hydrolysis, direct extraction (DCM *denotes* dichloromethane) and assay using oxime antiserum and dextran-coated charcoal (DCC) separation.

Above, right
Fig. 5. As for Fig. 4, but using ammonium sulphate separation.
Abbreviations in Figs. 5 and 6 are as in Fig. 4 legend.

Left
Fig. 6. As for Fig. 4, but using disuccinate antiserum and ammonium sulphate separation.

Scheme 2. Simplified radioimmunoassay for aldosterone released from the acid-labile aldosterone 18-glucuronoside conjugate in urine.

Pre-extraction of 5 ml urine performed with 25 ml water-washed dichloromethane.

Pre-extracted urine acidified to pH 1 with hydrochloric acid, and hydrolyzed overnight at 37°.

To 10,000 d.p.m. [³H-]aldosterone (50 Ci/mol) is added 0.5 ml of urine hydrolysate. *The same amount of labelled aldosterone is also added to a counting vial as a recovery standard.*

Urine extracted with 12 ml dichloromethane *(water-washed and dried over anhydrous sodium sulphate before use.)*

Extract washed with 1 x 2 ml 0.1N sodium hydroxide, 1 x 2 ml 0.1N acetic acid, then 1 x 2 ml distilled water.

Portion of extract (5 ml) evaporated under nitrogen, and residue redissolved in 5 ml methanol.

From the methanolic extract, 1.0 ml taken for recovery count, and 2 x 0.1 ml taken for radioimmunoassay.

STANDARDS prepared containing 0, 10, 20, 30, 50, 70, 100 pg aldosterone per tube.

To all tubes, 0.1 ml 5% propylene glycol in methanol is added.

Tubes evaporated *in vacuo* at 40°.

To all tubes is added 0.25 ml 1/16000 antibody dilution (in borate buffer containing 20,000 d.p.m. [³H-]aldosterone per ml, 2% methanol and 0.1% human γ-globulin).

Tubes mixed and incubated at 4° overnight.

To all tubes is added 0.25 ml 4 mg/ml 'Norit A' charcoal in borate buffer containing 0.05% dextran 'C'. Tubes mixed and centrifuged at 4°.

0.3 ml supernatant counted in 4.5 ml 'Instagel' scintillator.

Graph of $\frac{B}{B_O}$ *plotted against pg aldosterone/tube, where B = c.p.m. in assay tube and B_O = c.p.m. in zero tube.*

$$Output\ (\mu g/24\ h) = pg \times \frac{RECOVERY,\ STANDARD}{RECOVERY,\ SAMPLE} \times \frac{10}{0.5} \times \frac{TOTAL\ VOLUME}{10^6}.$$

Acknowledgements

We are grateful to Dr. J.K. McKenzie for a generous gift of antiserum and also to the Hormone Supply Officer of the National Institute of Arthritis, Metabolism and Digestive Disease, Bethesda, who also provided antiserum for this work.

References

1. Brodie, A.H., Shimizu, N., Tait, S.A.S. & Tait, J.F., *J. Clin. Endocr. 27* (1967) 997-1011.

2. Coghlan, J.P. & Scoggins, B.A., *J. Clin. Endocr. 27* (1967) 1470-1486.

3. Fraser, R. & James, V.H.T., *J. Endocr. 40* (1968) 59-72.

4. James, V.H.T., Rippon, A.E. & Arnold, M.L., *Acta Endocr. (Kbh)*, Supplement 138 (1969) 12.

5. Mayes, D., Furuyama, S., Kem, D.C. & Nugent, C.A., *J. Clin. Endocr. 30* (1970) 682-686.

6. Ito, T., Woo, J., Haning, R. & Horton, R., *J. Clin. Endocr. 34* (1972) 106-112.

7. Bayard, F., Beitins, I.Z., Kowarski, A. & Migeon, C.J., *J. Clin. Endocr. 31* (1970) 1-6.

8. Martin, B.T. & Nugent, C.A., *Steroids 21* (1970) 169-180.

9. Varsano-Aharon, N. & Ulick, S., *J. Clin. Endocr. 39* (1974) 375-379.

10. Gomex-Sanchez, C., Kem, D.C. & Kaplan, N.M., *J. Clin. Endocr. 36* (1973) 795-798.

11. MacKenzie, J.K. & Clements, J.A., *J. Clin. Endocr. 38* (1974) 622-627.

12. Pham-Huu-Trung, M.T. & Corvol, P., *Steroids 24* (1974) 587-598.

13. Varsano-Aharon, N. & Ulick, S., *J. Clin. Endocr. 37* (1973) 372-379.

Analytical case history

T-2

ASSAY STUDIES ON URINARY METADRENALINES

A.A.A. Aziz, J.P. Leppard and E. Reid
Wolfson Bioanalytical Centre, University of Surrey,
Guildford, GU2 5XH, U.K.

Requirement	*Normetadrenaline (normetanephrine, NM) and metadrenaline (metanephrine, M) individually in urine, down to 50 µg/l including conjugates.*					
Chemistry & metabolism	*Phenolic ring with (methyl)ethanolamine side-chain, pK 9.74 (M) or 9.56 (NM). Stability erratic at alkaline pH. Weak UV absorbance. Are metabolites of noradrenaline and adrenaline (which also occur in urine). Mainly in form of conjugates, largely sulphate in man.*					
End-step (The ref. letters relate to Fig. 4)	*Cellulose phosphate chromatography to separate NM & M [1] then fluorimetry as lutidines [2] — REFERENCE METHOD, C*	*VARIANT, C', of the REF. METHOD C; same end-step (TLC under study)*	*Cation-exchange HPLC with UV detector, as ATTEMPTED NOVEL ASSAY, H*	*VARIANT, H', of H with final fluorimetry*	*Reverse-phase HPLC with UV, as ATTEMPTED NOVEL ASSAY, h*	*GC-ECD on derivative [3] — REF. METHOD, G (alternative to C)*
Sample preparation	*Acid hydrolysis; Dowex-50; aq. NH₃ → concentrate*	*Charcoal in place of Dowex-50*	*As for C (charcoal also tried)*	*As for C*	*As for C*	*As for C*
Comments (For alternative approaches, see Scheme 1)	*Tolerably reliable but tedious; normal values fall within range expected*	*Seems valid and somewhat more convenient*	*Erratically over-estimates NM and M*	*Fair accord with C; tedious*	*Grossly over-estimates NM and M*	*Erratic accord (±) with C values*

A reasonably straightforward method for estimating the urinary outputs of normetadrenaline (NM) and metadrenaline (M), as indicators of noradrenaline and adrenaline 'status', would be useful in connection with the study of chronic stress (where any elevations might be small) besides pathological conditions where the levels are grossly elevated (as in phaeochromocytomas). Intricacy is a common feature of the diverse methods as published by numerous investigators [e.g. 2, 4, 5], most of whom shun earlier methods and yet do not report side-by-side comparisons. The following comments [6] are apt: "The small amounts of endogenous amines, the many steps in their analysis, the above-average technical skill required, the sensitivity of the fluorophor to environmental changes and the 'mysticism' associated with the procedures result in a methodology that is relatively difficult and temperamental ... Directions must be followed explicitly since what appears to be a minor modification may invalidate the procedures. Many papers do not contain sufficient details ...".

The present goal, which was hardly attained, was to develop an HPLC method for the separation and on-line estimation of NM and M, with a UV detector. It was axiomatic that the urine sample, hydrolyzed to liberate NM and M from conjugates, would have to be concentrated (say × 100) prior to HPLC, preferably or necessarily with concomitant removal of potentially interfering bioconstituents including noradrenaline and adrenaline. The trial of different sample preparation procedures, and the setting up of a reference method, are the main themes of the present article, and may be illuminating to other investigators faced with developing an assay method for basic trace-substances.

MEASUREMENT METHODS USED IN THE METHOD-DEVELOPMENT STUDIES

Fluorimetric determination, as outlined below, was the ultimate yardstick, but did not have to be used in all pilot work. Simpler approaches sufficed to assess recoveries in pilot work with authentic compounds in pure solution, if not with urine; but only the radioisotopic approach was both specific (such that spiked urine could be studied) and sensitive. Pilot work performed with unrealistically high levels of trace substances can give misleadingly good recoveries, since only a relatively small distortion will then result from any absolute loss such as may arise, for example, from tenacious adsorption on to glassware or chromatographic media.   The authentic amines now used were obtained (from Sigma) as hydrochlorides.

Radioisotopic method

For spiking of urine or authentic solutions of unlabelled NM or M, [7-^{3}H]NM and/or [7-^{3}H]M (New England Nuclear) was added in tracer amount. Although the working solutions of the radioisotopes, suitably in 0.1 M acetic, were kept at -20° if to be stored more than a few days, it became apparent late in the investigation that decomposition is a much more serious problem than is evident from the manufacturer's data sheets, and that occasional clean-up by TLC is only a palliative. Storage at liquid nitrogen temperature is advisable [P. Goodwin, personal communication]. A further hazard was adsorption on to the glass wall of dispensing syringes, minimized by silanization.

Determinations of radioactivity were made by liquid scintillation counting, suitably in a mixture containing 'Lissapol' [7].

Absorptiometric methods

NM and M show a good peak at 279 nm both in aqueous solution as cations (E = 0.245 if 0.1 mM, 1 cm light path) and in methanolic solution (E = 0.28). If, a conventional spectrophotometer is used in trials of sample preparation, difficulty may arise if the sample contains less than 10 mg/l. Concentrations of at least this value were employed in some pilot experiments, but confirmatory experiments were done with a more sensitive method at more realistic concentrations, below 1 mg/l.

Better sensitivity, albeit inferior to that of fluorimetric estimation, was obtainable by a colorimetric method devised in the present work as an outcome of having to detect spots on TLC plates. Whereas a 1 µg spot can just be detected by spraying with 4-aminophenazone and ferricyanide [8], 0.05 µg was found to be detectable by use of diazotized *p*-nitroaniline [5,9]. A solution of *p*-nitroaniline (0.63 g) in 5 ml of conc. HCl, diluted to 250 ml with water, serves for colorimetric determination of NM or M after diazotizing 5 ml at 0° with 0.5% NaNO$_2$ and making up to 10 ml. To 3 ml of NM or M in aqueous or methanolic 0.01N HCl, a 0.2 ml of 10% Na$_2$CO$_3$ solution is added to bring the pH to 9, followed by 0.3 ml of the diazo solution. The absorbance is measured at 510 nm without delay. As little as 0.1 µg/ml of NM or M can be estimated, but specificity cannot be expected to match that of fluorimetric assays; the method has been used merely for pure compounds.

Fluorimetric methods

From the large literature on fluorimetric estimation of catecholamines and metadrenalines, it is evident that these two groups of compounds must be pre-separated. Thereafter it is feasible to perform a differential estimation on a mixture of NM and M. Both give (cf. Art. E-3) lutidine fluorigens under suitable conditions at a pH value in the range 5-8, and a mere switch to a more acidic pH may suffice to confine the reaction to M [6, 10], although a switch of oxidizing agent has also been recommended [2]. The diversity of the literature, even in successive papers from a single laboratory, does not surprise us in view of difficulties we encountered in setting up a reliable method. Various agents can cause 'quenching', e.g. mercaptoethanol, or turbidity, e.g. methanol. The risk of 'rogue' samples must be minimized.

With scrupulous attention to sources of contamination such as glassware (routinely cleaned with nitric acid), plasticware, and dust, we have been able to assay NM and M reproducibly at pH 8.0 with a filter fluorimeter (Locarte Instruments Ltd.) by the method of Smith and Weil-Malherbe [11], using iodine as the oxidizing agent. At pH 3.0 with ferricyanide as the oxidizing agent in the presence of zinc sulphate [11], only M reacts; but differential assay has seldom been necessary in the present work, where NM and M were usually pre-separated. With either method as little as 20 ng/ml is measurable, provided that a suitable filter combination is chosen. Alternatively, NM + M and M alone may be estimated at pH 5.0 and 3.0 respectively with periodate as oxidizing agent in either case [6]; but in our hands NM has not reproducibly given as high a fluorescence as M in the pH 5.0 procedure. Other methods have been tried and eventually abandoned after unsuccessful attempts to optimize the conditions: one trouble has been the appearance of a precipitate, evidently associated with the use of zinc sulphate in the case of the catecholamine method of Sandhu and Freed [10] and with the combination cupric acetate-acetic acid-mercaptoethanol in the latest of the Weil-Malherbe methods [2].

TLC as an aid to method development

We do not rule out using TLC as a late step in NM and M assay; but this idea seemed unpropitious at the outset. Only gross elevations in output are claimed [8] to be demonstrable by applying solvent-extracted NM and M to silica gel plates running in an alkaline solvent (R_f's rather low), and spraying *(see above)*. Yet TLC has now proved useful, e.g. for detecting NM or M decomposition products: these run fast and diffusely in our preferred solvent, viz. *n*-butanol:glacial acetic acid: water (4:1:1) as used in a catecholamine assay which entailed fluorimetric estimation [12]. With cellulose [12] in place of silica gel, NM and M run poorly. As mentioned above, a diazo spray [9] is preferable; fluorescence-quenching detection may fail or even mislead. Inexplicably, endogenous or authentic NM and M show higher R_f's ($\sim$0.5 and $\sim$0.4) in the presence of urine-derived material than if pure.

APPROACHES EXPLORED FOR SAMPLE PREPARATION

The setting up of a satisfactory fluorimetry system represented merely one step towards the requisite setting up of a reference method for NM and M in urine. The other main need, applicable also to intended trial of HPLC, was a satisfactory way of preparing the sample, one aim being to remove catecholamines. Whilst the ultimate need for a sequence of sample-preparation steps [2] was not overlooked, the first need was to choose an initial step, hopefully applicable to a urinary hydrolysate notwithstanding the presence of salts and other potentially detrimental constituents. (Hydrolysis conditions are considered in a later Section.)

In pilot work with authentic NM and M, prior to trying urine, there was difficulty in achieving even tolerably good recoveries. As is outlined below, trial was made of two adsorbents, XAD-2 resin and charcoal, that have not hitherto been used in the metadrenaline field. However, most of the exploratory work was guided by published approaches, examples of which are shown in Scheme 1.

Solvent extraction

Solvent extraction is traditionally the preferred approach for isolation of organic compounds for microanalysis [18], at an alkaline pH in the case of basic substances, but is considered by Weil-Malherbe [2] to be of no advantage for catecholamines and their metabolites such as metadrenalines. As the leading advocates of this approach for metadrenalines, Anton and Sayre [6] have devised an elaborate series of solvent extractions, designated '(a)' in Scheme 1. In their hands the overall recoveries are of the order of 50%, with effective removal of the unwanted catecholamines. We have confirmed that, as judged by TLC, their initial extraction with isoamyl alcohol at neutral pH 'cleans up' urinary hydrolysates, with no loss of metadrenalines. Subsequent extraction of the latter with diethyl ether at pH 10, as described [19] by these authors, gave a poor yield when tried by us.

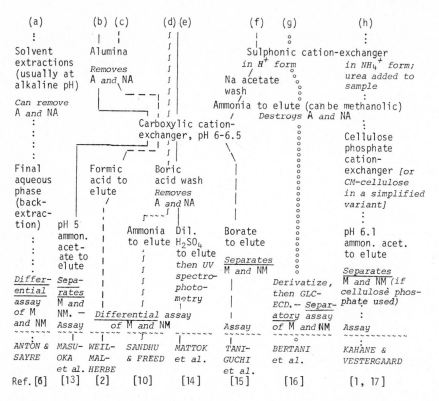

Scheme 1. Some published approaches for the assay of normetadrenaline (NM) and metadrenaline (M) in urinary hydrolysates, usually with fluorimetry for the final measurement. *Noradrenaline* (NA) *and adrenaline* (A) *interference has to be obviated. Other published approaches include Dowex-50 followed by paper chromatography* [9].

Disappointing results have likewise been obtained in our laboratory with other solvent systems, the trial of which (usually with authentic NM and/or M, in aqueous solution) is now summarized.

Ethyl acetate/Na$_2$SO$_4$ (to saturate)/pH 10 borate. - Even after the 4 successive extractions each with 1 vol. of solvent, as in Gutteridge's procedure [8; cf. 5], the amounts of NM and M extracted were only 54% and 55% respectively. Hydrolyzed urine gave poorer results. The published procedure, in which the extracted material is subjected to TLC, does not purport to be quantitative, or to be applicable to normal urine as well as phaeochromocytoma urine; the author does not state the recoveries.

Ethyl acetate/(NH$_4$)$_2$CO$_3$ (to saturate). - Even after 2 extractions each with 1 vol., both NM and M remained almost completely in the aqueous phase. Since the substances reported as extractable by this procedure [20] do not include metadrenalines, the present results do not imply disagreement with other laboratories.

Ethanol (0.1 vol. only)/K$_2$CO$_3$ (to saturate). - This extraction procedure, although reported by Bastos and colleagues [21] to be effective for basic drugs, gave only 20% recovery for NM, whilst somewhat better for M. Recoveries were very poor with a kindred procedure [22], viz. *chloroform : 2-propanol, 4:1 (1 vol. only)/NaHCO$_3$: K$_2$CO$_3$, 3:2 by wt. (to saturate).*

Adsorptive isolation

In the varied literature on assay of metadrenalines [2], there has been surprising
neglect of the possible usefulness of an adsorption-elution step. As shown by (b)
and (c) in Scheme 1, exposure to alumina has been used in several published metadrenaline assays as an initial preparative step; but the purpose has been to free
the metadrenalines from catecholamines by virtue of the propensity of the latter
to adsorb on to alumina because of their vicinal hydroxyl groups: thus it is not a
matter of adsorbing and eluting metadrenalines. Taking this into account, and
literature pointing to capricious behaviour of alumina, we have not tried alumina.
We have done a few experiments with a novel agent, titania (as beads; from AERE
Harwell, courtesy of Dr. A.R. Thomson); on loading at pH 10, even the best medium
(borate) left 30% unadsorbed, and 20% resisted elution with 0.01 M HCl. Whilst
further experiments with titania might have been more rewarding, our study of adsorbents has been virtually confined to two that had not previously been used in
the metadrenaline field, viz. XAD-2 resin and charcoal. Recently [23] the resin
XAD-4, similar in type to XAD-2, has been employed in a purification step for
plasma metadrenaline assay.

Trial of XAD-2 resin

This adsorptive resin of the 'Amberlite' series (Rohm & Haas) is effective for
many trace constituents of biological fluids [18, and this Volume, Art.G-1]. It
has now been tried as a 55 × 9 mm column, washed with methanol; omission of this
wash seemed to impair adsorption. The test solution, usually 10 ml of a solution
of M in 0.05 M potassium formate solution, was adjusted to an alkaline pH and
loaded slowly. Following a wash-through with water, the chosen elution procedure
was applied. (In a recent drug paper, 0.05 M formic acid in 40% methanol was used [24]).

Elution could not be achieved with a 1:1 mixture of methanol and water,
even with HCl added, nor with methanol alone, although NM and M dissolve readily
in these media. Fair success was achieved with a novel eluent, viz. 0.05 M tartaric acid in water (pH ⌐4): the recoveries in different experiments, after adsorption at pH 10, ranged from 43% to 104% for M in high load (⌐100 μg). However,
a single experiment with NM gave only 33%. After adsorption at pH 8 rather than
10, the best recovery of M was 77%. In one experiment where it was as low as 22%,
passage of dioxan brought off a further 60%. Thereafter a 1:1 mixture of aqueous
tartaric acid and dioxan was used as the eluent. (Dioxan must be removed before
fluorimetry, being a suppressor.) Incomplete recoveries seemed to be due to incomplete
adsorption rather than to tenacious retention by the resin. With M at pH 6, the
low final recovery (13%) was attributable to poor adsorption.

In subsequent experiments where the load of M was reduced to 5 μg, about
half of the M was recovered if the pH had been set at 10 in the adsorption step,
and one-third if set at 8. Subsequent trials were done at pH 10, with the risk
that the unionized forms of NM and M that predominate at this pH might deteriorate
during isolation - a risk that was minimized by having 2-mercaptoethanol present
(0.05%). The observed recoveries then ranged from 60% to 100% for M when present
in pure solution (even if only 0.2 μg was loaded) or, in one experiment, in hydrolyzed urine. For NM, half of a 0.2 μg load was recovered.

It was decided not to persevere with optimizing conditions for isolating
NM and M by use of XAD-2, necessarily at pH 10. It had already become evident
that NM and M are less amenable to isolation by XAD-2 than some of the various
compounds studied elsewhere (often with methanol as the eluent), and that the
variability might be difficult to overcome.

Trial of coated charcoal

There have been sporadic reports on sample preparation with the aid of charcoal, as
summarized elsewhere [18] together with an outline of pioneer literature from

Uppsala. Charcoal was advocated for adsorption analysis of amino acids as early as
1941 by Tiselius [24], who cited even earlier studies. An example of selectivity
is that, at acid pH, active charcoal ('Darco G-60') adsorbs pyrimidines (including
orotic acid) but not ureidosuccinic acid [25] or purines [26]; the pyrimidines
could be eluted with a conc. ammonia-ethanol-water mixture (10:25:65 by vol.) [25].
The Uppsala group later showed that, to facilitate elution, the active charcoal
could usefully be pre-treated with a 'saturator' such as n-hexanol. The usefulness
of charcoal thus partially deactivated, by 'coating' with n-octadecylamine [27], is
examplified by the preparation from urine of a concentrate containing hydroxyindoles
[28]; elution was with an acetone-water mixture (1:1). Uncoated charcoal suffices
to give good recoveries for some drugs in urine [29], and has been used in a convenient 'cartridge' form for a range of basic drugs [30]: since with diphenhydramine
the recoveries were variable on eluting with pure methanol, the latter was routinely supplemented with a trace of conc. HCl solution [30]. Charcoal coated with dextran or other macromolecular material has been widely adopted in radioimmunoassay,
but uncoated charcoal is sometimes preferable [31]; this application does not entail
an elution step, and therefore may have little relevance to sample preparation.

    The present study was conducted with charcoal (usually from Merck, 'Charcoal
activated GR', Batch 4123033) which had been boiled 2-3 h with a one-fold dilution of
conc. HCl, and washed with hot water till free from acid and dried at 250°. In a
pilot experiment with uncoated charcoal the recoveries of metadrenalines were so
poor (Table 1) that coated charcoal was used in all further work. The coating procedure [27] usually entailed stirring 15 g of charcoal with 50 ml of 1.5% stearic
acid (or other agent) in ethanol; the suspension was then diluted to 500 ml with
water. The filtered-off charcoal was dried and stored under nitrogen [cf. 24]. Where
paraffin wax was tried as a coating, it was applied as a 1% solution in light
petroleum, followed by washing in turn with ethyl acetate, ethanol and water. All
the experiments of Table 1 were done in a batch rather than a column mode, under
the general conditions stated in the heading.

    When some progress towards optimizing conditions had been made with authen-
tic solutions of NM and M, attention was turned to the endogenous NM and M of
urinary hydrolysates, which were found to need a larger amount of charcoal for
efficient isolation of the NM and M (Table 1). Stearic acid was adopted as coating
agent, being somewhat superior to octadecylamine in respect of final recovery. For
adsorption, pH 8 was adopted, and for elution the best yields were obtained with
acidified methanol (Table 1). With the conditions finally adopted, urinary hydrolysates have routinely given 60-70% recovery of endogenous NM and M as judged by
the recovery of added tracers. As can be inferred from Table 1, the non-recovered
material was largely adsorbed in the first instance, but resisted elution; a repeat of the elution step (not tabulated) was without avail.

    Coated charcoal was found to retain its efficiency for at least 4 months
even when stored in air (in a covered vessel); but the precaution was usually
taken of storing under nitrogen. A suspicion that the adsorptive efficiency of
stored charcoal had deteriorated turned out to be due to decomposition of the [^{3}H]
tracers to furnish non-adsorbable products, as noticed particularly with adrenaline;
but this does not fully account for lower recoveries observed with adrenaline as
compared with NM or M (see example in Table 1). Even where recoveries seemed satisfactory as judged by radioactivity measurements, it could not be taken for granted
that the product was still chemically intact. Examination of dried-down products
by TLC, e.g. with an isopropanol-n-butanol-formic acid-water system [32], has given
reassuring results for NM and M, provided that the solution (or urinary hydrolysate)
subjected to charcoal adsorption had been supplemented with 0.05 vol. of a 2-mercap-
toethanol solution (1% in 20% sodium sulphite). Early literature [cited in 1] bears
out the supposition that charcoal may encourage oxidation of phenolic compounds if
a precaution such as addition of mercaptoethanol is not taken. No such precaution
is needed if Dowex-50 is used instead of charcoal (see below).

Table 1. Trial of coated charcoal for sample preparation. Usually a portion of charcoal, coated as described in the text, was added as a suspension in pH 8.0 bicarbonate buffer to 10 ml of the buffer (0.035M) or of a buffered hydrolysate of urine, to adsorb added or (urine) endogenous metadrenalines. After shaking and standing (10 min), the charcoal was centrifuged off, washed with water, and eluted, usually with 10 ml of eluant. The eluate obtained by centrifugation and filtration was analyzed for NM and/or M by UV absorption, colour formation, or [^{3}H] where, as with urine, tracer had been added initially. *The representative experiments tabulated are more comparable within each group than between groups.*

Variable investigated	Auth (-entics) or urine	Coating agent & mg charcoal if not 10 mg	Adsorption pH	Eluting agent *Proportions are by vol.*	NM+M, or NM/M(adrenaline) individually, % UNADSORBED	ELUTED
Uncoated 'active'	Auth, 200 µg [1]	None 50	10	CHCl$_3$:iPrOH, 5:1 EtOH:conc.NH$_3$, 4:1	<1 <1	1 [2] 20
Coating agent	Auth, 5 µg [3]	Octadecane Octadecylamine Paraffin wax Stearic acid	10	EtOH:conc.NH$_3$, 4:1	<1/<1 <1/<1 <1/<1 <1/<1	43/54 45/40 28/30 50/56
Adsorption pH	Auth, 5 µg	Stearic acid	1 4 6 7-10	MeOH:0.1 M HCl, 9:1	65 25 2 <1	*Elution not tried*
Amount of charcoal	Urine [4]	Stearic acid 10 20 50 100 200 300	8	*ditto*	84/85(87) 84/77(43) 43/28(43) 25/16(24) 10/11(23) 8/10(20)	9/16(7) 13/16(9) 25/57(26) 60/75(31) 53/90(24) 40/92(23)
Coating agent	Urine	Octadecylamine 100 Stearic acid	8	*ditto*	<1 <1	61/68 [5] 76/67
Eluting agent	Urine	Stearic acid 100	8	*ditto* MeOH:conc.NH$_3$, 4:1	*Not determined*	82/84 68/67 [6]
Adsorption pH	Urine	Stearic acid 100	1 8	MeOH:0.1 M HCl, 9:1	96 ± 1 [7] 20 ± 0.5 [7]	*Elution not tried*
Source of charcoal	Urine [8]	Stearic acid 100 *Merck* [9] *Sigma* *Fisons*	8	*ditto*	10 18 11	66 55 58

NOTES:
[1] *Coated charcoal with similar high load gives good eluate recovery.*
[2] *Poor eluate recoveries were also obtained with a range [29] of other solvents.*
[3] *With higher loads in other experiments, different coating agents behaved comparably and stearic acid was of no special advantage.*
[4] *Experiments with other urine samples bore out the desirability of using 100 rather than 10 mg of charcoal for* urine, *and gave better eluate recoveries (footnote* [8] *is relevant). Mercaptoethanol was usually added (see text).*
[5] *Each of the 4 values was the mean of 5-6 results which agreed well.*
[6] *The alkaline eluting agent caused some degradation, as shown by TLC.*
[7] *S.E.M., from 4 observations.*
[8] *Some deterioration of the tracers (see text) may account for the unimpressive eluate recoveries; presumably some counts not due to NM or M escaped elution.*
[9] *In general, the preceding experiments were performed with Merck charcoal. 'Norit A' also worked, but there was difficulty in removing fine particles.*

Besides the foregoing experiments in which charcoal was used in a batch mode for the sake of handling a number of samples simultaneously, other experiments were done with columns (12 × 5 mm approx.) of charcoal (100 mg) admixed with 200 mg of Celite that had been washed with the eluent; before the charcoal-Celite suspension in pH 8 bicarbonate buffer was put in the column, a 3 mm layer of Celite alone was introduced. The mixed suspension was stirred in the column with a rod whilst settling to a bed. The test solution (10 ml) was then applied, and henceforth the flow of liquid was assisted by gentle pressure from a peristaltic pump. Elution of NM and M was effected by methanol:0.1 M HCl (9:1 by vol.), preceded by a water wash and in some experiments by passage of 1 ml of 1% SDS solution. The latter was remarkably effective in removing urinary pigments, even with batch rather than column operation, but was not routinely used because occasionally it led to some premature elution of NM and M. Yet, in a pilot experiment which included the SDS washing step, excellent recoveries of NM (81%) and M (81%) were obtained with the acidic eluent, of which 6 ml sufficed; a further 15% and 8% respectively were accounted for as unadsorbed or readily washed off the charcoal. Another pilot experiment (without SDS), not pursued, pointed to the feasibility of eluting NM and M separately, through use of a longer column of charcoal (20 × 10 mm). An alternative to SDS as a way of removing urinary pigments is an initial treatment with charcoal at pH 1 (the pH of urinary hydrolysates prior to neutralization); only with the subsequent charcoal step at alkaline pH are NM and M adsorbed. However, mere freezing and thawing of the urine initially *(see below)* suffices to remove pigments; moreover, with SDS there may be a complication due to some alteration (complexing ?) of NM or M as revealed by higher R_f's in TLC. A detergent effect is demonstrable in HPLC [33].

In summary, charcoal used in a batch or column mode appears to be a reliable means of isolating NM and M from hydrolyzed urine in fair yield, for subsequent analytical steps which are considered later in this article. Our recommendations concerning conditions include: pre-coating of the charcoal with stearic acid (a step known to facilitate elution in the case of amino acids and peptides; trace-supplementation of the hydrolysate with 2-mercaptoethanol; adsorption of the NM and M at pH 8; and elution with acidified methanol. (An acidic phenol-containing eluent [27] might have been effective, but phenol is hard to remove subsequently and interferes in fluorimetry and colorimetry.) Adrenaline and noradrenaline put through the charcoal procedure seem to be absent from the dried-down eluate, as judged by TLC with colorimetric detection.

Promising though charcoal was, its very novelty for the present application to metadrenalines called for continued study of more orthodox approaches so that a known reference method could be set up.

Isolation by cation-exchange

Whilst the pK values for NM (9.56) and M (9.74) [34] are rather close to allow of facile separation by cation-exchange chromatography, this approach has been a popular means of isolating them conjointly [2]. Some of the ion-exchange procedures shown in Scheme 1 as possible steps (with 'conventional' operation, not HPLC) in assay of NM and M have now been tried out on authentic compounds, usually in high amount (∿50 μg) such that any inadvertent losses due to irreversible adsorption should be relatively small. In the following column-chromatographic experiments, the fractions were normally collected in tubes containing sufficient formic acid to bring the pH to near 1 in the interests of stability.

Trial of a carboxylic cation-exchanger

The assay methods shown as (b)-(f) in Scheme 1 entailed use of a carboxylic resin such as Biorex-70 (BioRad Labs., Bromley); a reported [10] advantage over sulphonic resins is its freedom from fluorogens. A demerit of such resins is temperature-sensitivity [15]; moreover, urinary electrolytes sometimes impair retention of NM

and M [2, 10]. In our hands, Biorex-70 resin gave erratic results both for adrenaline,as eluted (presumably as a complex) by boric acid [10, 13],and for M as eluted
by dilute formic acid [2] or by borate - an eluent which is claimed to separate NM
and M [15]. In the light of our subsequent experiences with charcoal, addition of
2-mercaptoethanol might have been beneficial insofar as the troubles encountered
with Biorex-70 were suggestive of oxidative decomposition, not to be blamed on the
resin.

Trial of a sulphonic cation-exchanger

In early trials of a sulphonic cation-exchanger (Dowex-50), separation of adrenaline
and M was attempted, by elution with borate buffers. At pH 8.7 there was quite
efficient elution of adrenaline, and at pH 10 there was partial elution of M. Less
alkaline pH values might be feasible, as was indicated by trial of pH 6.5 followed
by pH 8.7 ammonium formate buffers (with dioxan present, 35% v/v, in the hope of
minimizing any adsorptive losses).

These trials of Dowex-50 in a chromatographic mode were not, however, pursued.
As is outlined later, the further work with Dowex-50 was guided by methods (b)-(h)
in Scheme 1, and entailed use of short columns, aimed at concentrating up the metadrenalines rather than removing catecholamines chromatographically [17]. — In fact,
batchwise rather than column operation is not precluded [9].

Trial of a cellulose phosphate cation-exchanger

For separation of noradrenaline, NM and related compounds in tissue extracts, Levin
[35] used cellulose phosphate paper with, surprisingly, electrolyte-free eluents. We
have yet to ascertain whether NM and M are separable on such paper, but have been
successful with a cellulose phosphate column procedure, as applied by Kahane & Vestergaard [1] to Dowex-50 concentrates from urinary hydrolysates, i.e. (h) in Scheme 1.

P-11 cellulose phosphate (Whatman/Reeve Angel, Maidstone; Batch 2111795
was used) is put through the recommended pre-treatments [2] and, in the NH_4^+ form, is
made up as a 450 × 6 mm bed, to fill a plastic column (acrylic; Wright Scientific,
Kenley). The solution containing NM and M (corresponding to 25 ml of original urine)
is loaded at pH 6.1 and slowly chromatographed with a gradient of pH 6.1 ammonium acetate buffer. Good yields of M and NM as separate peaks (in that order), suitably
located by scanning for [³H] if tracer addition were made initially, are obtainable
if, and only if, the authors' instructions [1] are meticulously followed. Fluorimetric determinations at pH 8 (*see above;* the authors use a pH 7 method) may then be
made on the individual or pooled 3 ml fractions, the collection of which is best
done with a siphon-operated fraction collector (manufactured by Central Ignition,
London N19 4PX). The usual precaution of keeping the tube contents acidic may be
omitted, the fluorimetry being done with minimum delay.

This cellulose phosphate procedure, preceded by a Dowex-50 step which will
destroy catecholamines, has furnished us with the desired reference method as is
now amplified. Any catecholamines that may escape destruction in the initial Dowex-
50 step would, as judged by a trial run with [³H]adrenaline, elute from cellulose
phosphate well before M. Any urinary pigments that are loaded on to cellulose
phosphate along with NM and M are removed in the wash-through, being unretained.

ADOPTION OF A REFERENCE METHOD

Before success had been achieved with the reference method [1] now to be considered,
a GC-ECD method was sought as an alternative. The method of Bertani *et al.* [16],
i.e. procedure (g) in Scheme 1, did not give satisfactory peaks in our hands, even
with authentic NM or M for the derivatization and with the benefit of written advice
from Dr. L.M. Bertani. Difficulties in preparing the TFA derivatives were overcome,
but NM tended to give multiple peaks and M sometimes gave no peak. Other authors

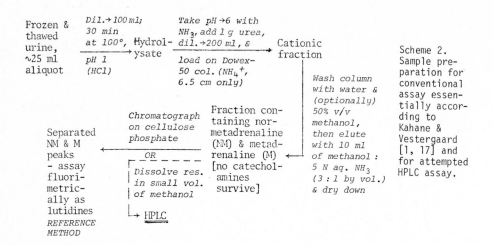

Scheme 2. Sample preparation for conventional assay essentially according to Kahane & Vestergaard [1, 17] and for attempted HPLC assay.

have been content with GC separation of NM and M in admixture. We have, however, had fair success with an attractive GC-ECD method [3] that was described to us in advance of publication and does separate NM and M. As will be shown later, our NM and M values obtained by this method, with an initial Dowex-50 step rather than a solvent extraction procedure as described to us [3], do not tally closely with those obtained by the cellulose phosphate procedure, in which we have confidence. We are, however, not confident that in setting up the unpublished GC method we have been as successful as its originators in optimizing the conditions.

    We have, then, adopted the tedious but fairly reliable assay method that hinges on cellulose phosphate chromatography [1], with minor variants that will be outlined. A possible variant which is too wide a departure from the published method to be adopted for reference purposes is the use of coated charcoal (with mercaptoethanol present; *see above*) in place of Dowex-50; insofar as it has been validated *(see below)*, it does offer promise of being trustworthy. The following scrutiny and amplification deals in turn with each step in our reference method, an outline of which is set down in Scheme 2.

Storage and hydrolysis of the urine

Any diurnal variation in NM or M output [8, 15] is probably outweighed by large day-to-day variations between and within individuals [15]. Yet it is a sensible precaution to use 24-h collections wherever possible, with initial addition of 5 N HCl (say 10 ml) to the storage vessel to obviate deterioration. On thawing urines that had been stored at -20°, we observed a pigmented sediment. Its removal (by centrifugation) entails no loss of NM or M, and gives cleaner extracts as can be shown by TLC, possibly with some gain in the reliability of the fluorimetric estimations. We recommend, therefore, that even fresh urines be frozen and thawed, and the sediment removed.

    Only exceptionally [2, 8] has an enzymic method been used, with [11] or without prior acid hydrolysis, for hydrolysis of metadrenaline conjugates, these being mainly sulphates in the human. The enzymic approach may call for prior removal of inhibitory anions from the urine and may have other disadvantages [2] which seem to surpass possible disadvantages of acid hydrolysis [18]. Accordingly, a conventional acid hydrolysis (Scheme 2) has been adopted in the present work, with the stipulated [17] 4-fold dilution of the sample. The evidence from earlier studies [11, 15] that there is quite adequate survival of NM has now been reinforced by 'hydrolyzing' pure NM and then estimating it fluorimetrically or colorimetrically. In an experiment where [³H]M was isolated from urine with or without the hydrolysis step, the recoveries were 68% and 88% respectively.

Dowex-50

For the concentration/desalting step (Scheme 2) the resin was Dowex X2 50-W, 100-200 mesh (batch 8OC 1240; bought from Sigma, London, in the hydrogen form), prewashed and freed from fines on a bulk scale [15]. We feel it unsafe to salvage and re-cycle the resin (or the cellulose phosphate) after use for a urine sample. The resin column, of width only 9 mm if for a normal-size urine aliquot (25 ml), is converted *in situ* to the NH_4^+ form which, when the neutralized hydrolysate is loaded, resists conversion to the Na^+ form provided that the neutralization has been done with ammonium rather than sodium hydroxide [17]. This neutralization is coupled with a further dilution, and with addition of urea in the interests of good recovery from the resin [17].

In several respects the procedure [17] departs from the earlier procedure [15; denoted as (f) in Scheme 1] on which it is based, and which employed a long resin column in the H^+ form. With the NH_4^+ form, amino acids are not retained, whereas the H^+ form retains amino acids which may then be brought off with 0.1 M sodium acetate [15] - a procedure which Kahane & Vestergaard [17] found to entail the risk of some premature elution of metadrenalines, as we have confirmed. Whereas these authors eluted the NM and M with 5 M aqueous ammonia, and then took care to dry down only partially (in a vacuum desiccator over H_2SO_4), we favour the variants indicated in Scheme 2, for the sake of rendering the sample suitable for attempted HPLC analysis *(see later)* as well as for continuation through to fluorimetric analysis. An aqueous methanol wash removes some UV-absorbing material that could interfere with HPLC. The ammoniacal elution is done with a methanolic medium, to facilitate complete drying down.

A measure of the recovery of endogenous NM and M from urine, after hydrolysis and Dowex-50 treatment, is obtainable by [³H] measurements to ascertain the recovery of the tracers added initially. In 10 experiments with urine, the average recovery (with S.E.M.) was 61±6%, which we regard as acceptable although lower than claimed [17].

Radioactivity measurements do not themselves guarantee that the compounds have remained chemically intact. More rigorous checking has indicated that neither the exposure to ammonia nor, contrary to an expressed warning [17], the *complete* drying down have much adverse effect on NM or M. In one of the TLC experiments performed to check this, the NM and M were exposed to the further 'insult' of a 5-week storage period in acid solution at 4°. The results (Table 2) showed an acceptable recovery of [³H]NM and [³H]M in the expected TLC positions. Moreover, the chromatographic pattern with cellulose phosphate is normal even where there has been several months' storage of the dried-down Dowex-50 eluate (kept desiccated under N_2 with exclusion of light) — such storage being a convenient analytical stratagem to which the Dowex-50 step lends itself. We have verified by TLC (with the diazo spray) that adrenaline, as a representative catecholamine, does not survive the ammoniacal elution step [15, 17].

Cellulose phosphate step and final fluorimetry

If the published description [1] of the preparation and use of the cellulose phosphate is followed meticulously, the NM and M are obtainable in good yield as discrete peaks, each occupying no more than 6 ml of eluate. The fluorimetric estimations may be performed on the contents of individual tubes or on a pool based on the distribution of [³H] counts. Whilst it may be valid to rely on independent standards made up in ammonium acetate eluting buffer, not put through the column, the

Table 2. Survival tests with authentic NM and M, in relation to handling/storage of the material isolated from urinary hydrolysates by use of Dowex-50. An 0.1 M acetic acid solution of NM or M (as hydrochloride; 15 µg, in 0.3 ml) with a tracer amount of the [³H] compound was taken for each test, with duplicates throughout. For Dowex-50 conditions, see Scheme 2. Evaporations were done over a desiccant *in vacuo* at room temperature [17]. Immediately prior to TLC examination (with the butanol-acetic system) the test solutions were dried down, and the residue taken up in methanol for loading. From the position on the TLC plate corresponding to NM or M, the separated material was eluted by methanol and counted.
For the NM and M run as the controls, without prior exposure to ammonia, there was good recovery (near 90%) recovery of the counts in the expected positions. It was not the purpose of the experiment to check survival in the dry state rather than in solution.

Whether put through Dowex-50	Whether in 5 M aq. NH₃ as (mock) eluate	Whether dried down fully	Form in which stored at 4° for 5 weeks	Recovery of counts, as % of counts in control spot	
				NM	M
No	Yes (finally)	Yes (then TLC immediately)	As stock soln., *prior* to foregoing	118	83
No	Yes	Yes	In 4 N formic acid	-	102
Yes	Yes	No (partial, to remove NH₃)	In 4 N formic acid	110	74

spiking of aliquots of the actual NM- and M-containing fractions with standard is our preferred approach to ensure a 'fluorigenic environment' identical with that of the NM and M derived from the urine. We do in fact find that in the presence of the ammonium acetate eluting buffer the fluorimetric reading for NM at pH 8 is barely one-fifth that of M, whereas in the absence of this buffer it is nearly one-half. The latter difference could reflect the choice of filters, this choice needing careful investigation which, as is evident from the literature, will not lead to a general solution applicable to any fluorimeter in any laboratory.— Each laboratory must optimize, and recognize two constraints: over-enthusiastic 'mono-chromation' of the incident beam can make a satisfactory output signal unachievable, and inadvertent heating of the sample can cause disastrous signal fading. Notwithstanding the low signal given by NM under our conditions, reliability is good. The values obtained for normal urine are of the order of 0.25 mg of NM and 0.15 mg of M for 24 h, and fall within the wide range of reported values [4].

POSSIBLE APPLICABILITY OF HPLC

All HPLC runs were done at room temperature, with degassed solutions. The availability of HPLC apparatus capable of mixing 'eluent B' into 'eluent A' for gradient elution (Varian, Model 4200) was a boon in the methodological explorations with urinary material. However, trials with authentic material were usually done isocratically to save the delay after each run due to the requisite 'purging' with pure 'B' and re-equilibration with 'A' — this re-equilibration being especially important with ion-exchange packings. The purging step (say 20 min) turned out to be especially important in the reverse-phase studies, as an unexplained insurance against 'rogue' chromatograms. Such purging may also give sharper ion-exchange peaks.

A 50 mm pre-column was always incorporated in the assembly where urinary material was to be run. The UV detector (Cecil Instruments, Cambridge) had a home-made 15 µl cell, and was usually set at 279 nm. Since the mode of HPLC operation was constant-flow rather than constant-pressure, the chart records of absorbance allowed of peak-area measurements, which gave better quantitation than peak-height measurements.

Sample preparation

The need to treat the urinary hydrolysate so as to obtain a salt-free concentrate
containing NM and M was usually met by application of the above-mentioned Dowex-50
procedure as outlined in Scheme 2. When aliquots (5-10 μl) were to be applied to
HPLC columns, the residue from the dried-down eluate was dissolved in methanol
(usually 0.4 ml), rejecting any insoluble material such as was often present if the
urine had not been frozen and thawed so as to throw pigmented material out of solution initially. The methanolic concentrates could be stored for at least a few
days at 4° without risk to NM or M, although storage in dry form *(see above)* seems
safer. Injection was by syringe (septum-less stopped-flow); a loop is under trial.

   In anticipation of discussion *(below)* of problems due to unwanted UV-absorbing material in Dowex-50 concentrates subjected to ion-exchange HPLC, attempted
remedies are now mentioned. None in fact led to NM and M peaks free from contaminants.
(a) Washing of the Dowex-50 column with aqueous methanol prior to elution (Scheme 2)
reduced the need for a similar wash in the HPLC run.
(b) Passage of the Dowex-50 product through an anion-exchanger, Dowex-1, is inno-
cuous (90% recovery of [³H]NM/M) and may even effect a modest reduction in the contamination of the HPLC peaks.
(c) Charcoal adsorption (with precautionary addition of mercaptoethanol), as recently applied (with uncoated charcoal) in the HPLC analysis of serum for anticonvulsants [36], appeared acceptable as an alternative, or preamble, to the Dowex-50
procedure for HPLC sample preparation, but does not give purer peaks.
(d) Initial washing of the urine with *n*-heptane was of no advantage.

Trials with various HPLC packings

Certain adsorptive packings and a pellicular cation-exchanger were tried and abandoned because of failure to obtain NM and M as separate peaks or even as a single
sharp peak, as has been summarized elsewhere [37]. A 'Micropak-CH' reverse-phase
packing did allow of separation, with an iso-propanol : water system; but before
it could be tried on a urinary concentrate it underwent deterioration such as has
also been encountered with two other types of packing.

   Two types of bonded-phase porous packing, both microparticulate (10 μm),
proved sufficiently promising to warrant thorough efforts to optimize conditions,
as outlined below and more fully described elsewhere [37]. Both, however, were
short-lived even when, on switching to replacements, better preservation was
sought by extra precautions such as minimizing the alkalinity of the eluents and
storing the columns with some organic solvent (methanol or acetonitrile) present.
As a prophylactic against microbial attack, cation-exchange media were supplemented with sodium azide (to 0.05%) in the later experiments.

Cation-exchange separations

Success in separating NM and M by cation-exchange was achieved when Partisil-SCX
(Whatman/Reeve Angel) came on the market, available only as pre-packed columns (a
policy recently relaxed). Fig. 1 shows that pH 5.5 is suitable; with slight alkalinity there was an inexplicable lengthening of retention time and a worsening of
'tailing'. Subsequent gradient runs, with formate replacing citrate in the interests of forestalling microbial growth, have indicated that with urinary concentrates, in place of authentic compounds, the use of a pH even 2 units below or
above 5.5 may aggravate the problem of swamping of the NM and M by other UV-absorbing bioconstituents. This problem has not been overcome by a stratagem that has
been devised to flush out irrelevant UV-absorbing material which otherwise results
in uninterpretable patterns in the NM-M region. This stratagem, as shown in Fig.2,
consists of initial passage of water with a small admixture of methanol.

The positions shown in Fig. 2 for NM and M have been established partly by ascertaining where increments in UV absorption occur if a sample is spiked with NM and M and re-run. Since, however, retention times show some variability, confirmatory evidence has been obtained, without re-running, by a more direct approach that entails adding tracer amounts of labelled NM and M before loading, and collecting HPLC fractions for off-line [^{3}H] measurement. In such runs, the NM and M peaks have accounted for at least 80% of the [^{3}H] applied to the column.

At first sight, Fig. 2 implies successful flushing out of irrelevant material and isolation of NM and M as clean peaks. This is illusory since, as is shown later, UV quantitation gives grossly excessive values for 'NM' and 'M'. Trial runs have been performed [37; cf. Fig. 1] with a range of cationic UV-absorbing substances known to be present in urine. Taking account of their known daily outputs in urine [38], only two qualify as possible contaminants: tyramine — which arises by the action of intestinal bacteria [39] — runs close to NM (sometimes slightly slower, and sometimes slightly faster), and 3-methoxytyramine almost coincides with M. Serotonin likewise runs with M, but would not have survived the initial acid hydrolysis [11]. Octopamine may be present in a small peak that occurs much earlier than NM [37], and in the run of Fig. 2 it was deliberately added as a useful marker and internal standard; its daily output [40] is low compared with that of metadrenalines. Unidentified amines, evidently not amphoteric since Dowex-1 fails to remove them, presumably account for the broad peaks which follow 'M' in Fig. 2 and, in part, for the 'NM' and 'M' peaks. As is amplified later, they do not respond in the fluorimetric assay for NM and M. The pattern does show some variations from one urine to another.

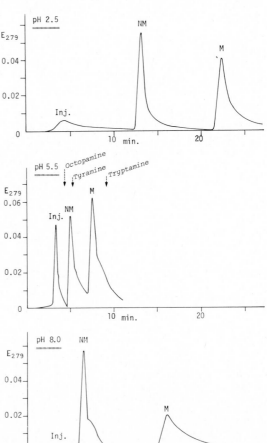

Fig. 1. Isocratic HPLC method trial with authentic normetadrenaline (NM) and metadrenaline (M), each 5 μg, on PARTISIL-SCX (250 × 4.6 mm column). The eluent was 0.2 M sodium citrate buffer, at a flow rate of 50 ml/h. *The positions of certain other authentic compounds are also shown for the favoured pH (5.5). The influence of pH on the separation behaviour in this trial was hardly in accordance with expectation.*

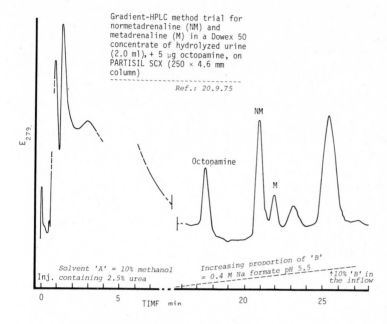

Gradient-HPLC method trial for
normetadrenaline (NM) and
metadrenaline (M) in a Dowex 50
concentrate of hydrolyzed urine
(2.0 ml), + 5 µg octopamine, on
PARTISIL SCX (250 × 4.6 mm
column)

Ref.: 20.9.75

Solvent 'A' = 10% methanol
Inj. containing 2.5% urea

Increasing proportion of 'B'
= 0.4 M Na formate pH 5.5
↑10% 'B' in the inflow

Fig. 2.
Illustrative
run with a
'cationic
concentrate'
from normal
urine, using
a micro-
particulate
cation-
exchange HPLC
packing.
Flow rate:
1 ml/min.
*Results obtain-
able with a
shallower gra-
dient [37; col-
umn erroneously
stated to be
only 2.2 mm i.d.]
are outlined in
the text. The
possible helpful-
ness of urea in
minimizing adsorp-
tion [17] is un-
proved, as is the
benefit of using
20% methanol for
the flush-out;
'B' may induce pre-
cipitation of urea
in the cell ! 'HS'
Pellionex was
used in the pre-
column ('HC' was
too retentive)
since loose Par-
tisil was still
unobtainable.*

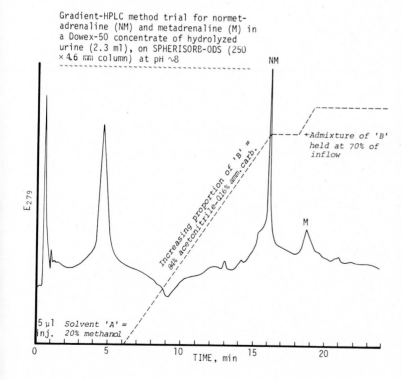

Gradient-HPLC method trial for normetadrenaline (NM) and metadrenaline (M) in
a Dowex-50 concentrate of hydrolyzed
urine (2.3 ml), on SPHERISORB-ODS (250
× 4.6 mm column) at pH ∼8

Increasing proportion of 'B' =
94% acetonitrile-0.16% amm. carb.

←Admixture of 'B'
held at 70% of
inflow

5 µl   Solvent 'A' =
inj.   20% methanol

Fig. 3.
Illustrative
run, as above
but with a
reverse-phase
packing (10 µm).
*The % values
signify ml per
100 ml of mix-
ture, the other
constituent
being water.
The pre-column
contained the
same packing
as the main
column.*

The gradient in Fig. 2, albeit shallow, was steeper than in earlier runs, for the sake of reducing the long running time. A gradient of only half the steepness was of some benefit in splitting up the crude 'NM' and 'M' peaks [37]: NM was then present in a spike which appeared on the descending portion of the peak, and M was present in the second of two peaks which seemingly corresponded to the single 'M' peak of Fig. 2. Whilst the 'NM' and 'M' values were lower than with the steeper gradient, they were 2-4 times higher than those established by the reference method.

It is conceivable that use of a longer column and of isocratic elution (following the mandatory 'flush-out' with 'A') might have split off NM and M as homogeneous peaks, so small as to be only just measurable. This time-consuming mode of operation has not been tried out with urinary extracts, nor has much effort been devoted to possible variations such as measuring at a wavelength other than 279 nm, although one experiment did point to some gain in selectivity by working at 260 nm. (At 250 nm or lower, the formic acid in the eluent would have interfered.) Discouragement became acute when the column was found to have lost resolution and even retentive power, evidently due to bleeding of the bonded phase. With a replacement column which was used only for several runs with authentic compounds, never above pH 7.5, there was similar but faster deterioration. Meanwhile, our efforts had been largely switched to an ODS reverse-phase packing that had just come on the market.

Reverse-phase (ODS) separations

Encouraging results were obtained on trying 'Spherisorb-ODS' (PhaseSep), a bead preparation which was dry-packed. For 'flushing out' irrelevant UV-absorbing material from urinary extracts, aqueous methanol ('eluent A') was again helpful. For separation of authentic NM and M, an aqueous acetonitrile system, containing ammonium carbonate proved to be effective ('eluent B'). Fig. 3 shows a gradient run in which urine-derived peaks containing NM and M were brought off by an isocratic step with a 70 : 30 mixture of 'B' and 'A'. Such peaks were, however, excessively large, giving 'NM' and 'M' values of the order of 10 times the true values. Little improvement resulted from performing the isocratic step with a weaker mixture, 35 : 65, as illustrated elsewhere [37], although this modification resolved the metadrenaline region into multiple peaks of which the first contained NM and the last contained M. Other modifications such as a Dowex-1 step in the sample preparation were of no help, nor did trial of authentic cationic bioconstituents give firm clues as to the identity of the interfering material in the 'NM' peak (some octopamine present ?) and the 'M' peak [37]. Only with a rich mixture, say 70 : 30, are 3-methoxytyramine and tryptamine readily eluted, well clear of M; either could serve as an internal standard.

Like the Micropak and Partisil columns, the Spherisorb column developed symptoms of severe deterioration. A fresh column deteriorated very quickly although used (only for authentic compounds) with the ammonium carbonate omitted from eluent 'B' or else replaced by ammonium bicarbonate. The latter additive seemed to give the worst of both worlds: it was still detrimental to the packing, presumably because of its slight alkalinity, and yet did not give individual peaks, adequately sharp, for NM and M. To get tolerably good peaks, with a low baseline, it seems obligatory to use ammonium carbonate[*], and to purge with neat 'B' at the end of each run. For column storage, if not in 'A', salt-free 'B' is desirable.

With Spherisorb in good condition, the separation conditions now developed for NM and M are sufficently efficacious to argue against the generalization [41] that Spherisorb-ODS is inefficient for separating organic bases. The trouble lies in the evident heterogeneity of our urinary extracts, besides the tendency of the -ODS to strip off (even at near-neutral pH) in spite of its linkage to the silica base by C-Si rather than C-O-Si bonds. (Partisil-SCX likewise has C-Si bonds.)

---

[*]*This reduced tailing (adsorption on unreacted silanol groups?) of indoles on C_{18} at pH $\gg 7$ [46].*

COMPARISON OF POSSIBLE APPROACHES

The strategy of the investigation, and the tactical successes and set-backs, are now recapitulated.

(a) A fluorimetric method had to be chosen for the end-measurement in the trial of possible reference methods. The choice fell on an early method which its originator had subsequently abandoned in favour of an 'improved' method [2] — an outcome which, in the context of the enormous literature on the fluorimetry of metadrenalines, speaks for itself.

(b) A separate but interrelated problem was the choice of an approach for preparing the samples, with a view in the first instance to fluorimetric assay of the NM and M once separated from interfering bioconstituents and possibly from each other. Cellulose phosphate chromatography [1] proved effective in isolating NM and M, as separate fractions, subject to prior work-up which hinged on a cation-exchange concentrating/desalting step [17] applied to the urinary hydrolysate (Scheme 2). Other multi-step approaches to sample preparation (Scheme 1), including solvent extraction, were tried or at least considered and, except for GC, were rejected for various reasons.

(c) 'Coated' charcoal appeared promising as an alternative way of concentrating/desalting, novel in the present context.

(d) The investigation of (b) and (c), initially with authentic NM and M rather than urine, was aided by TLC, by a colorimetric method (less sensitive and specific than fluorimetry), and by the availability of [^{3}H]-labelled NM and M which continued to be of help when urine came to be assayed. A freezing step turned out to be helpful for removing unwanted pigmented material from the urine.

(e) Efforts to set up a GC reference method (not novel) met with partial success *(see below)*.

(f) With a microparticulate cation-exchanger, the NM and (if not 'lost') the M in urinary concentrates were separable by HPLC, but so impure that gross over-estimates were obtained by on-line UV estimations although not by off-line fluorimetric estimations done to check the method *(see below)*.

(g) With a reverse-phase (-ODS) packing, NM and M separated by HPLC were hopelessly impure. In this and other work with bonded-phase packings, disastrous bleeding has occurred sooner or later.

Fig. 4 documents the conclusion that the values obtained for 'NM' and 'M' in normal urine by the above HPLC methods, viz. (f) (denoted H in the Figure) and (g) (denoted h), are hopelessly high compared with those obtained by the cellulose phosphate reference method (denoted C). Where an H plot exists for NM but not for M, the reason is inexplicable loss of M such as occasionally happens in various types of manipulation, suggestive of lability greater than that of NM; in any future HPLC work, it may be advantageous to supplement the eluents with 2-mercaptoethanol. Usually, however, NM and M show 'concordant disagreement' in the method comparisons of Fig. 4.

The fair agreement between the reference values and those obtained through cation-exchange HPLC by off-line fluorimetry (denoted H'), the latter measurement method being unresponsive to tyramine or 3-methoxytyramine, accords with the guess that these bioconstituents are contaminants of the 'NM' and 'M' peaks respectively. The wide range of possible contaminants so far investigated [37] has not included *N*-acetylhistamine [39] or *N,N*-dimethyltryptamine [38].

As is also evident from Fig. 4, use of the 'charcoal variant' (denoted C') of the reference method did not entail any systematic error with normal urines, and gave low but conceivably true values for two phaeochromocytoma urines. The GC method (denoted G), in our hands, showed erratic disagreement with the reference method C, with low values for the phaeochromocytomas; our GC conditions are, however, not ideal in that the NM and M peaks tend to be superimposed on a descending but still high baseline.

CONCLUDING COMMENTS

The present investigation of methods hardly lends encouragement to anyone who seeks to set up an HPLC method for an amine present in urine at a concentration of the order of 100 µg/l (including conjugates). However, some improvement may be possible

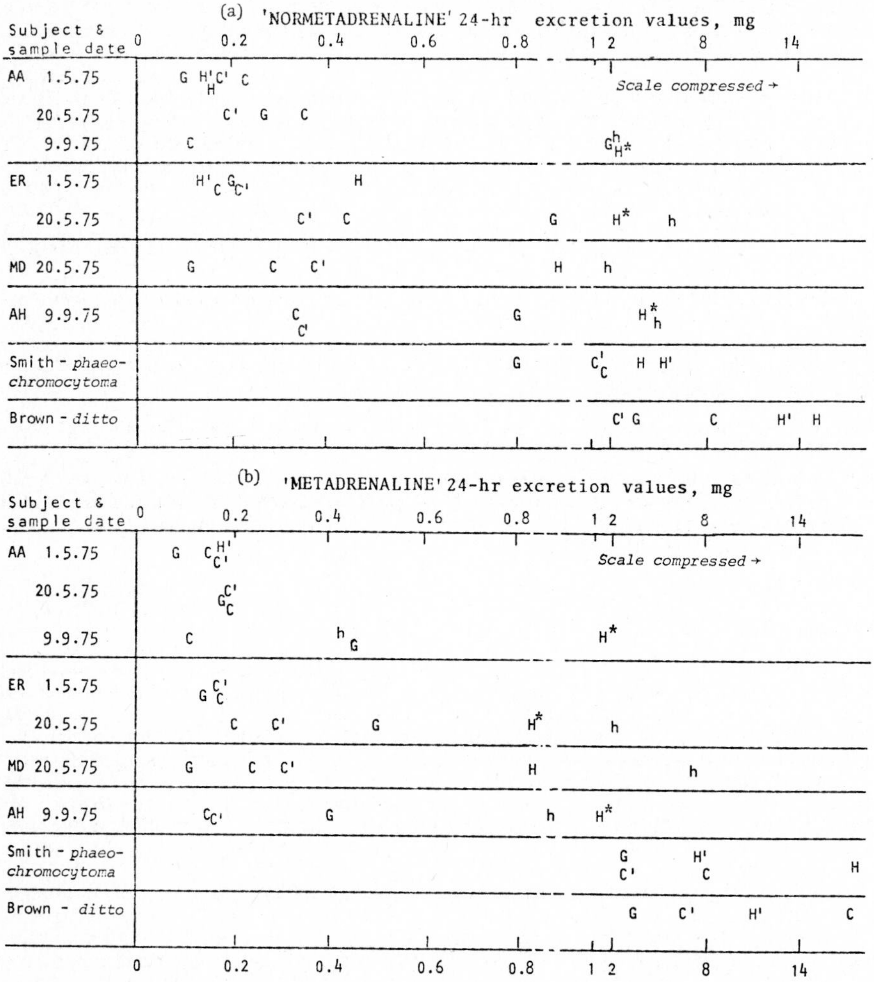

(a) 'NORMETADRENALINE' 24-hr excretion values, mg

Subject & sample date	0	0.2	0.4	0.6	0.8	1 2	8	14
AA 1.5.75		G H'C' C H					*Scale compressed →*	
20.5.75		C' G C						
9.9.75		C				G^h_H*		
ER 1.5.75		H'_C G_{C'}		H				
20.5.75			C' C			G	H* h	
MD 20.5.75		G	C C'			H h		
AH 9.9.75			C C'		G		H* h	
Smith - *phaeo-chromocytoma*						G	C'_C H H'	
Brown - *ditto*							C' G C	H' H

(b) 'METADRENALINE' 24-hr excretion values, mg

Subject & sample date	0	0.2	0.4	0.6	0.8	1 2	8	14
AA 1.5.75		G C_{C'}H'					*Scale compressed →*	
20.5.75		G_CC'						
9.9.75		C	h G			H*		
ER 1.5.75		G_CC'						
20.5.75		C C'	G		H*	h		
MD 20.5.75		G	C C'			H	h	
AH 9.9.75		C_{C'}	G		h	H*		
Smith - *phaeo-chromocytoma*						G C'	H' C	H
Brown - *ditto*						G	C' H'	C

| | 0 | 0.2 | 0.4 | 0.6 | 0.8 | 1 2 | 8 | 14 |

Key to methods:

C = Dowex/cellulose phos./fluorimetry   H = Dowex/ion-exch. HPLC, on-line UV (*= *steep gradient*)
C'= Charcoal/   "   /   "   H' = " /   "   " /fluorimetry
G = Dowex/GC-ECD   h =   " /reverse-phase HPLC, on-line UV

Fig. 4. Comparison of different methods, including the reference method (C), for assay of NM and M in urine. *The mean C values for the normal urines are 0.27 and 0.17.*

in our 'best' although still inadequate cation-exchange HPLC conditions, as applied to urinary 'cationic concentrates' which could be of help as starting material in other analytical connections. It is unfortunate that only sulphonic-type cation-exchange HPLC packings are at present commercially available; one wonders if an exchanger with carboxyl or phosphate groups might give cleaner metadrenaline peaks.

Knox's group have reported [33] a promising reverse-phase approach where a detergent facilitates metadrenaline separation, perhaps by a mechanism related to the ion-pair approaches which Schill describes earlier in this Volume and which could render metadrenalines easier to solvent-extract. A perchlorate-containing system has already proved efficacious in separating authentic metadrenalines by ion-pair HPLC [42].

The metadrenalines in 'NM' and 'M' peaks emerging from an HPLC column might be specifically measurable, if not too impure, by use of a polarographic in place of a UV detector [43]. On-line fluorimetry is precluded because of the reaction sequence needed to form lutidines for the fluorimetry.

Even the 'established' non-HPLC methods now selected have entailed performing exploratory studies, and overcoming troubles. This article may, then, help others who seek to establish, for organic bases, an assay method which inescapably involves sample preparation aimed at getting a concentrate with partial purification. Those blessed with access to MS will not find MS to be an easy short-cut for metadrenalines [44, 45].

Acknowledgements
The work was supported by the Medical Research Council. Skilled and enthusiastic help was given by Dr. A.D.R. Harrison (who did the GC work, and has made many useful suggestions), Miss B.E. Brockway, Mrs. M.T. Goodall, Mr. R.J. Merritt, and Mrs. H. Spencer. Prof. M. Sandler and colleagues kindly described their GC method and provided phaeochromocytoma urines. Prof. J.H. Knox and colleagues gave valuable guidance (to J.P.L.) on the practice of HPLC at the outset of the work. The suppliers of HPLC packings have been helpful in connection with stability problems. Acknowledgement is made to the Ministry of Higher Education of the Republic of Iraq for a Research Studentship held by the first author.

References

1. Kahane, Z. & Vestergaard, P., *Clin. Chim. Acta 25* (1969) 453-458.

2. Weil-Malherbe, H., in *Methods of Biochemical Analysis,* Supplemental Vol.: *Analysis of Biogenic Amines and Their Related Enzymes* (Glick, D., ed.), Interscience, New York (1971) pp. 119-152.

3. Bubb, F.A., Weg, M.W. & Sandler, M., *unpublished experiments (personal communication).*

4. Loraine, J. A. and Bell, E.T., *Hormone Assays and their Clinical Application,* 3rd edn., Livingstone, Edinburgh (1971) pp. 266 & 281.

5. Kopin, I.J., in *The Thyroid and Biogenic Amines* (Rall, J.E. & Kopin, I.J., eds.) [Vol. 1 of *Methods in Investigative and Diagnostic Endocrinology* (Berson, S.A., ed.)], North-Holland, Amsterdam (1972) pp. 489-496.

6. Anton, A.H. & Sayre, D.F., as for ref. 5, pp. 398-436. *(See also ref. 19.)*

7. Wood, P., English, J., Chakraborty, J. & Hinton, R., *Lab. Pract. 24* (1975) 739-740.

8. Gutteridge, J.M.C., *Clin. Chim. Acta 21* (1968) 211-216. *(See also, for TLC, ref. 32.)*

9. Stott, A.W. & Robinson, R., *J. Clin. Path. 19* (1966) 487-490.

10. Sandhu, R.S. & Freed, R.M., *Stand. Meths. Clin. Chem. 7* (1972) 231-245.

11. Smith, E.R.B. & Weil-Malherbe, H., *J. Lab. Clin. Med. 60* (1962) 212-223.

12. Takahashi, S. & Gjessing, L.R., *Clin. Chim. Acta 36* (1972) 369-378.

13. Masuoka, D.T., Drell, W., Schott, H.F., Alcaraz. A.F. & James, E.C., *Anal. Biochem. 5* (1963) 426-432.

14. Mattok, G.L., Wilson, D.L. & Heacock, R.A., *Clin. Chim.Acta 14* (1966) 99-107.

15. Taniguchi, K., Kakimoto, Y. & Armstrong, M.D., *J. Lab. Clin. Med. 64* (1964) 469-484.

16. Bertani, L.M., Dziedzic, S.W., Clarke, D.D. & Gitlow, S.E., *Clin. Chim. Acta 30* (1970) 227-233.

17. Kahane, Z. & Vestergaard, P., *J. Lab. Clin. Med. 70* (1967) 333-342.

18. Reid, E., *Analyst 101* (1976) 1-18.

19. Anton, A.H. & Sayre, D.F., *J. Pharm. Exp. Ther. 153* (1966) 15-29.

20. Horning, M.G., Gregory, P., Nowlin, J., Stafford, M., Lertratanangkoon, K., Butler, C., Stilwell, W.G. & Hill, R.M., *Clin. Chem. 20* (1974) 282-287.

21. Bastos, M.L., Kananen, G.E., Young, R.M., Monforte, J.R. & Sunshine, I., *Clin. Chem. 16* (1970) 931-940.

22. Aggarwal, V., Bath, R. & Sunshine, I., *Clin. Chem. 20* (1974) 307-309.

23. Wang, M.-T., Yoshioka, M., Imai, K. & Tamura, Z., *Clin. Chim.Acta 63* (1975) 21-27.

24. Tiselius, A., *Arkiv Kemi, Mineral., Geol. 15B Pt. 6* (1941) pp. 1-5.

25. Wu, R. & Wilson, D.W., *J. Biol. Chem. 223* (1956) 195-205.

26. Heinrich, M.R. & Wilson, D.W., *J. Biol. Chem. 186* (1950) 186.

27. Asatoor, A. & Dalgliesh, C.E., *J. Chem. Soc.* (1956) 2291-2298.

28. King, L.J., Parke, D.V. & Williams, R.T., *Biochem. J. 98* (1966) 266-277.

29. Meola, J.M. & Vanko, M., *Clin. Chem. 20* (1974) 184-187.

30. Hindmarsh, K.W., Hamon, N.W. & LeGatt, D.F. *Clin. Chem. 21* (1975) 1852-1853.

31. Binoux, M.A. & Odell, W.D., *J. Clin. Endocr. Metab. 36* (1973) 303-310.

32. Passon, P.G. & Peuler, J.D., *Anal. Biochem. 51* (1973) 618

33. Jurand, J., in *High Pressure Liquid Chromatography in Clinical Chemistry* (Dixon, P.F., Gray, C.H., Lim, C.K. & Stoll, M.S., eds.), Academic Press, London (1976) 125-130.

34. Kappe, T. & Armstrong, M.D., *J. Med. Chem. 8* (1965) 368-374.

35. Levin, J.A., *Anal. Biochem. 51* (1973) 42-60.

36. Adams, R.F. & Vandemark, F.L., *Clin. Chem. 22* (1976) 25-31.

37. Leppard, J.P., Harrison, A.D.R. & Reid, E., *as for* ref. 33. 131-141.

38. Diem, K. & Lentner, C. (eds.), *Scientific Tables,* 7th edn., Geigy, Basle (1970) pp. 668-670.

39. Perry, T.L., Hestrin, M., MacDougall, L & Hansen, S., *Clin. Chim. Acta 14* (1966) 116-123.

40. Manghani, K.K., Lunzer, M.R., Billing, B.H. & Sherlock, S., *Lancet ii* (1975) 943-946.

41. Twitchett, P.J. & Moffat, A.C., *J. Chromatog. 111* (1975) 149-157.

42. Persson, B.-A. & Karger, B.L., *J. Chromat. Sci. 12* (1974) 521-528.

43. Kissinger, P.T., Felice, L.J., Riggin, R.M., Pachia, L.A. & Wenke, D.C., *Clin. Chem. 20* (1974) 992-995.

44. Miyazaki, H., Hashimoto, Y., Iwanaga, M. & Kubodera, T., *J. Chromatog. 99* (1974) 575-586.

45. Durden, D.A., Davis, B.A. & Boulton, A.A., *Biomed. Mass Spect. 1* (1974) 83-95.

46. Graffeo, A.P. & Karger, B.L., *Clin. Chem. 22* (1976) 184-187.

T-3 ASSAY OF METHAQUALONE IN BLOOD

Stanley S. Brown
Division of Clinical Chemistry
Clinical Research Centre
Watford Road, Harrow, Middlesex HA1 3UJ, U.K.

Requirement   *Assay of the unchanged drug in serum or heparinized plasma at about the range of therapeutic levels, viz. 1-10 mg/litre.*

Chemistry &   *Lipophilic, acid-soluble, quinazoline derivative with characteristic*
metabolism   *UV adsorption spectrum; volatile enough (as free base) for GC. Resistant to chemical hydrolysis or oxidation. Subject to hepatic microsomal hydroxylation, predominantly to hydroxymethyl compounds. Many conjugates excreted in urine; some may circulate in plasma, possibly with enterohepatic recirculation.*

End-step   *UV spectrometry for 'toxic' levels, provided blanks are low; fluorimetry (after reduction to dihydro-derivative) or GC (flame ionization or possibly nitrogen detector) for sub-therapeutic levels.*

Sample   *Extraction with solvent of low polarity, e.g. hexane. Back-extraction*
preparation   *into acid, and return to solvent, so as to eliminate phenolic metabolite(s).*

Comments   *The therapeutic dose of methaqualone is large enough, and the volume of distribution small enough, to make direct methods of assay quite sensitive and practicable. Lipids and neutral lipophilic drugs may come through in the GC unless there is efficient back-extraction.*

Methaqualone [1] was first synthesized in 1951 as a potential analgesic drug with a structural similarity to the active principle, febrifugine, of the ancient Chinese anti-malarial *Ch'ang Shan*. Although its structure appears relatively complex, it is readily prepared (Fig. 1) from simple starting materials - anthranilic acid, o-toluidine and an acetylating agent. The reaction is reversed by strong acid or alkaline hydrolysis, and this affords a means of colorimetric analysis of pharmaceutical products, by diazotisation and coupling.

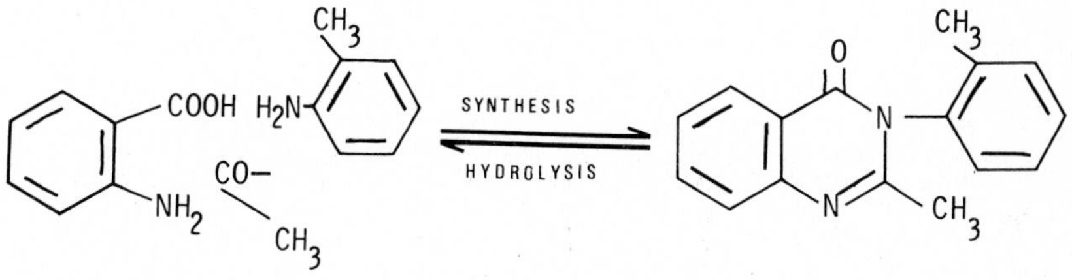

Fig. 1. Scheme of synthesis and hydrolysis of methaqualone.

It can be seen that methaqualone is both a cyclic amide and a pyrimidine derivative, and therefore has a formal structural resemblance to the piperidone hyponotics and to the barbiturates. It proved to have an hypnotic-sedative property in man at dosage levels of about 5 mg/kg, and was thus promoted in many countries, from the late 1950's onwards, as a desirable alternative to the barbiturates. The last twenty years have seen the rise, decline, and virtual fall of methaqualone. Its socio-pharmacologic case history [2] is even more fascinating than its analytical case history. In some countries, notably Germany, it has found its way into the pharmacopoeia because of its inclusion in compound preparations, which cover the treatment of a whole range of ailments. This is not just a point of academic interest; doubtless the pharmacokinetics of methaqualone are influenced by the concurrent or prior administration of many other drugs, especially if they are liable to affect hepatic microsomal oxidation.

ANALYTICAL CHEMISTRY

The relatively unusual structure of methaqualone confers on it some characteristic physical and chemical properties and make it amenable to a variety of analytical techniques. It is a high-melting lipophilic solid which is insoluble in neutral or aqueous alkaline solution, but readily soluble in acids because of the weak basicity of the $N(1)$ atom. Crystalline salts such as the hydrochloride or picrate are readily obtained. Some preparations of methaqualone for oral administration are formulated with the free base, but most with the hydrochloride; this particular point is the subject of bioavailability data described below.

The $N(3)$ substituent prevents tautomerism, so that methaqualone is stable enough for satisfactory GC running on a wide variety of stationary phases [3-5]. Polarographic or chemical reduction of methaqualone yields the 1,2-dihydro derivative, which like its congenor anthranilic acid displays intense ultra-violet fluorescence [6]. This presupposes that methaqualone, like other oxoquinazolines, has strong UV absorption; in fact the spectrum of methaqualone in polar solvents or in acids is sufficiently characteristic to be useful for qualitative or quantitative assay in biological materials. The problem here is one of sensitivity, and differential extraction techniques have been worked out in attempts to reduce interference from 'biological blanks' or from metabolites of the drug. Hepatic oxidative metabolism appears to be non-specific in character and the pattern of metabolites probably varies both between individuals, and within individuals over a period of time (methaqualone is as effective an 'inducer' as phenobarbitone).

Preliminary chromatographic methods of purification may be necessary if methaqualone is to be adequately distinguished by spectrophotometric assay from potentially interfering substances. In practice, spectrophotometric methods are barely sensitive enough for the determination of therapeutic levels of methaqualone, but they have been widely applied in toxicological studies involving gross overdosage [1]. IR and NMR spectra have occasionally been used to confirm the identity of methaqualone in forensic investigations. MS (or mass fragmentography) has been applied both for the elucidation of the structure of some methaqualone metabolites and also for quantitative pharmacokinetic studies [7-9].

Thus a whole range of analytical methods can be used to assay the drug in biological materials. The technique of choice for a given application will depend not only on the level to be expected, but also on the instrumentation which is at hand. The therapeutic dose of methaqualone is large enough, and the volume of distribution small enough, to make direct methods of assay quite sensitive and practicable. No particular endogeneous metabolites interfere, although lipids, e.g. cholesterol, and neutral lipophilic drugs, e.g. glutethimide, may come through unless there is efficient back-extraction. The World Health Organization [10] in fact recommends GC; this of course offers a very convenient means of distinguishing methaqualone from its metabolites.

The problem presented by the occurrence of such metabolites is by no means unique to methaqualone, but the general difficulties are well exemplified in this context. The principal metabolites are phenolic or hydroxyl (i.e. benzyl) derivatives (Fig. 2). The phenolic compounds can be largely eliminated by suitable back-extraction, but separation may not be so readily achieved with the neutral hydroxymethyl compounds. The extent of the interference which can be suffered by conventional photometric assays can be demonstrated (Fig. 3) from some published data [11]. Simple extraction of serum specimens with polar solvents such as chloroform yields a mixture of strongly UV-absorbing materials, with spectra essentially indistinguishable from that of methaqualone itself. However, extraction of the same material with a less polar solvent, e.g. hexane, and back-extraction with acid, so as to recover the methaqualone free from phenolic impurities, affords a much better correlation between the results of spectrophotometric assays and the corresponding GC assays. It is surprising how few comparative data of this kind have been published.

PHARMACOKINETIC APPLICATION

Data which illustrate the usefulness of a typical GC assay for methaqualone in plasma are shown in Table 1 and refer to a published study [12]. Several other reports [13, 14, 15] describe pharmacokinetic applications of different assays for methaqualone. The main object of the experiment [12] was to determine the rise and fall of plasma methaqualone levels in normal fasting subjects after therapeutic doses of different preparations of methaqualone. The chief interest lay in discovering whether the free base or the hydrochloride was more rapidly absorbed. The results clearly indicated that the latter was more quickly absorbed than the former, at least with the two formulations which were used in this study. What is perhaps of more interest is to bring out, from the data, the extent of variation of rate of absorption between different subjects.

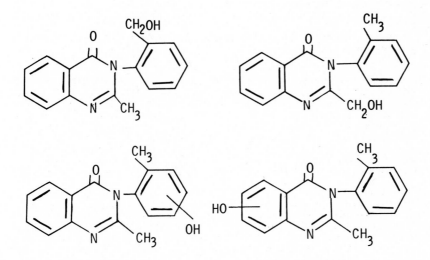

Fig. 2. Structure of principal metabolites of methaqualone.

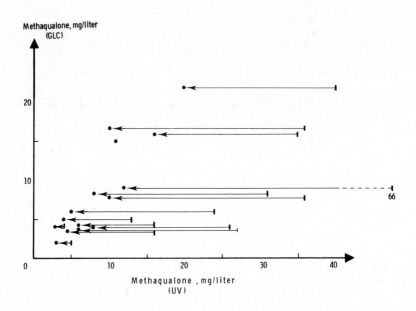

Fig. 3. Assay of sera in cases of methaqualone abuse. Relationship between results of GC and UV methods; the circles refer to hexane extraction and the bars to chloroform extraction. [Data derived from ref. 11, and Figure reproduced with permission, from *Ciba Found. Symp. 26* (1974), 133 ('The Poisoned Patient: the Role of the Laboratory')]

The upper part of Table 1 shows the change in plasma methaqualone levels in normal fasting subjects after the ingestion of a 300 mg dose of methaqualone hydrochloride with 200 ml of water. An estimate of the subjective response, and its approximate onset and duration, was made in each case - of course before the plasma methaqualone levels were available. In this Table, the subjects have been ranked A to H in order of the apparent speed of absorption of the drug, i.e. in relation to the plasma levels 30 min after ingestion. Only in one subject, H, was the level near the limit of detection by this assay. Substantially higher levels were seen in all the other subjects, and the range of levels at this time stood in the ratio of 1 to 20. All except one of the subjects (G) reported a distinct but relatively transient response to the drug after 30 min, manifesting itself as incoordination ('tipsiness') or drowsiness. At 1 h after ingestion, the plasma levels were much closer, in the range 2-5 mg/litre; thereafter the levels fell off slowly, but were still measurable 8 h after ingestion.

The same 8 subjects were then tested again after an interval of 1 month, and on this occasion received a dose of 250 mg of methaqualone base. Now (Table 1, lower part), they were ranked according to the peak level which was reached after 1 h, since in all except the first of them (Subject A) the level at time 30 min was quite low. Thus the picture contrasts markedly with that following the absorption of methaqualone hydrochloride. It is particularly interesting that Subject A again headed the list whereas Subject H was again at the bottom of the list. Concerning pharmacological response to methaqualone base, none of the subjects was really affected by the drug, which is in marked contrast to the previous experi-

Table 1. Plasma methaqualone levels in healthy subjects following ingestion of
the drug. *To ensure strict comparability, the 'hydrochloride' specimens and
the 'base' specimens from a given subject were extracted and analyzed (in random
order) in a single GC run. The C.V. for between-batch repeat analyses was 13%
(mean level, 2.6 mg/litre, N = 14 pairs).*

Subject								Subjective response

Subject	0.5	1.0	1.5	2.0	3.0	5.0	8.0	Subjective response
Methaqualone hydrochloride (2 x 150 mg)								
A	3.9	4.8	3.3	3.2	1.7	1.0	0.7	Marked effect at 0.25 h
B	3.7	4.6	4.7	2.8	2.0	1.6	1.1	Marked effect at 0.3 h
C	3.3	4.6	3.6	2.8	2.2	1.6	1.0	Marked effect at 0.25 h
D	2.8	4.9	2.6	2.1	1.4	0.4	0.2	Marked effect at 0.3 h
E	1.7	3.7	4.0	3.6	2.0	1.1	0.8	Mild effect at 0.5 h
F	1.0	2.9	2.4	3.6	2.1	1.2	1.7	Marked effect at 0.25 h
G	0.4	2.0	2.4	3.1	2.9	1.4	0.9	Little effect at all
H	0.2	2.6	3.0	3.4	1.4	0.9	0.6	Slight effect at 0.75 h
Methaqualone base (250 mg)								
A	3.2	4.2	2.4	1.6	1.6	1.1	0.2	Some effect at 0.75 h
E	0.2	3.2	3.5	3.4	1.9	1.0	0.7	No effect
G	0.2	2.3	1.9	2.4	1.6	1.0	0.9	Little effect at all
F	0.7	2.1	1.9	1.9	1.4	0.9	0.9	Slight effect at 0.5 h
C	0.2	1.8	3.2	4.0	2.6	1.3	1.0	Little effect at all
B	0.2	0.8	1.3	1.3	1.3	1.1	1.1	Slight effect at 0.75 h
H	0.2	0.2	0.8	1.0	2.3	1.1	0.8	Little effect at all

The column header reads: Plasma methaqualone (mg/litre) at time (h):

ment. Yet all of the subjects, except B and H at the bottom of the Table,
achieved quite respectable levels of plasma methaqualone after a period of 1 to 2 h.

The fact that the base and hydrochloride gave such different pharmacokinetic
pictures is not really surprising. After all, they are substantially different
substances, one being a weak base and the other a quaternary salt, even though they
must follow very similar metabolic patterns after the initial absorption stage. It
could be argued that the differences in rate of absorption and in pharmacological
effect were connected not with the free base or salt form, but rather with the
pharmaceutical character of the tablet formulation; this is a plausible hypothesis,
although perhaps somewhat unlikely. The point now stressed is that the data demonstrate the value of pharmacokinetic measurements based on a relatively simple and
reasonably specific assay.

References

1. Brown, S.S. & Goenechea, S., *Clin. Pharmacol. Therap. 14* (1973) 314-324.
2. Falco, M., *Methaqualone: a Study of Drug Control.* Drug Abuse Council, Inc., Washington, D.C. (1975).
3. Berry, D.J., *J. Chromatog. 42* (1969) 39-44.
4. Mitchard, M. & Williams, M.E., *J. Chromatog. 72* (1972) 29-34.
5. Douglas, J.F. & Shahinian, S., *J. Pharm. Sci. 62* (1973) 835-836.
6. Brown, S.S. & Smart, G.A., *J. Pharm. Pharmacol. 21* (1969) 466-468.
7. Bogentoft, C., Ericsson, O., Danielsson, B., Lindgren, J.E. & Holmstedt, B., *Acta Pharm. Suecica 9* (1972) 151-154.
8. Holmstedt, B. & Lindgren, J.E., *Ciba Found. Symp. 26* (1974) 105-124 *('The Poisoned Patient: the Role of the Laboratory').*
9. Bonnichsen, R., Dimberg, R., Mårde, Y. & Ryhage, R., *Clin. Chim. Acta 60* (1975) 67-75.
10. World Health Organization. *Technical Report 556, Detection of Dependence-Producing Drugs in Body Fluids,* World Health Organization, Geneva (1974), p.22.
11. Bailey, D.N. & Jatlow, P.I., *Clin. Chem. 19* (1973) 615-620.
12. Goenechea, S., Brown, S.S. & Ferguson, M.M., *Arch. Toxikol. 31* (1973) 25-30.
13. Alván, G., Lindgren, J.E., Bogentoft, C. & Ericsson, O., *Eur. J. Clin. Pharmacol. 6* (1973) 187-190.
14. Smyth, R.D., Lee, J.K., Polk, A., Chemburkar, R.B. & Savacool, A.M., *J. Clin. Pharmacol. 13* (1973) 391-400.
15. Morris, R.N., Gunderson, G.A., Babcock, S.W. & Zaroslinski, J.F., *Clin. Pharmacol. Therap. 13* (1972) 719-723.

Analytical case history

T-4
ASSAY OF CHLORPROMAZINE AND SOME OF ITS METABOLITES IN BIOLOGICAL FLUIDS

S.H. Curry

Department of Pharmacology and Therapeutics
The London Hospital Medical College
Turner Street, London, E1 2AD, U.K.

Many attempts have been made to assay a wide range of phenothiazine drugs in biological fluids. The subject has been reviewed a number of times. The earliest work (soon after the introduction of chlorpromazine) concerned spot tests for examination of urine for the presence of drug-related material. More sophisticated chromatographic and spectrophotometric techniques were later applied when knowledge of the routes of metabolism and excretion had developed, but it was not until 1967 that the discovery of a method suitable for the specific assay of any of the unmetabolized drugs in plasma of patients receiving clinical doses was announced. Since then, the use of GC with an electron-capture detector (ECD) has become the standard technique for chlorpromazine (see Appendix). The position may be summarized as follows.—

Requirement	*Assay sensitive to ∿10 ng/ml, for plasma and urine, detecting unchanged drug and certain metabolites separately.*
Chemistry & metabolism	*Phenothiazines with amine side-chains. Metabolism by hydroxylation, sulphoxidation, N-oxidation and demethylation. Conjugates occur in both plasma and urine.*
End-step	*GC with ECD.*
Sample preparation	*Solvent extraction. Derivatization if necessary.*
Comments & alternatives	*Sensitivity ∿10 ng per assay tube; assay adequate for most purposes; almost no drug interference; various alternatives available discussed in text.*

I plan in this presentation to outline the history of chlorpromazine assay over the last 25 years, and to show the way in which analytical developments have matched clinical needs.

Chlorpromazine was introduced into clinical medicine around 1950. It is still widely used as the first choice anti-psychotic phenothiazine. The drug has been extensively studied, and, in particular, its metabolites and their assay have been the subject of over one hundred papers [1-3]. It has a remarkably large number of metabolites, perhaps as many as 200. Most of the available physicochemical techniques have been applied to its analysis, and various approaches have proved applicable in various situations. Much of the work has exploited the increased polarity of the metabolites over the unchanged drug, which facilitates selective solvent extraction, and the GC approach (Table 1).

Initial work was aimed at detecting chlorpromazine (and other phenothiazine drugs) in urine. Soon after the drug was introduced it was realized that defaulting, i.e. failure of patients to consume prescribed medicines, was to be a major problem in its clinical application. Tests were needed to determine the degree of defaulting. The tests developed made use of the fact that phenothiazine drugs are converted to coloured semiquinone radical ions when dissolved in strong

Table 1. Relative GC retention times and solvent extraction properties of
reference compounds. Conjugates of hydroxylated compounds are studied as
aglycones after hydrolysis.

Compound*	Demethylation	Sulphoxidation	Hydroxylation	Amine oxidation	Relative retention time, min	Extracted readily from plasma into:-
			Metabolic changes			
CPZ					1	Heptane/ether/DCM
Nor$_1$CPZ	✓				1.17	Heptane/ether/DCM
Nor$_2$CPZ	✓				1.25(2.00)$^\Delta$	Heptane/ether/DCM
CPZSO		✓			2.98	Heptane/ether/DCM
Nor$_1$CPZSO	✓	✓			3.90	-
Nor$_2$CPZSO	✓	✓			4.87(6.35)$^\Delta$	-
7-OH CPZ			✓		1.62†	Ether/DCM
7-OH Nor$_1$CPZ	✓		✓		2.08	Ether/DCM
7-OH Nor$_2$CPZ	✓		✓		1.77	Ether/DCM
7-OH CPZSO		✓	✓		4.62	-
7-OH Nor$_1$CPZSO	✓	✓	✓		6.19	-
7-OH Nor$_2$CPZSO	✓	✓	✓		5.65	-
CPZNO				✓	2.19$^\#$	Ether/DCM
CPZNOSO		✓		✓	3.06$^\#$	-

* See text *(Appendix, Section A)* for abbreviations; DCM is dichloromethane.

† 7-OH compounds as silyl derivatives.

$^\#$ Partially decomposed to CPZ, CPZSO and other compounds on GC columns.

$^\Delta$ As imines with iso-valeraldehyde.

sulphuric acid. These tests have been of inestimable value in detecting defaulters.
However, it must be appreciated that they are very non-specific. Any phenothiazine drug and its metabolites is detected, so that, at best, mixtures of drug-
derived material are assayed.

   The second phase of chlorpromazine analysis had a very specific aim. In
the mid-fifties it was fashionable to screen drug metabolites for the action of
the precursors. With this in mind Brodie and his colleagues devised a method for
detection of chlorpromazine and its first metabolite, chlorpromazine sulphoxide,
in blood and urine of pretreated animals [4]. This method, though highly specific,
was not sufficiently sensitive for the study of human plasma, and chlorpromazine
sulphoxide proved to have little activity.

   The third phase consisted of lengthy and sophisticated studies, using a
wide range of techniques, but principally various forms of paper and thin-layer

chromatography, with a view to detection and identification of more and more chlorpromazine metabolites in urine. This had several objectives but chiefly: (1) the study of drug metabolism for its own sake; and (2) the refinement of the earlier spot tests with a view to better techniques for detecting drug defaulting. The quantitative counterpart of this was the very important observation that 5-10% of a daily dose appears in a 24-h urine sample as ether- or dichloromethane-extractable phenothiazine material - a very small amount of unmetabolized chlorpromazine plus various metabolites of intermediate lipophilicity. The remainder of the dose is excreted in urine and bile as highly polar conjugates. This observation provides the basis for the most convenient drug defaulting test at present available *(see later)* [5, 6].

It was in 1965 that attention was first focussed on plasma levels of chlorpromazine in man [7]. This occurred in the very early days of the current wave of interest in plasma levels of drugs. At first, interest centred around the unchanged drug. This was extensively studied for basic pharmacokinetic features, and for the relation between pharmacokinetics and clinical effects, using the then new GC method. This method revolutionized the study of chlorpromazine biochemistry, providing for the first time a sensitive, specific and readily-applicable method for assay of the drug. The relation between clinical rating and plasma levels will be considered later [8-22].

The gas-chromatographic method has been applied more recently to the solvent-extractable metabolites of chlorpromazine [23-27]. It is now realized that, at best, only a small number of compounds are of pharmacological interest. In plasma, the virtually inactive chlorpromazine sulphoxide is almost always detected. Demonomethylchlorpromazine, dedimethylchlorpromazine, 7-hydroxychlorpromazine and chlorpromazine *N*-oxide sometimes occur, but they have reduced potency, and their concentrations are lower than those of chlorpromazine. It is therefore unlikely that they contribute greatly to the action of chlorpromazine. Indeed, patients manifesting clinical responses have been shown to have virtually zero concentrations of the metabolites. This does not alter the fact that these compounds, if given directly, might possibly show clinical action. It has in fact been suggested that 7-hydroxychlorpromazine might combine the antipsychotic action of chlorpromazine with the antidepressant action of desipramine.

The relation between chlorpromazine kinetics and response is complex. In particular, clinical improvement occurs against a background of an overall rise in plasma chlorpromazine caused by dosing at a rate greater than that of elimination, followed by an overall fall as enzyme induction occurs. This makes the dubious concept of 'steady-state' inapplicable, especially as wild fluctuations in plasma chlorpromazine occur within the overall pattern. There is also a high degree of inter-patient variation, not only as regards recorded levels, but in response to particular levels. Additionally, relapse does not necessarily occur on cessation of treatment even when plasma chlorpromazine falls very low. Nevertheless, it is now possible to make specific recommendations in regard to plasma monitoring, and these will now be noted, as the logical end-point of a 25-year saga of chlorpromazine assay.

MONITORING OF PLASMA

Concurrent studies of clinical effect and concentrations in plasma have been mostly conducted with the unmetabolized drug. One report showed chlorpromazine sulphoxide to be virtually inactive. Two other reports have been concerned with the relation between response, and 7-hydroxychlorpromazine and demonomethylchlorpromazine, taking chlorpromazine sulphoxide concentrations into account. One of these two reports concerned a heterogeneous group of eight patients, and statistical analysis is impossible. In the other report, the only statistically significant finding was an inverse relation between plasma chlorpromazine sulphoxide and response.

Thus, although future monitoring of metabolites in plasma may be in order, at present monitoring can reasonably be confined to chlorpromazine. Results can be compared with the data in Table 2. The members of a group of 57 patients in a long-stay schizophrenic population, all showing some response to chlorpromazine, were rated on a seven-point scale for illness at the time of assessment. The scale is shown in the Table. They were sampled three times, just before a dose, and 2 and 4 h later, and the chlorpromazine in their plasma was estimated. They were grouped in five subgroups according to plasma level range. Their mean scores indicate the best response in the 100.1 - 500 ng/ml group (p <0.05), and prudence suggests that during therapy patients should optimally have a mean overall plasma concentration in the range 35 - 350 ng/ml, thus including some of the patients in the group with a mean score of 5. Of course, there are patients who need and tolerate high concentrations, there are patients who tolerate only low concentrations, and there are patients who obtain no benefit from their chlorpromazine at any concentration in plasma. Monitoring of plasma chlorpromazine is at best an indication of whether or not a patient is receiving adequate amounts of the materials shown to be associated with clinical success in other patients.

Table 2. Severity of illness as a function of chlorpromazine concentration.

Illness scale: (1) Normal, not ill at all; (2) borderline mentally ill; (3) mildly ill; (4) moderately ill; (5) markedly ill; (6) severely ill; (7) among the most extremely ill patients.

Concentration range[*], ng/ml	Mean dose, mg t.d.s.	n	Score Mean	Score SEM
<10	238	4	5.8	0.9
10.1 - 35	83	21	5.2	0.1
35.1 - 100	115	22	5.0	0.1
100.1 - 500	206	8	4.3	0.2
>500	875	2	6.5	0.5

[*] *No differences amongst groups in age, sex or weight.*

MONITORING OF URINE

There is very little unchanged chlorpromazine in urine. Fig. 1 shows the relation between urinary output of solvent-extractable chlorpromazine metabolites (excretion, mg/day) and dosage (mg/day) in 20 patients. Again, the degree of variation is considerable; but, generally speaking, these data agree with analogous data from other workers, in showing that 5-10% of the dose appears in urine in this form. Less than this percentage, when found in repeated measurements, probably indicates defaulting, although a high or a low percentage (in particular) could indicate an unusual metabolic pattern. A high percentage will, very occasionally, indicate overdosing. Urinary excretion is far more satisfactory than plasma monitoring for detecting these problems, as a patient can be consuming his prescribed drugs, but be metabolizing them too rapidly.

PARENTERAL PHENOTHIAZINES

There is one special aspect of chlorpromazine monitoring. It has been shown that there are certain patients, some of them defaulters, but others known to be satisfactory tablet-takers, who fail to achieve clinically useful plasma levels of chlorpromazine regardless of dose. The satisfactory tablet-takers have absorption problems. These patients are often more satisfactorily treated with long-acting fluphenazine or flupenthixol injections, and monitoring reveals their problem. This results from conversion of chlorpromazine in the intestine into inactive products which are absorbed into the blood but cleared rapidly in urine [28-30].

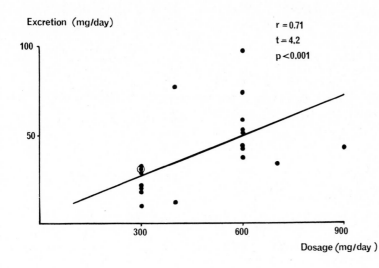

Excretion (mg/day)

r = 0.71
t = 4.2
p < 0.001

Fig. 1.
Urinary excre-
tion (mg/day)
of mixed
solvent-
extractable
chlorpromazine
metabolites
in relation
to chlorproma-
zine dosage
(mg/day).

Dosage (mg/day)

APPENDIX: Methods

A: REFERENCE MATERIALS

The key methods applicable in chlorpromazine monitoring are scattered among a wide
range of publications, and this paper provides an opportunity to summarize them.
The reasons for the use of particular procedures are to be found in the original
papers.

Samples of chlorpromazine hydrochloride are available from the manufacturers.
Samples of chlorpromazine model metabolites (arising by hydroxylation, sulphoxidation, demethylation and *N*-oxidation) are available from Dr. A.A. Manian, National
Institute of Mental Health, Rockville, Maryland, U.S.A. These metabolites will be
referred to in this paper by means of abbreviations: CPZ is chlorpromazine; pre-
fixes Nor_1, Nor_2 and 7-OH indicate demonomethyl-, dedimethyl-, and 7-hydroxy-
respectively; suffixes SO and NO indicate sulphoxide and amine (side chain) oxide
respectively. Thus (e.g.) 7-OH Nor_2 CPZSO is 7-hydroxydedimethyl-chlorpromazine
sulphoxide (II) (CPZ is I):

B: MATERIALS

All reagents, solvents, gases etc., should be of the highest available grade. No
specific recommendation can be made in regard to tubes and pipettes, because of
local differences in availability, except to say that at some stages in the methods,
plastic (polycarbonate) centrifuge tubes are needed. These tubes must seal tight to
avoid leakage, they must not absorb CPZ or its metabolites from the aqueous or solvent solutions used, and they must be translucent. Pipettes of plastic can also be
used if they meet these criteria. Glass tubes and pipettes (if used) must be chosen
with similar considerations in mind. Unless disposable hardware is used, a washing

system must be set up which adequately removes all traces of the compounds without changing the tube or pipette characteristics. Tubes, etc., once chosen should be reserved for CPZ assay.

C: STANDARD SOLUTIONS

Absolute standards are prepared from weighed quantities of the reference materials dissolved at known concentrations in solvents suitable for GC-EC. In this laboratory, the routine is to weigh 10 mg quantities, dissolve them in 2-3 ml methanol, and dilute to 10 ml with methanol. These solutions are stable for long periods if stored at 4° in the dark. Working dilutions are prepared as and when required, in methanol, plasma, 0.1 M HCl or 0.1 M NH_4OH.

D: GC-ECD

Any GC-EC instrument with a Ni-63 or Sr-90 detector can be used, provided it is known to give 'clean' signals to one nanogram (10^{-9} g) samples of CPZ and its metabolites. Conditions are as follows:

Column: 8-9 ft., 3.5 mm i.d., 3% OV-17 on Chromosorb W HP 80-100 mesh at 265° (purchased, or laboratory-prepared by standard methods).
Direct on-column injection, or injection port at 280°.
Detector in pulsed or continuous DC mode depending on instrument characteristics.
Dry, high purity N_2 as the carrier gas at 40 psig giving a flow rate of 60-80 ml/min.
The retention time of CPZ is approximately 4 min in this system (see Table 1 for other retention times).

E: SAMPLES

Collect blood samples (usually sufficient to yield 4-5 ml plasma or more if necessary) by venepuncture into oxalate or citrate tubes and centrifuge on the day of collection. Separate plasma and store at 4° in the dark for the minimum possible time before assay.

F: EXTRACTION AND ASSAY OF CPZ AND ITS DEMETHYLATED AND SULPHOXIDIZED ANALOGUES (CPZ, CPZSO, Nor_1CPZ, Nor_2CPZ)

To 2 ml of plasma in a 25 ml stoppered polycarbonate centrifuge tube add 1 ml of M NaOH and 10 ml *n*-heptane containing 1.5% amyl alcohol. Shake the tube mechanically for 30 min and centrifuge. Transfer a 9 ml aliquot of the organic layer to a 15 ml glass-stoppered centrifuge tube containing 2 ml of 0.05 M HCl. Shake mechanically for 10 min and centrifuge. Transfer a 1.8 ml aliquot of the aqueous layer to a 15 ml tapered glass-stoppered centrifuge tube. Make alkaline with 0.2 ml of M NH_4OH and extract with 100 µl of toluene containing 15% amyl alcohol and 0.1% isovaleraldehyde. Shake mechanically for 15 min and centrifuge. Remove the aqueous layer by aspiration. Collect the organic layer in the tapered part of the tube by a series of centrifugation and aspiration steps. Examine 10 µl samples of the organic layer by GC.

Compare the signals produced with those from ten 2 ml samples from a series of 5 solutions containing the reference compounds of interest at 0, 20, 50, 125 and 250 ng/ml (of each compound) in blood-bank plasma sampled in duplicate. A standard curve prepared for each compound by plotting peak height against original concentration in plasma can be used for reading unknown concentrations directly.

G: EXTRACTION AND ASSAY OF HYDROXYLATED DERIVATIVES (7-OH CPZ, AND Nor_1 AND Nor_2 ANALOGUES)

To a second 2 ml plasma sample in a 50 ml glass-stoppered centrifuge tube add 1 ml of M NH_4OH and 10 ml of peroxide-free diethyl ether. Shake the tube mechanically for 10 min and centrifuge. Transfer a 7 ml aliquot of the ether to a glass-stoppered tube containing 2 ml of 0.1 M HCl. Shake the tube mechanically for 10 min and centrifuge. Transfer a 1.8 ml aliquot of the aqueous layer to a glass-stoppered tube containing 4 ml of ether. Add NH_4OH to bring the pH of the aqueous layer to 9. Shake the tube mechanically for 10 min and centrifuge. Transfer a 3 ml aliquot of the ether layer to a tapered centrifuge tube and evaporate to dryness on a water bath at 35° in a stream of nitrogen. Redissolve the residue in 50 μl of heptane containing 1% bis-(trimethylsilyl)-acetamide (BSA). Examine 10 μl samples of the organic layer by GC.

Compare the signals produced with those from ten 2 ml samples from a series of 5 solutions containing the reference compounds of interest at 0, 20, 50, 125 and 250 ng/ml in blood-bank plasma sampled in duplicate. A standard curve prepared by plotting, for each compound, the peak height against the original concentration in plasma can be used for reading the unknown concentrations directly.

H: ASSAY OF CPZNO AND CPZNOSO

Divide a plasma sample into two 2 ml sub-samples. Reduce one sub-sample (A) by addition of 0.5 ml 2N HCl, and 1 ml of aqueous sodium metabisulphite (M), or by bubbling SO_2 gas through for 2-3 min. Add 1.5 ml of water to the other sample (B). Extract and assay both tubes as described under F (*above*) assessing CPZ and CPZSO signals. In these extracts, the CPZ$_{(A-B)}$ reading and the CPZSO$_{(A-B)}$ readings indicate, by difference, the concentrations of CPZNO and CPZNOSO in the original plasma samples before separation and reduction. If desired, a series of CPZNO and CPZNOSO samples at 0, 50, 125 and 250 ng/ml can be taken through this procedure, in a way analogous to that described for CPZ in F (*above*).

I: ASSAY OF NON-CONJUGATED CPZ METABOLITES IN URINE

Adjust a 2 ml urine sample to pH 9-9.5 by addition of 1 ml of saturated $NaHCO_3$ solution (or equivalent) and extract three times, with 3, 2 and 2 ml of dichloromethane. At each extraction shake 15 min, centrifuge, and remove 2 ml of the dichloromethane to a clean tube. Evaporate the pooled dichloromethane extracts to dryness on a water bath at 50° in a stream of nitrogen. Redissolve the residue in 0.2 ml of 0.1 M HCl. Add 3 ml of 50% (v/v) H_2SO_4. Lightly stopper the tube, and heat on a water bath at 50° for 60 min. Cool to room temperature. Transfer the solution quantitatively to a 5 ml volumetric flask and make up to volume with 50% H_2SO_4. Read the absorbance at 400, 550, and 700 nm in a spectrophotometer, using a background cancellation method if there is a substantial reading at 400 and 700 mμ. The absorbance at 550 nm is related to the amount of dichloromethane-extractable metabolites originally present. The concentration is obtained from a calibration graph prepared from CPZ solutions in urine at 0, 10, 50, 100, 250 and 500 μg/ml, sampled in duplicate.

J: PRECISION AND ACCURACY

The precision and accuracy of these methods depends to some extent on the skill of the operator conducting the experiment in each case. The best that will be obtained will be a perfectly correct answer calculated from identical readings obtained in replicate assays of any one blood-bank plasma solution of the particular derivative(s) of interest. In practice, replicates should never differ by more than ±10% of their mean. The statistical aspects of the assay were considered in detail in the original publications.

References

1. *BIBLIOGRAPHY, Psychopharmacology Service Centre Bulletin 2* (1963) 71-106.

2. Usdin, E., *CRC Critical Reviews in Clinical Laboratory Sciences 2* (1971) 347-391.

3. *The Phenothiazines and Structurally Related Drugs* (I.S. Forrest, C.J. Carr & E. Usdin, eds.), Raven Press, New York (1974).

4. Salzman, N.P. & Brodie, B.B., *J. Pharmac. Exp. Ther.* 118 (1956) 46-54.

5. Bolt, A.G., Forrest, I.S. & Serra, M.T., *J. Pharm. Sci.* 55 (1966) 1205-1208.

6. Turner, W.J., Turano, P.A. & March, J.E., *Clin. Chem.* 16 (1970) 916-921.

7. Curry, S.H. & Brodie, B.B., *Fed. Proc.* 26 (1967) 761.

8. Curry, S.H., *Anal. Chem.* 40 (1968) 1251-1255.

9. Curry, S.H., *Agressologie* 9 (1968) 115-121.

10. Rivera-Calimlim, L., Castaneda, L. & Lasagna, L., *Clin. Pharmac. Ther.* 14 (1973) 978-986.

11. Sakalis, G., Chan, T.L., Gershon, S. & Park, S., *Psychopharmacologia (Berl.)* 32 (1973) 279-284.

12. Spirtes, M., *Clin. Chem.* 18 (1972) 317-318.

13. Flint, D.R., Ferullo, C.R., Levandoski, P. & Hwang, B., *Clin. Chem.* 17 (1971) 830.

14. Curry, S.H. in *The Phenothiazines and Structurally Related Drugs* (I.S. Forrest, C.J. Carr & E. Usdin, eds.), Raven Press, New York (1974) pp. 335-345.

15. Efron, D.H., Harris, S.R., Manian, A.A. & Gaudette, L.E., *Psychopharmacologia* 19 (1971) 207-210.

16. Lehr, R.E. & Kaul, P.N., *J. Pharm. Sci.* 64 (1975) 950-953.

17. Christoph, G.W., Schmidt, D., Janowsky, D.S. & Davis, J.M., *Clin. Chim. Acta* 38 (1972) 265-270.

18. Kawashima, K., Dixon, R. & Spector, S., *Eur. J. Pharmacol.* 32 (1975) 195-202.

19. Whelpton, R. & Curry, S.H., *J. Pharm. Pharmacol.* 27 (1975) 970-971.

20. Kaul, P.N., Conway, M.W. & Clark, M.L. in *The Phenothiazines and Structurally Related Drugs* (I.S. Forrest, C.J. Carr & E. Usdin, eds.), Raven Press, New York (1974) pp. 391-398.

21. Sakalis, G., Curry, S.H., Mould, G.P. & Lader, M.H., *Clin. Pharmac. Ther.* 13 (1972) 931-946.

22. Hammar, C-G., Holmstedt, B. & Ryhage, R., *Anal. Biochem.* 25 (1968) 533-543.

23. Mackay, A.V.P., Healey, A.F. & Baker, J., *Brit. J. Clin. Pharmac.* 1 (1974) 425-430.

24. Loga, S., Curry, S.H. & Lader, M.H., *Brit. J. Clin. Pharmac.* 2 (1975) 197-208.

25. Curry, S.H. & Evans, S., *Psychopharmacology Communications* 1 (1975) *in press.*

26. Curry, S.H. & Evans, S. (1976), *submitted for publication.*

27. Whelpton, R. & Curry, S.H., *J. Chromatog.* (1976) *in press.*

28. Curry, S.H. & Adamson, L., *Lancet* 2 (1972) 543-544.

29. Adamson, L., Curry, S.H., Bridges, P.K., Firestone, A.F., Lavin, N.I., Lewis, D.M., Watson, R.D., Xavier, C.M. & Anderson, J., *Diseases of the Nervous System* 34 (1973) 181-191.

30. Curry, S.H., Lewis, D.M., Samuel, G. & Mould, G.P. in *The Future of Pharmacotherapy: New Drug Delivery Systems* (F.J. Ayd, ed.), International Drug Therapy Newsletter, Baltimore (1973) pp. 53-60.

Analytical case history

T-5   PROBLEMS IN THE ANALYSIS OF *N*-OXYGENATED PRODUCTS
        OF THE PHENOTHIAZINES

David A. Cowan
Department of Pharmacy, Chelsea College,
Manresa Road, London, SW3 6LX, U.K.

Dimethylaminoalkyl phenothiazines (e.g. chlorpromazine, promazine and methotrime-
prazine) are N-oxidized chemically and metabolically to the corresponding N-oxides.
Alternatively, they are demethylated and then N-oxidized to form the secondary and
primary hydroxylamines. These hydroxylamines are unstable and the phenothiazine
nucleus may be liberated and itself N-oxidized. It is likely that these N-oxygena-
tion products have great biochemical significance. The labile nature of these N-
oxygenated products makes their analysis difficult and it is important to under-
stand the physico-chemical characteristics of the compounds concerned to ensure
significant results. See Fig. 10 for the analytical method adopted.

Chlorpromazine is a tertiary amine and is oxidized on the alkyl nitrogen atom to
form the *N*-oxide as a major metabolite. It is also *N*-demethylated and the resultant *nor*$_1$-chlorpromazine and *nor*$_2$-chlorpromazine may be *N*-oxygenated to form the
secondary and primary hydroxylamines respectively. The hydroxylamines can lose the
entire side-chain to liberate the phenothiazine nucleus which may be *N*-oxidized on
the aromatic nitrogen atom to form various products.

Many aromatic and aliphatic *N*-hydroxy compounds are known to be both chemically and metabolically active, and certain aromatic hydroxylamines have been impli-
cated in the induction of tumours and the oxidation of haemoglobin [1, 2].

ANALYSIS OF
N-OXIDES

We have inves-
tigated the
N-oxides of
chlorpromazine
(Fig. 1, $R^1 = Cl$,
$R^2 = H$), proma-
zine ($R^1 = H$,
$R^2 = H$) and
methotrimepra-
zine ($R^1 = -OCH_3$,
$R^2 = CH_3$). The

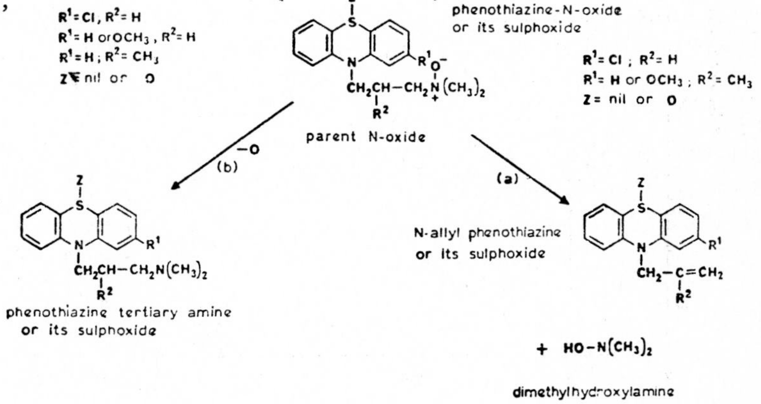

Fig. 1. Routes
of thermolysis
of some 10-
alkyl-dimethyl-
amino-pheno-
thiazine-*N*-
oxides and
their sulph-
oxides.

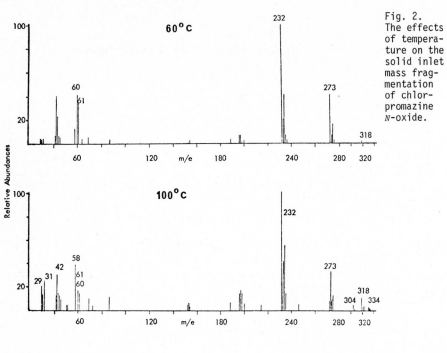

Fig. 2.
The effects
of tempera-
ture on the
solid inlet
mass frag-
mentation
of chlor-
promazine
N-oxide.

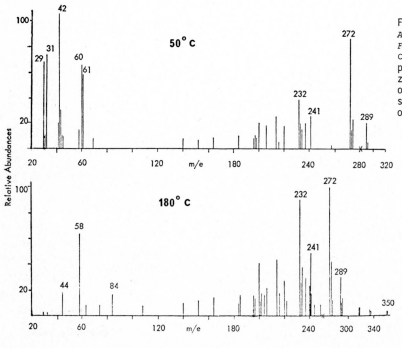

Fig. 3.
As for
Fig. 2:
chloro-
proma-
zine-N-
oxide-
sulph-
oxide.

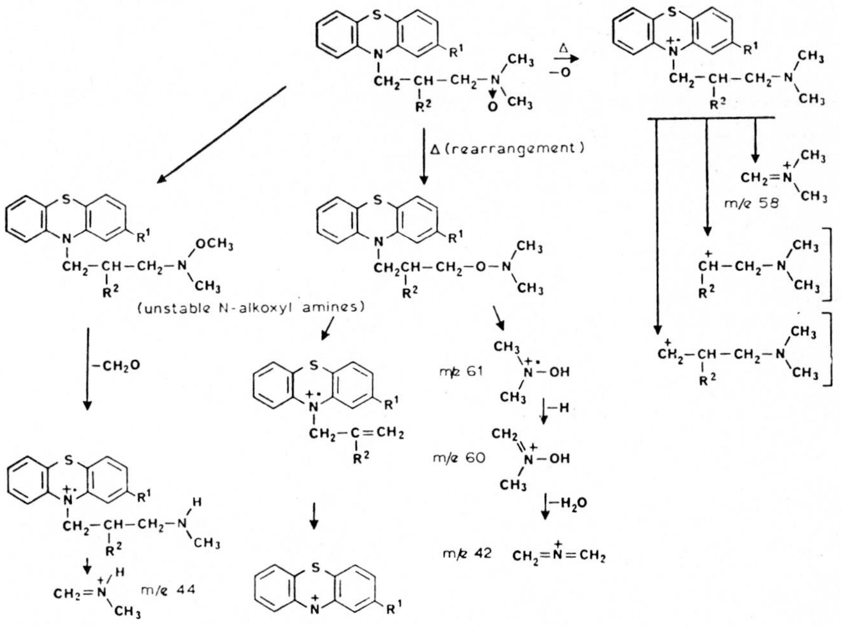

Fig. 4. Routes of thermolysis and fragmentation of some 10-alkyl-dimethyl-aminophenothiazine-N-oxides in the mass spectrometer ion source.

major product in most cases is the N-allyl Cope elimination product with the concomitant liberation of dimethylhydroxylamine. It was considered that this liberation of dimethylhydroxylamine would allow identification of these N-oxides by solid-inlet MS. Alternatively, the N-oxide can lose either formaldehyde and demethylate to the secondary amine or simply lose oxygen, reverting to the parent tertiary amine.

GC analysis of the elimination and reduction products of the N-oxides of both chlorpromazine and methotrimeprazine gave errors which were too large to allow use of the method.

The solid inlet mass spectra of each N-oxide investigated were found to vary with temperature [3]. For example, the spectra of chlorpromazine N-oxide run at probe temperatures of 60° and 100° (Fig. 2) show a reduction in the relative intensity of the peaks at m/e 60 and 61 and an increase in the peak at m/e 58 with increased temperature. This is even more pronounced in the spectra of the N-oxide sulphoxide of chlorpromazine (Fig. 3) where the peaks at m/e 61, 60 and 42 disappear at higher probe temperatures to be replaced by peaks at m/e 58 and 44.

The routes of thermolysis and fragmentation are indicated in Fig. 4. At probe temperatures of less than 100° the allyl derivative and dimethyl hydroxyl-amine are produced, the latter giving ions at m/e 61, 60 and 42. At elevated

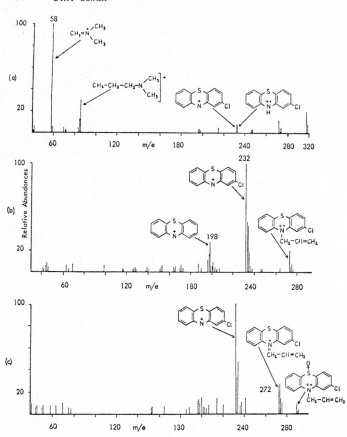

Fig. 5. Comparison of the GC mass spectra of chlorpromazine and the elimination products of its *N*-oxide and *N*-oxide sulphoxide.
(a) Chlorpromazine.
(b) *N*-oxide elimination product.
(c) *N*-oxide sulphoxide elimination product.

probe temperatures oxygen is lost and the presence of the intense ion at *m/e* 58 indicates the formation of the parent tertiary amine. In addition, a Meisenheimer-type rearrangement probably occurs to form the unstable *N*-alkoxylamine which loses formaldehyde to produce the secondary amine. The loss of formaldehyde in the ion source is indicated by the presence of ions at *m/e* 29 (M-1), 30 (M‡), and 31 (M+1). The secondary amine fragments to give the intense ion at *m/e* 44. A similar pattern is observed for the *N*-oxide sulphoxides. Thus we found that these *N*-oxides can be identified by solid-inlet MS provided that the conditions are carefully controlled.

We then examined the behaviour of the *N*-oxides in GC-MS. The spectrum of chlorpromazine of Fig. 5a agrees closely with the solid-inlet mass spectrum published by Gilbert and Millard [4]. The mass spectrum of the largest GC peak was recorded for the *N*-oxide (Fig. 5b) and *N*-oxide sulphoxide (Fig. 5c). These peaks and thus these spectra correspond to the respective Cope elimination products. A similar pattern is observed for methotrimeprazine (Fig. 6). Note the molecular ions corresponding to the allyl (Fig. 6b) and allyl sulphoxide (Fig. 6c) elimination products. However, both promazine *N*-oxide and promazine *N*-oxide sulphoxide eliminate under the GC conditions to produce phenothiazine (Fig. 7). The variability in the behaviour of these compounds will make their assay from biological fluids by a direct GC technique rather unreliable.

We found that cathode-ray polarography provided an answer [5]. The polarograms of chlorpromazine *N*-oxide (Fig. 8) and of chlorpromazine *N*-oxide sulphoxide

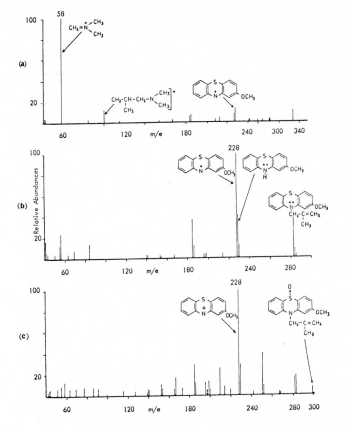

Fig. 6. Comparison of
the GC mass spectra of
methotrimeprazine and
the elimination pro-
ducts of its *N*-oxide
and *N*-oxide sulphoxide.

(a) Methotrimeprazine.
(b) *N*-oxide elimination
product.
(c) *N*-oxide sulphoxide
elimination product.

show that these compounds have virtually identical peak potentials (E_p) but the
reduction wave peak height, AB, of the *N*-oxide sulphoxide is twice that of the
same concentration of either chlorpromazine *N*-oxide or chlorpromazine *S*-oxide.
Linear calibration curves were obtained (Fig. 9) by plotting the logarithm of the
peak height against the negative logarithm of the concentration over the range of
10^{-5} to 5×10^{-8} M. The technique was applied to the analyses of the *N*-oxide, the
sulphoxide and the *N*-oxide sulphoxide of chlorpromazine in biological fluids.

PROCEDURE FOR SEPARATION AND ANALYSIS (Fig. 10)

Methyl orange solution is added to the biological fluid and the pH adjusted to 4.
Extraction with a benzene-dichloroethane mixture separates the parent chlorpromazine
and its *N*-oxide from the sulphoxides. The addition of *n*-heptane to the organic extract to reduce the proportion of dichloroethane to about 3% enables the chlorpromazine to be separated from its *N*-oxide. The organic extract is evaporated under
reduced pressure using a rotary film evaporator in subdued lighting. The residue is
dissolved in buffer with the aid of a small amount of ethanol if necessary and the
solution is then polarographed. The parent chlorpromazine may be analyzed by GC.

Half of the aqueous solution of the dye complexes is made alkaline to break
the complexes and any sulphoxide or *N*-oxide sulphoxide is extracted into dichloroethane. This organic extract is evaporated, the residue re-dissolved in buffer and

Fig. 7. Comparison of the
GC mass spectra of:
(a) promazine,
(b) the elimination pro-
ducts of its *N*-oxide and
N-oxide sulphoxide,
(c) the phenothiazine
nucleus.

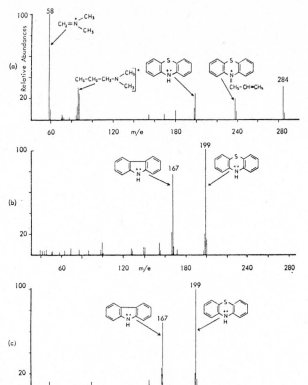

polarographed. The observed
polarographic peak current
is proportional to the concentration of chlorpromazine
sulphoxide and *N*-oxide sulphoxide in the sample (x).
The remaining half of the
aqueous solution of dye complexes is treated with sulphur dioxide so that any
chlorpromazine *N*-oxide sulphoxide present is converted
to the amine sulphoxide.
After extraction as before,
the polarographic peak
current (y) is proportional
to the original chlorpromazine sulphoxide plus the
chlorpromazine sulphoxide
from any *N*-oxide sulphoxide
in the original sample. Thus
the difference in peak
current (x-y) is proportional to the total concentration of chlorpromazine *N*-
oxide sulphoxide.

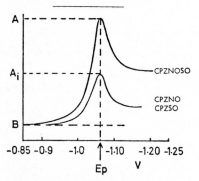

Fig. 8. Cathode ray polarograms of chlorpromazine-*N*-
oxide (CPZNO), chlorpromazine-
s-oxide (CPZSO) and chlorpro-
mazine-*N*-oxide sulphoxide
(CPZNOSO) in Britton-Robinson
buffer pH 5.

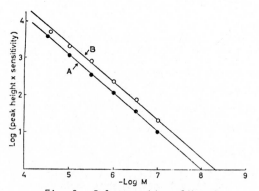

Fig. 9. Polarographic calibration
curves for the determination of chlorpromazine oxides in Britton-Robinson
buffer pH 5. (A) = curve for chlor-
promazine-*N*-oxide and chlorpromazine
sulphoxide; (B) = curve for chlorpro-
mazine-*N*-oxide-sulphoxide.

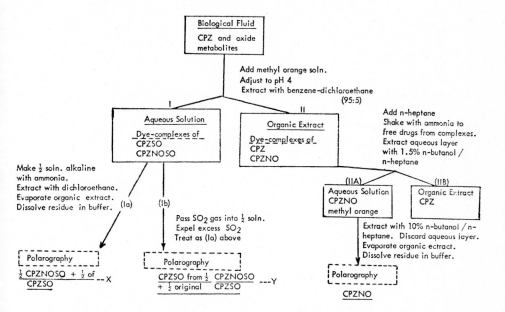

Fig. 10. Scheme for the separation and analysis of the *N*-oxides and sulphoxides of chlorpromazine in biological samples.

The recoveries from urine and plasma were found to be better than 95% in each case. This polarographic method is thus both sensitive and able to quantify both *N*-oxides and *N*-oxide sulphoxides in biological samples.

ANALYSIS OF HYDROXYLAMINES

Chlorpromazine may be *N*-demethylated prior to *N*-oxidation to form *N*-hydroxy*nor*$_1$ chlorpromazine or *N*-hydroxy*nor*$_2$ chlorpromazine. On GC examination both these compounds give a peak corresponding to the 2-chlorophenothiazine nucleus. This is comparable with the side-chain elimination of promazine *N*-oxide to produce the phenothiazine nucleus.

These hydroxylamines and their sulphoxides were thus determined indirectly by GC analysis of the elimination product. Since all the hydroxylamines give only a single peak corresponding to 2-chlorophenothiazine, initial solvent extraction is necessary to distinguish between these metabolites.

ANALYSIS OF PINK SPOT

We had previously observed a pink spot on the thin-layer plates of urine and blood extracts of patients receiving chlorpromazine. This pink spot was visible without treatment with any spray reagent. We found that, on incubation *in vitro* with fortified liver homogenates, 2-chlorophenathiazine and phenothiazine were metabolized to give products which, by TLC, gave pink spots before spraying. These pink spots were readily reduced by ascorbic acid to 2-chlorophenothiazine hydroxylamine and phenothiazine hydroxylamine respectively, showing that they were strong oxidizing agents. This was further confirmed by the liberation of iodine from hydriodic acid by the pink product of 2-chlorophenothiazine and by the production of blue colour with acidified potassium dichromate and diethyl ether. These pink compounds could be

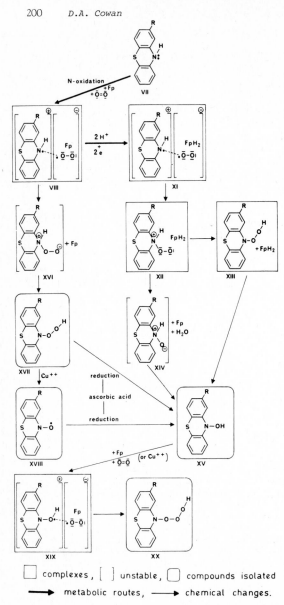

Fig. 11. The formation of nitr-oxide, *N*-hydroperoxides, *N*-oxy-hydroperoxide and hydroxylamines as a result of the metabolic *N*-oxidation of phenothiazines.

reduced to the hydroxylamines or back to the parent nucleus. They gave no e.s.r. signal alone but the pink compound from 2-chloro-phenothiazine reacted with di-cyano-t-butyl azide — a free radical inducing agent - to give a compound having a characteristic spectrum identical with that of 2-chlorophenothiazine nitroxide. Heating the pink compound of 2-chlorophenothiazine formed the symmetrical 2-chlorophenothiazine-*N*-peroxide. The mass spectra of the pink compounds indicated the presence of two oxygen atoms in each compound which itself was neither the sulphoxide nor the sulphone. As a result of all this and other evidence, it was concluded that the two oxygen atoms must be linked to the nitrogen atom of the molecule by the hydroperoxide linkage.

Beckett [6] has postula-ted (Fig. 11) the involvement of flavoprotein and molecular oxygen in this *N*-oxidation to produce the *N*-hydroperoxide as the result of metabolic *N*-oxidation of pheno-thiazines. Transfer of one elec-tron from the nitrogen lone pair via the flavoprotein to the mole-cule oxygen in the complex will yield complex VIII. This may be reduced metabolically to produce the hydroxylamine or dissociate to the hydroperoxide. The hydro-peroxide may give the nitroxide, this reaction being catalyzed by trace heavy metals in aqueous solution. The nitroxide may then be reduced, possibly during incubation, to the hydroxylamines. The further oxida-tion to form an oxyhydroperoxide is also postulated although conclusive evidence is lacking. Work is continuing to clarify the mechanisms further and to quantify these active compounds.

CONCLUDING COMMENTS

Because the phenothiazine drugs and all these metabolites are photosensitive and readily oxidized, all assays are carried out in the dark or in subdued lighting. In addition an atmosphere of nitrogen is used whenever possible and, since the majority of these compounds are thermolabile, solvent evaporation is carried out under reduced pressure using a rotary film evaporation or by bubbling nitrogen gas through the solvent at room temperature. During extraction of the compounds the use of strong acid or base is always avoided.

Taking these precautions has enabled us to analyze biological samples and to distinguish the labile *N*-oxygenated metabolic products of phenothiazine drugs.

Acknowledgement

I acknowledge the collaboration of Dr. E. Essien of the University of Ife, Nigeria and of Dr. W. Franklin Smyth of the Chemistry Department of Chelsea College for his work on the polarography of the phenothiazine *N*-oxides.

References

1. Weisburger, J.H. & Weisburger, E.K., *Pharmacol. Rev. 25* (1973) 188-189.

2. Gorrod, J.W. & Jenner, P., *Int. J. Clin. Pharmacol. 12* (1975) 180-185.

3. Essien, E.E., Cowan, D.A. & Beckett, A.H., *J. Pharm. Pharmac. 27* (1975) 334-342.

4. Gilbert, J.N.T. & Millard, B.J., *Org. Mass Spectrom. 2* (1969) 17-31.

5. Beckett, A.H., Essien, E.E. & Smyth, W. Franklin, *J. Pharm. Pharmac. 26* (1974) 399-407.

6. Beckett, A.H., *Xenobiotica 5* (1975) 449-452.

T-6

DETERMINATION OF TWO BENZODIAZEPINE ANTICONVULSANTS
IN THE PLASMA OF RHESUS MONKEYS WHEN GIVEN INTRAVENOUSLY,
SINGLY OR TOGETHER OR IN COMBINATION WITH A BENZHYDRYL⁻
PIPERAZINE ANTICONVULSANT

J.M. Clifford
G.D. Searle & Co.,
High Wycombe,
Bucks., HP12 4HL, U.K.

Requirement — *SC-13504, diazepam and clonazepam and their metabolites when together in blood plasma, down to 5-10 ng/ml.*

Chemistry & metabolism — *Chemical structures of and data on the three compounds are shown below and in Table 4 respectively. The reduction of the -NO₂ of clonazepam occurs as a metabolic step.*

End-step — *Differential pulse polarography.*

Sample preparation — *Differential solvent extraction; Fig. 5 shows possibly advantageous further steps.*

Comments & alternatives — *Interference of diazepam with clonazepam metabolites and* vice-versa. *Loss of selectivity due to metabolic reduction of the -NO₂ group. Sensitivity is not as good as GC-ECD for diazepam and clonazepam or nitrogen detection (AFID) for SC-13504; however, the method reported has only one analytical end-step.*
This pilot study showed that attempts were made to measure too many parameters. The ratio diazepam/desmethyldiazepam in plasma and the measurement of plasma SC-13504 after treatment with the various combinations should yield sufficient data for single-dose studies.

Patients with epilepsy are frequently treated with more than one anticonvulsant drug. The addition of one or more such drugs may improve seizure control but at the same time lead to the onset of drug side-effects or even increase seizure frequency: in both cases the measurement of plasma levels of the anticonvulsants can assist in the management of the patients' condition. Contradictory findings have been reported on the interaction of diphenylhydantoin with the benzodiazepines. Vajda *et al.* [2] showed that the addition of chlordiazepoxide or diazepam therapy to cardiac patients receiving diphenylhydantoin as an antiarrhythmic agent resulted in a rise in plasma levels of diphenylhydantoin, whilst Houghton and Richens [3] reported that the serum half-life of diphenylhydantoin decreased and the ratio of the main metabolite

DIAZEPAM 1mg/kg

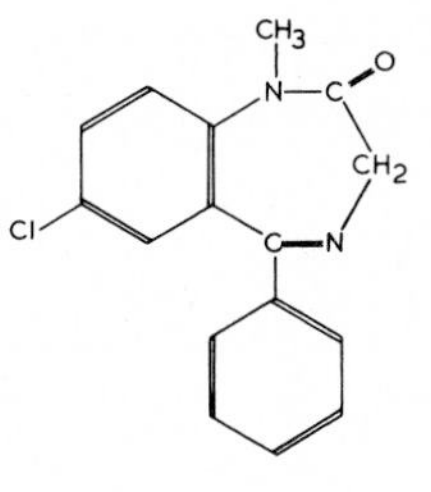

CLONAZEPAM 1mg/kg

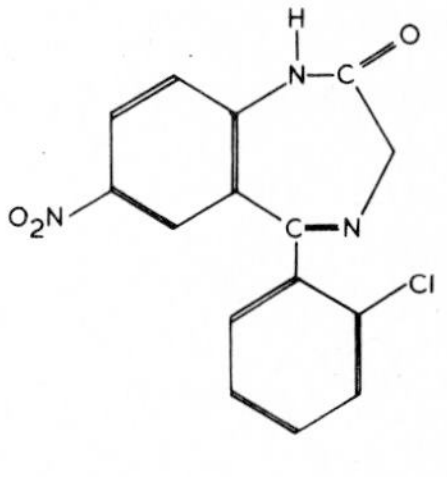

SC-13504 4mg/1kg

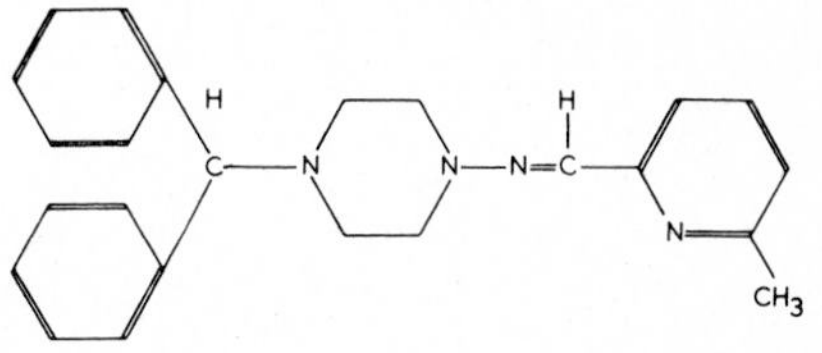

Table 1. Plasma levels of anticonvulsants required for the control of seizures.

COMPOUND	HUMAN EPILEPTICS: Steady-state plasma level, µg/ml	BABOONS — CONTROL OF I.L.S.-INDUCED MYOCLONIC SEIZURES: Plasma level after single i.v. dose, µg/ml [from ref. 8]
Ethosuximide	40-100 (spect.)*	80-90 (GC)
Phenobarbitone	20-45 (GC)	10-20 (GC)
Phenytoin	10-25 (GC)	35-40 (GC)
SC-13504	-	2-3 (polar)
Diazepam	0.25-1 (GC)	1.5-4 (GC)
Clonazepam	0.29-0.75 (GC)	0.25-0.75 (RIA)

* In parentheses: method of analysis (spect. = spectrophotometric, polar = polarographic).

of diphenylhydantoin to unchanged diphenylhydantoin increased on the addition of diazepam to the phenytoin treatment.

As in neither of these studies were the plasma levels of the benzodiazepines measured, and as interaction data on the benzodiazepines are meagre [4], it was decided to conduct a pilot study to test the feasibility of measuring plasma levels of two benzodiazepines used in epilepsy, diazepam and clonazepam, in the presence of a benzhydrylpiperazine, SC-13504. The method chosen was selective solvent extraction and differential pulse polarography, as all these compounds have a reducible azomethine moiety which could be used for quantification of the parent compounds [1]. SC-13504 has been shown to be an effective anticonvulsant in animal models of epilepsy [5-7], and in this study the drug was given singly or together with diazepam and clonazepam to 6 normal male rhesus monkeys by the intravenous route.

The sensitivity of the polarographic determination has been found adequate for measuring plasma levels of a number of anticonvulsants given chronically to human epileptics or of those found after single-dose administration to photosensitive baboon models of epilepsy [8] (Table 1). Although the polarographic sensitivity of standard solutions is very good, careful prior separation procedures are needed to maintain such sensitivity. Any biotransformation of a drug or compound near to the electroactive centre will alter the $E_{\frac{1}{2}}$ and give some selectivity; this coupled with careful selective solvent extraction can obviate the need for chromatographic techniques. Differential solvent extraction depends on the partitioning characteristics of these compounds and their metabolites at different buffer pH's. Data for diazepam and two of its metabolites have been reported by Zingales [9] (Table 2). A sensitivity comparison between GC and polarography is shown in Table 3.

METHOD (cf. Table 4)

Plasma samples from rhesus monkeys were obtained at 5, 15, 30, 60, 120 and 300 min after intravenous treatment with SC-13504 alone, diazepam and clonazepam alone, and SC-13504 plus either diazepam or clonazepam. The single dosages given were 4 mg/kg for SC-13504 and 1 mg/kg for diazepam and clorazepam; these were given in a random order. The plasma was kept at -20° until re-thawed to 37° just prior to analysis. A differential solvent extraction based on the findings of Barrett et al. [10] was developed for diazepam and clonazepam and some of their metabolites, and utilized for SC-13504: these compounds were extracted from plasma adjusted to pH 7.4 with phosphate buffer into petroleum ether b.p. range 40-60°, or into diethyl ether (Fig. 1), and then quantified by differential pulse polarography [1].

Table 2. Partition characteristics of diazepam and two of its metabolites. The values represent % extracted into toluene-*n*-heptane-isoamyl alcohol. [Adapted from ref. 9].

	BUFFER pH				
	2	4	7.4	9	12
Diazepam	65	78	95	100	100
N-desmethyl-diazepam	20	50	80	100	90
3-Hydroxy-diazepam	85	90	100	100	100

Table 3. Comparison of detection limits of anticonvulsants by differential pulse pola-polarography and GC-ECD.

ANTI-CONVULSANT	GC SENSITIVITY	POLAROGRAPHIC SENSITIVITY
Diazepam	10-20 ng/ml blood[*]	50-70 ng/ml plasma 10 ng/ml std. solution
Desmethyl-diazepam	20-40 ng/ml blood[*]	10 ng/ml std. solution
Clonazepam	0.5-1.0 ng/ml blood[†]	50-70 ng/ml plasma 10 ng/ml std. solution
SC-13504	6 ng/ml std. solution	30 ng/ml plas-plasma

[*] *measured as the benzophenone,*
[†] *measured as N-1-methylated derivative.*

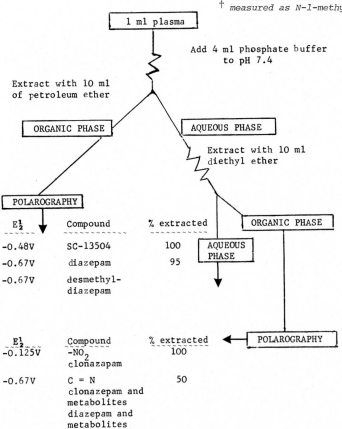

Fig. 1. Selective solvent extraction technique prior to polarographic determination of plasma levels of diazepam, clona-zepam and SC-13504.

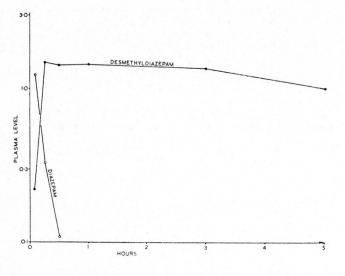

Fig. 2. Plasma
levels (µg/ml)
after i.v. adminis-
tration of diazepam
(1 mg/kg) to a
rhesus monkey.

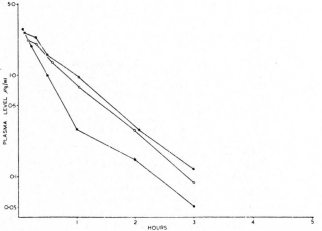

Fig. 3. Plasma
level of >C=N-group
in SC-13504 after
i.v. administration
to rhesus monkeys.
*Uppermost
curve:*
SC 13504 alone.
Middle curve:
SC 13504
  + clonazepam.
Bottom curve:
SC 13504
  + diazepam.

RESULTS

The method was found to be practical for determining diazepam and desmethyldiazepam
or SC-13504 alone and in the presence of diazepam and clonazepam. The disposition
of diazepam and desmethyldiazepam in a rhesus monkey after intravenous administration as measured by their plasma levels (Fig. 2) reflected the findings of Coutinho
et al. [11] in cynomologus monkeys given [^{14}C]diazepam orally.

Three rhesus monkeys received either SC-13504 alone, SC-13504 with diazepam,
or SC-13504 with clonazepam. The plasma levels of SC-13504 with these treatments
are shown in Fig. 3. The polarographic potential scans are shown from both a petroleum ether extraction (Fig. 4a) and a diethyl ether extraction (Fig. 4b) of plasma
from a monkey receiving both SC-13504 and diazepam. It was also observed that a

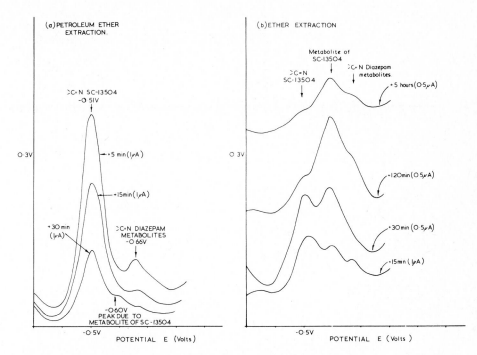

Fig. 4. Polarographic potential scans on material extracted by (a) petroleum ether or (b) diethyl ether from the plasma of a rhesus monkey given SC-13504 (4 mg/kg) and diazepam (1 mg/kg) i.v.

Table 4. Some relevant chemistry for bioanalysis of diazepam, clonazepam and SC-13504.

PARAMETER	DIAZEPAM	CLONAZEPAM	SC-13404
Relative molecular mass	285	316	370
Melting point	132-134°	238-240°	130-132°
pK_a	3.3	1.5 and 10.5	5.3
Partition coefficients: (i) $CHCl_3$/buffer at pH 7 (ii) *n*-octanol/phosphate buffer	1000 454	– 257	733 –
Protein binding	90% human albumin 96% human plasma	47% human albumin	

polarographic reduction wave from the ether extract which was considered due to an unknown metabolite of SC-13504 occurred earlier after treatment with SC-13504 together with diazepam of clonazepam than with SC-13504 alone.

DISCUSSION

The extraction method used was satisfactory for measuring SC-13504, diazepam and desmethyldiazepam; but the measurement of plasma levels of clonazepam metabolites

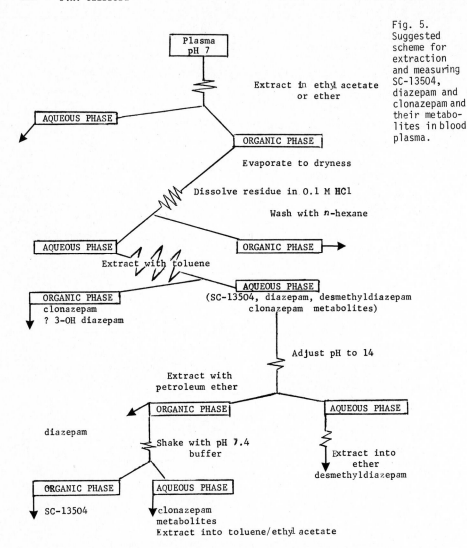

Fig. 5.
Suggested scheme for extraction and measuring SC-13504, diazepam and clonazepam and their metabolites in blood plasma.

was not so successful, especially in the presence of the metabolites of diazepam. A hypothetical scheme has therefore been elaborated, based on the method of Noestoft and Larsen [12] which would, it is thought, improve the selectivity of such a method for determination of the benzodiazepine metabolites (Fig. 5); but this has yet to be tested.

Acknowledgements

The analysis of the plasma samples by Malcolm Smyth of Chelsea College, London and the useful discussions on this methodology with him and Dr. Franklin-Smyth are gratefully acknowledged.

References

1. Smyth, M.R., Franklin-Smyth, W., Palmer, R.F. & Clifford, J.M., *Analyst* (1976) *in press.*

2. Vajda, F.J.E., Prineas, R.J. & Lovell, R.R.H., *Br. Med. J. 1* (1971) 346.

3. Houghton, G.W. & Richens, A., *Br. J. Clin. Pharmacol. 1* (1974) 344-345.

4. Kutt, H., *Epilepsia 16* (1975) 393-402.

5. Craig, C.R., *Arch. Int. Pharmacodyn. Therap. 165* (1967) 328-336.

6. Joy, R.M. & Edmonds, H.L., *Neuropharmacology 13* (1974) 145-147.

7. Killam, E.K., *Proc. West. Pharmacol. Soc. 17* (1974) 33-36.

8. Meldrum, B.S., Horton, R.W. & Toseland, P.A., *Arch. Neurol. 32* (1975) 289-294.

9. Zingales, I.A., *J. Chromatog. 75* (1973) 55-78.

10. Barrett, J., Franklin-Smyth, W. & Hart, J.P., *J. Pharm. Pharmacol. 26* (1974) 9-17.

11. Coutinho, C.B., Cheripko, J.A., Carbone, J.J., Manning, J.E. & Boff, E., *Xenobiotica 3* (1973) 681-690.

12. Noestoft, J. & Larsen, N.E., *J. Chromatog. 93* (1974) 113-122.

Analytical case history

NIFLUMIC ACID IN PLASMA AND URINE

T-7

T. Cowen and J.R. Salmon
*Squibb International Development Laboratory,
Moreton, Merseyside L46 1QW, U.K.*

Requirement   *A specific assay for plasma and urine samples containing levels
between 0 and 30 μg/ml, as encountered in bioavailability comparisons
of different formulations.*

Chemistry &   *Niflumic acid is a substituted 2-amino-nicotinic acid with high UV
metabolism   absorbance and no fluorescence. Metabolized extensively by hydroxylation.*

End-step   *HPLC on a C_{18} reverse-phase column with UV detection at 286 nm.*

Sample   *Extraction into diethyl ether from samples buffered to pH 4. The
preparation   ether evaporate is dissolved in the HPLC solvent and chromatographed.
100% recovery.*

Comments &   *Few or no interferences; metabolites well separated. Capable of per-
alternatives   forming 60 assays per day per instrument. HPLC assay was chosen
after problems with UV and GC assays previously developed within the
company.*

Body-fluid assays for pharmaceuticals may be required for several reasons. For
example, the bioavailabilities of different formulations containing the same drug
may have to be compared. Alternatively it may be required, in the clinic, to
tailor each individual's dosage regime according to both therapeutic effect and
body-fluid levels. This presentation deals with some of our experiences, within
the Squibb laboratories, in developing body-fluid assays for use in bioavailability
studies with the drug, niflumic acid.

Niflumic acid is a
nicotinic acid derivative
substituted in the 2 position by *m*-trifluoro methyl-
aniline. It falls into the
class of anti-inflammatory
drugs. It is both well absorbed and extensively
metabolized. Metabolism
occurs largely by hydroxylation in both the 5 and
the 4 positions in the
molecule [1]. These meta-
bolites are also subse-
quently conjugated with
either sulphate or glucuronic acid. Radioactive tracer experiments, using $[^{14}C]$-
labelled material, have shown that the parent molecule and the metabolites are
relatively slowly eliminated [2]; most of the drug is excreted in the conjugated
form. —

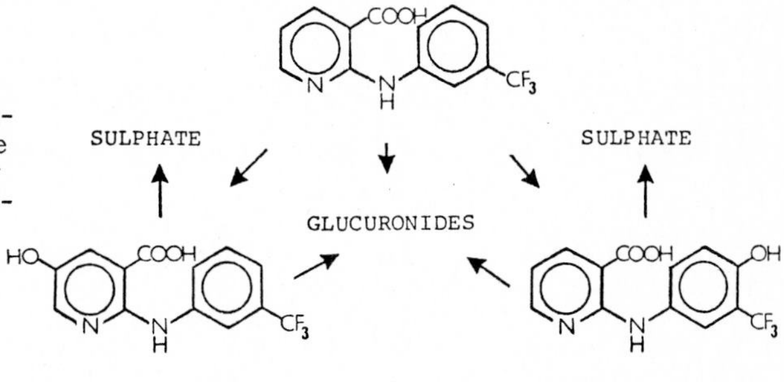

    URINE: 40% of dose after 48 h; 75% conjugated.

    FAECES: 30% of dose after 72 h; 25-50% conjugated.

Development of assay methods for drugs in body fluids can, in many cases, depend upon the situation in which they are required. If the requirement is for a relatively small number of assays, <100, then highly sophisticated methods such as GC-MS can often be considered. However, many bioavailability studies, especially double-blind cross-over studies, can easily generate 1000 or more samples. In these situations the type of assay developed is largely governed by speed and ease of use. Thus in many cases an assay involving a suitably simple extraction followed by either UV or fluorescence measurement often represents the ideal.

The relevant physical properties one needs to consider in these cases are UV spectrum, fluorescence spectrum and pH-partition behaviour. Niflumic acid has a high UV absorbance which lends itself to either a simple UV assay or a chromatographic assay with UV detection: λ_{max} 286 nm; $E_{1\ cm}^{1\%}$ = 1070.
There is no native fluorescence. The isoelectric point lies at pH 4 when the aqueous solubility is, typically, a few $\mu g/ml$.

ASSAYS PREVIOUSLY DEVELOPED

Several assay procedures had already been developed within the company. These methods were re-evaluated for use with bioavailability studies being carried out during 1975. The first procedure (Fig. 1) was a UV assay which had previously been used with dog plasma samples [3]. The procedure involved extraction of niflumic acid into diethyl ether at about pH 1. The drug was then back-extracted into sodium hydroxide, in which solution the UV absorbance was measured. The method required an extracted standard because the pH was wrong for optimum partition and some metabolites were co-extracted. Additional problems with variable blanks showed the procedure to be very sensitive to haemolysis.

In order to confer greater specificity on the method, a GC method was developed (Fig. 2). This involved chromatographing niflumic acid as its trimethyl-silyl ester [4]. Serum samples were extracted at pH 2 with ether. The ether layer was removed and evaporated. The residue was then treated with BSA as silylating reagent in carbon disulphide. Di-n-butyl phthalate was added as internal standard (Fig. 3).

This procedure also suffered from several drawbacks. Firstly, the recovery was low because the pH used for extraction was not optimal. This necessitated the use of through-process standards. Secondly, the chromatography was prone to interference which gave rise to poor baseline stability and extraneous peaks.

HPLC ASSAY

Further work with niflumic acid formulations resulted in a bioavailability study for which about 600 plasma and urine samples would require assay. Re-evaluation of the previously mentioned procedures showed them to be neither reliable nor rapid enough for this particular application.

Thoughts were turned towards the possible use of HPLC as a means of developing a rapid, interference-free assay. A reversed-phase separation was the first method of choice. Our laboratory had developed methods for chemically bonding stable C_{18} coatings onto silica gels such as 'Merckosorb' and 'Partisil'. These were packed into 250 × 4.6 mm i.d. columns using a balanced density slurry. These columns provide a great deal of versatility in the range of sample types that can be separated.

Most of our work on reversed-phase columns involves the use of acetonitrile/water mixtures. In general these give greater efficiency than methanol/water mixtures. Occasionally, with difficult separations, it is advantageous to use acetonitrile/methanol/water mixtures. The conditions finally chosen, with a C_{18} treated 'Partisil 10' column as above, were elution with a 40 : 60 (v/v) mixture of acetoni-

trile and 0.017 M, pH
7, phosphate buffer,
run at 1 ml/min; the
sample (5 µl) was
applied with a SGE
10BL RD3 syringe
and septum injector,
and peaks were mea-
sured at 286 nm with
a UV detector (Cecil
Insts., Model 212).

Niflumic acid
was eluted within
four min using this
system (Fig. 4). It
was shown to be well
separated from known
metabolites which
appeared at or near
the solvent front.

The extrac-
tion procedure was
modified to improve
the recovery (Fig.
5). A 1 ml sample
of plasma or urine
is buffered to pH 4
then saturated with
potassium chloride.
This is extracted
with ether (8 ml).
An aliquot of the
ether layer (5 ml)
is taken and eva-
porated to dryness.
The residue is dis-
solved in the HPLC
eluting solvent
ready for injec-
tion onto the
column. Injec-
tions (5 µl) of
sample solution
and of a suitable

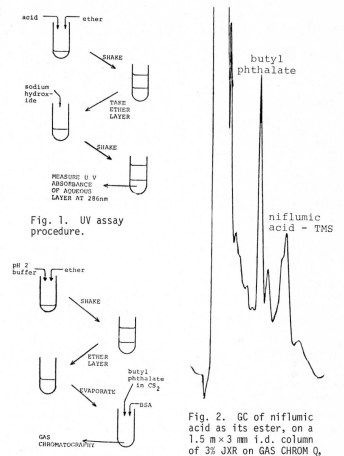

Fig. 1. UV assay
procedure.

Fig. 3. GC assay. 'BSA'
denotes *N,O*-bis(trimethylsilyl)acetamide.

Fig. 2. GC of niflumic
acid as its ester, on a
1.5 m × 3 mm i.d. column
of 3% JXR on GAS CHROM Q,
run at 215° with 40 ml/
min nitrogen.

standard solution, prepared in the HPLC solvent, are made and the niflumic acid
content determined by peak height measurement. Inclusion of an internal standard
was not found necessary since replicate injections generally gave agreement within
±1%. The procedure was shown to give 100% recovery of niflumic acid spiked into
plasma or urine samples. No interfering components were found when blank plasma
and urine samples were examined. Urine samples generally showed much lower niflumic acid contents (Fig. 6) because of extensive metabolism. Modification of the
eluting solvent enables further separation of the metabolites. Thus it may be
possible to look for these specifically.

Many problems were found when large numbers of samples were processed
through the same column. These were usually associated with the build-up of
sample debris at the head of the column. This could usually be overcome by
washing the column successively with methanol and chloroform. When the back-
pressure became excessive, it was found necessary to repack the column head.

Fig. 4 *(on right)*. HPLC separation of niflumic acid *(arrow)* in a
plasma extract on a C_{18} column. *For conditions, see text.*

Injections were made into the centre of a porous teflon plug which
was separated from the column packing by a 5 mm layer of glass
beads (Fig. 7). When necessary the teflon plug and the glass beads
were replaced. This usually restored the column's performance to
its previous level.

The performance of the assay is summarized in Table 1.
Precision was estimated from results from a series of operators
over several days. Replicate injections from the same solution
gave agreement within ±1%.

Some typical results are illustrated. Fig. 8 shows differences observed when subjects are fasted or fed prior to taking a
capsule formulation. Fig. 9 shows differences between a good
formulation and one that did not release niflumic acid very efficiently.

(on left)

Fig. 6. HPLC separation of
niflumic acid *(arrow)* in a
urine extract. *The early
material (twin peak) is
attributable to metabolites.*

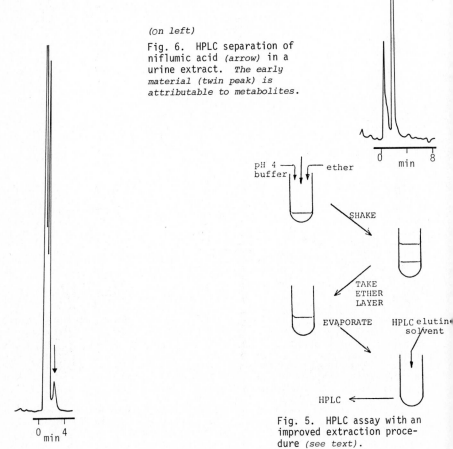

Fig. 5. HPLC assay with an
improved extraction procedure *(see text)*.

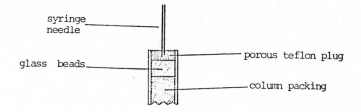

syringe needle

glass beads

porous teflon plug

column packing

Fig. 7.
Head of
column
assembly,
showing
mode of
injection
(see text).

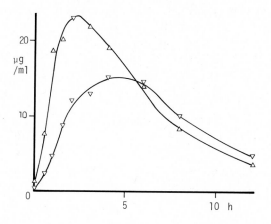

Fig. 8. Plasma levels
following ingestion of a
capsule formulation by
fasted (Δ) or fed (∇)
subjects.

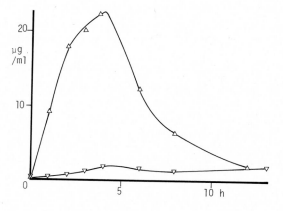

Fig. 9. Plasma levels
in a comparison of two
formulations, Δ and ∇.

Table 1.   Performance characteristics of the HPLC assay.

FEATURE	CAPABILITY
applicability	niflumic acid in human plasma and urine
efficiency	101% recovery
bias	+0.6 µg/ml
precision	±0.7 µg/ml S.D.
range	0-30 µg/ml
specificity	separates known metabolites
assay time	up to 60 samples per day manually

References

1. Cohen, A.I., Weliky, I., Lan, S.J. & Levine, S.D., *Biomed. Mass Spectrom. 1* (1974) 1-4.

2. Lan, S.J., Chando, T.J., Weliky, I. & Schreiber, E.C., *J. Pharmacol. Exp. Ther. 186* (1973) 323-330.

3. Heald, A.F., Squibb *internal communication.*

4. Evans, J.R., Squibb *internal communication.*

Analytical case history

T-8

HALQUINOL IN ANIMAL FEEDS: AN EXERCISE IN ASSAY DESIGN

J.E. Fairbrother
Squibb International Development Laboratory,
Moreton, Merseyside L46 1QW, U.K.

Requirement *Assay of halquinol (chlorhydroxyquinoline) in pig feeds down to*
120 µg/g; values must include chelated complexes; must be specific
in presence of other feed additives.

Chemistry *A mixture of mono- and dichloro-substituted oxines; strong UV absor-*
bance. Halquinol chelates strongly with most metal ions especially
transition metals (Cu, Zn, Mn are common additives to most feeds). Cu
chelate has rather low solubility and is very stable. Several
chelates show high fluorescence yield.

End-step *GC, after silylation.*

Sample *Chloroform-extracted material in n-hexane transferred to an aqueous*
preparation *phase and back-extracted into dichloromethane.*

Comments & *Bearing on assay development for drugs in body fluids, some problems*
alternatives *were now encountered:*
- extraction from the feed including all chelated material;
- separation from co-extracted interfering substances without allowing
  chelates to re-form.
- specific quantitation of the three individual components with good
  recovery and precision (halquinol is even lost by chelation with
  metal in the needle of the syringe used for GC).
Consideration is given in the text to other conceivable approaches.

In this presentation I wish to share our experiences and frustrations in the development of an assay procedure for halquinol in pig feeds.

Although this may seem a strange case study to examine in the context of drug
assay in body fluids, I think the lessons to be learned are quite pertinent. As will
become evident, we started our work in this area of feed assay with very little previous experience. We knew a reasonable amount about our drug substance but we were
eventually to learn much more. We came to feel that those who seek to develop assays
without enough background study are often destined to waste a good deal of time.

Halquinol is a mixture of
chlorinated oxines. As in the case
of oxine, its parent compound, it
is a very strong chelating agent
and many of the chelates formed
are relatively insoluble.

The feeds we initially
examined were piglet creep and
grower rations. Halquinol was
added at a level of 600 g/ton
(∿590µg/g) in order to control
scouring in young pigs. These
feeds contain various meal materials and added supplements and
medicaments (Table 1).

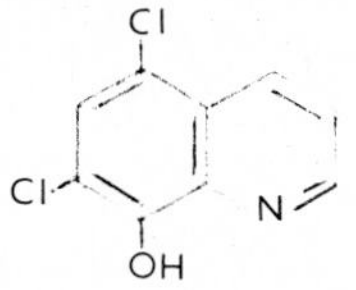

57 – 74 %

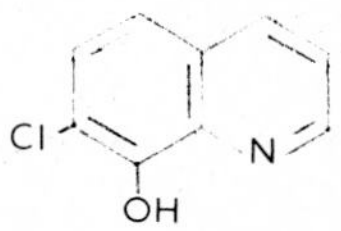

∌4 %

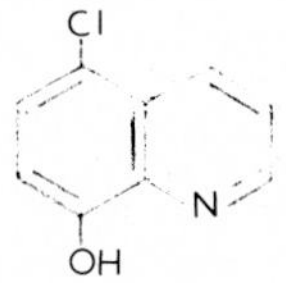

23 – 40 %

ASSAY IN FEED (600 μg/g)

Initially we wanted a simple assay to measure compounding accuracy of halquinol in feed, and our attempts were directed towards the development of a rapid and uncomplicated procedure. Possible approaches are now summarized.

Spectrophotometry

Several years earlier we had success-fully used UV spectrophotometry to determine halquinol in a milo pre-mix containing 2% halquinol. The halquinol was extracted with chloro-form and the absorbance measured at 365 nm. When such a procedure was scrutinized, very high and variable blank values for the feed were obtained.

Table 1. Pig grower rations.

Meals	Minerals & Vitamins	Medicaments
Wheat	Ca	Cu (200 ppm)
Barley	P	Arsanilic Acid
Fish	Fe	Dimetridazole
Meat	Zn	Nitrovin
Bone	Cu	Carbadox
Soya	Mn	Virginiamycin
Peanut	Vitamins A,D Vitamin B (group)	

Halquinol had also been determined in the milo pre-mix using the green colour of the halquinol-Fe chelate formed on the addition of $FeCl_3$ in acetone/$CHCl_3$. High and variable blanks were again obtained.

Polarography

The basis was a continuous liquid/liquid extraction system originally designed for the determination of halquinol in blood. It depended on partitioning between iso-octane and an aqueous pH 6 phase containing EDTA. Samples of feed were extracted with dilute acid. The acid extracts were more strongly acidified to break the che-late, EDTA was added, and the pH was adjusted to 6. This solution was then parti-tioned with iso-octane in a liquid/liquid continuous extractor for three hours. The iso-octane extract was cooled and partitioned with 1 N HCl.

The HCl extract was examined polarographically, and showed peaks at -0.78 and -0.88 volts corresponding to the dichloro- and monochloro - components. Recove-ries of about 60% were obtained, and problems were encountered with the formation of a foam at the interface between the iso-octane and aqueous layers; the foam could not be adequately suppressed even with silicone anti-foam. Attempts to use the same system with manual separation in separating funnels gave emulsions which could not be completely broken even on centrifuging.

Chelatometry

Attempts to quantitatively precipitate halquinol as its copper chelate were unsatis-factory due to other interactions of the Cu with extracted components from the feed.

Our lack of success gave us much frustration; but with hindsight our initial work on the UV assay which gave such high blank values was far too superficial, and we moved on to try other approaches far too quickly.

Fluorimetry (Fig. 1)

Fluorimetry had been tried before, and we had estab-lished the sensitivity and selectively of the fluori-metric response of the Mg and Al chelates.

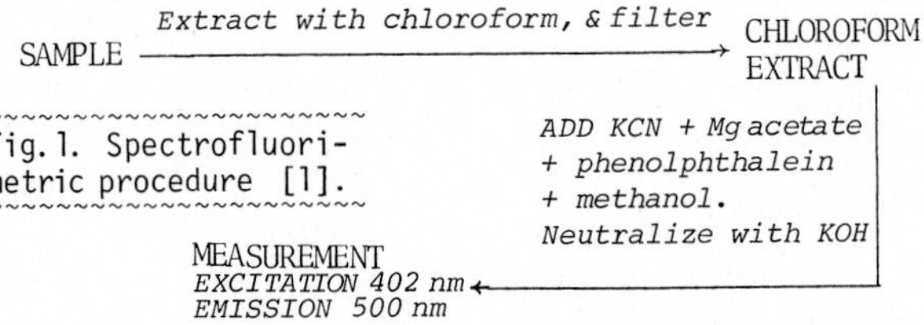

SAMPLE —— *Extract with chloroform, & filter* ——→ CHLOROFORM EXTRACT

Fig. 1. Spectrofluori-metric procedure [1].

ADD KCN + Mg acetate
+ phenolphthalein
+ methanol.
Neutralize with KOH

MEASUREMENT
EXCITATION 402 nm
EMISSION 500 nm

Low recoveries were obtained by fluorimetry. This was puzzling until it was realized that the chloroform extracts of the feed were slightly acidic and that this greatly reduced the fluorescence yield of the Mg/halquinol chelate. The neutralization of this non-aqueous extract was achieved by incorporating phenol-phthalein into the solution, without causing interference in the procedure.

The trace metals extracted from the feed, particularly Cu, prevented some of the halquinol from forming the Mg chelate. This was overcome by suppressing the Cu and the other heavy metal ions with cyanide.

ASSAY IN FEED (120 μg/g) [2]

Shortly after the development of this procedure a new and more extensive use of the product was introduced, namely the inclusion of 120 g halquinol per ton of feed as a growth-promoter. This involved a wider range of grower and finisher rations.

UV spectrophotometric assay

In the fluorimetric assay the feed gave blank values too high by ∿30%, and also the relative proportions of halquinol to copper caused greater extraction problems. The previously rejected UV spectrophotometric procedure was re-evaluated. Chloroform was still found to be the best solvent for the extraction of halquinol from the feed whilst extracting a minimum of interfering substances. It was found that in chloroform solution the conversion of halquinol to the Cu chelate was rapid. The copper chelate although less soluble than halquinol at least did not crystallize from solution in chloroform, as had been found with diethyl ether, acetone, dioxan and ethyl acetate.

It was decided to try to clean up the chloroform extract and also to break up the chelate by back-extracting the halquinol into strong acid. However, *shaking* the chloroform extract with 2 N sulphuric acid gave emulsions and an unfavourable partitioning of the halquinol. Efforts to overcome these problems established that although halquinol is a mixture of volatile phenols it was possible to rotary-eva-porate the chloroform extracts without significant loss of halquinol. The residue could then be dissolved in *n*-hexane and the halquinol partitioned between the hexane and 2 N sulphuric acid (15 : 85) with quantitative transfer of the halquinol to the acid layer. To form the Mg chelate for fluorimetric determination required neutralization of this solution; hence UV absorption was examined as an alternative. Measurement of absorbance at 258.5 nm gave a measure of the halquinol in the acid extract; but interference from co-extracted feed components was of the order of 10%. The absorption curve for the feed blank showed a very broad absorption peak, where-as that for halquinol was relatively sharp; thus it was possible to compensate for the feed blank by subtracting the absorption obtained at 290 nm. Using this pro-cedure gave acceptable recoveries (∿95%).

We now had a workable assay; but it did not show the individual components of halquinol, and could in no way be considered a stability assay.

GC assay

A number of GC procedures had been described for substituted oxines, and it was found that by silylation of halquinol a separation of its main components 5,7-di-chloro-oxine and 5-chloro-oxine could be achieved on a column of 5% JXR on Gas Chrom Q at 175° (Fig. 2a). This system did not separate the 5-chloro and 7-chloro oxines; but the low level of 7-chloro-oxine in halquinol rendered this relatively unimportant, and it was decided to attempt to determine the combined mono-chloro oxines. Chloroform extraction of halquinol from the feed gave a considerable degree of conversion of the halquinol into the Cu chelate, and the chelate did not present the free hydroxyl group of halquinol for silylation.

Accordingly, the lengthy back-extraction procedure used in the above UV assay was tried. The final acid extract was treated with EDTA and neutralized to pH 7, and the halquinol back-extracted into dichloromethane. It was found that the copper chelate was more rapidly dissociated in perchloric acid than in sulphuric acid, and therefore perchloric acid was adopted.

The dichloromethane was rotary-evaporated and the residue silylated with BSA. This procedure gave low recoveries, and it was found that this was due to loss of halquinol by volatilization during the evaporation of the dichloromethane. This problem was overcome (Fig 3) by adding the BSA before evaporation.

This procedure gave good recoveries of dichloroxine (∿94%) and monochloroxine (∿104%) from feed, and the combined results agreed with those obtained by the UV assay procedure (Table 2). In some cases, however, recoveries of 80-90% have been obtained from certain feeds with both the UV and GC procedures. This could be due to protein binding, and alternative extraction procedures are currently being examined to overcome this problem.

Possible variants

More recently [3] it has been found that the 5-chloro and 7-chloro-oxine can be resolved after silylation on a column of 5% OV225 at 165° (Fig. 2b),

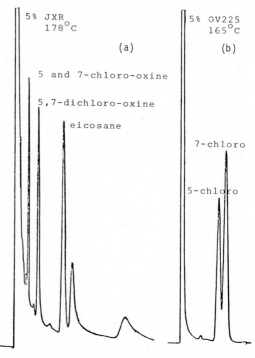

Fig. 2. GC of halquinol (BSA-silylated), with the oven set at (a) 178°, (b) 165°.

Table 2. Comparison of UV and GC assay values (μg/g) for halquinol added as a spike to feeds.

Sample	UV assay, *TOTAL*	GC assay		
		TOTAL	*Monochloro* components	*Dichloro* components
1	110	115	30	85
2	105	107	29	78
3	112	116	39	77
4	94	92	34	58

and that the GC method can be improved by changing the GC conditions to allow separate determination of the 7-chloro-oxine component.

A simpler approach might be the HPLC determination of halquinol in the chloroform extract obtained directly from the feed. This approach is now being evaluated.

References

1. Fairbrother, J.E. & Heyes, W.F., *Analyst 98* (1973) 797-801.

2. Cowen, T. & Heyes, W.F., *Analyst 101* (1976), *in press*.

3. Wood, P.R., *private (Squibb) communication*.

T-9

THE DETERMINATION OF IRGASAN(R) DP300 IN BIOLOGICAL FLUIDS

D.R. Hoar and D.J. Sissons
Unilever Research Colworth/Welwyn Laboratory,
Colworth House, Sharnbrook, Bedford, MK44 ILQ, U.K.

Requirement	*Irgasan(R) DP300 in blood, urine and bile at 25 µg/l; both free and conjugated forms must be measured.*
Chemistry & metabolism	*Diphenyl ether containing 3 chlorine atoms and a hydroxyl group. The parent compound is stable to acid but the conjugate, the glucuronide in the rat, is easily hydrolyzed by acid.*
End-step	*GC with ECD.*
Sample preparation	*Free form extracted from buffered solution with diethyl ether. Conjugate hydrolyzed by 60% sulphuric acid and then extracted with hexane/acetone.*
Comments	*Method has sensitivity of 2 µg/l but background blank level limits practical sensitivity to 10 µg/l.*
	In comparison with enzymic hydrolysis (entailing final extraction at an acid pH), acid hydrolysis of the conjugate is an improvement in respect of speed and effectiveness. Radiochemical checking shows reproducible recoveries, 95-105% for free form and 80-95% for conjugate.

Diverse analytical techniques have been used for the separation, detection and estimation of trace substances in extracts of biological origin. Many methods, whilst extremely sensitive to standard solutions, lack specificity when applied to biological substrates. The determination of low levels of germicides in biological fluids is no exception, and requires an effective clean-up procedure and/or a highly specific detection system.

The germicide Irgasan DP300, 2-hydroxy-2',4,4'-trichlorodiphenyl ether (Ciba Geigy), has found increasing use in recent years in toilet preparations. It has been shown [1] to be rapidly metabolised *in vivo* and to be excreted predominantly as the glucuronide. Any procedure for the determination of DP300 in biological fluids must therefore be capable of estimating both free and conjugated forms of the germicide. This paper gives details of the development of such a procedure which was initially devised for the analysis of human and rat blood but was subsequently applied to urine and to fish tissues and bile.

ASSAY METHODS
Determination of free DP300

1. Add 2 ml of pH 2.2 phosphate/citrate buffer to 1 ml of K-EDTA stabilized blood.
2. Freeze the homogenized mixture in a dry-ice bath at -20° and allow to thaw at room temperature.
3. Extract the mixture successively with 3 × 10 ml diethyl ether, shaking vigorously for 2-3 min on each occasion.
4. Carefully evaporate the bulked extract to 1 ml for GC analysis.

Determination of total DP300

1. Carefully add 5 ml of 60% sulphuric acid (60 ml concentrated acid diluted to 100 ml with water) to 1 ml K-EDTA stabilized blood. Mix well between incremental addition to avoid 'spitting'.
2. Heat for 30 min in a water bath at 60°.
3. Cool the mixture and extract successively with 3 × 10 ml hexane/acetone mixture (9:1 by vol), shaking vigorously for 2-3 min on each occasion.
4. Carefully evaporate the bulked extract to 1 ml.
5. Shake the extract with 1 ml of pH 6.0 phosphate/citrate buffer and allow phases to separate.
6. Analyze the upper hexane layer by GC.

GC analysis

A Pye series 104 gas chromatograph fitted with a 2.1 m × 4 mm i.d. glass column containing 2.5% w/w of both SE30 and QF1 and 0.02% w/w Epikote resin on 80-100 mesh Aeropak 30 was used with a ^{63}Ni electron-capture detector under the following conditions: column temp., 215°; detector temp., 300°; carrier gas: nitrogen at 60 ml/min; purge gas: nitrogen at 40 ml/min.

METHOD DEVELOPMENT

Extraction of free DP300

DP300 is readily soluble in hexane, and this solvent forms the basis of at least one method [2] for the extraction of free DP300 from blood. Complete recovery of DP300 from water can be demonstrated with a single hexane extraction. However when added to 1 ml of whole blood *in vitro*, the recovery of DP300 in a single extraction with 10 ml of hexane was only 50%. Exhaustive extraction increased this recovery only to 65%, which suggested that DP300 was rapidly fixed in blood, even *in vitro*. This was probably due to protein binding; hence a standard freeze-thaw step was introduced to minimize this effect. The use of a more polar solvent coupled with exhaustive extraction was, however, preferable; but care had to be taken not to co-extract any additional more polar interfering material that would require an extra clean-up step prior to GC analysis. Stretz and Stahr [3] overcame the problem of releasing bound forms of insecticide residues in blood by the addition of 60% (w/v) sulphuric acid prior to extraction with hexane/acetone (9:1 by vol). We compared this technique to exhaustive extraction with either hexane or diethyl ether, and obtained the data presented in Table 1.

The results confirmed the unsuitability of hexane as extracting solvent, but indicated that either direct extraction with diethyl ether or extraction following the addition of strong acid were suitable for complete recovery of DP300 added *in vitro*. When these procedures were applied to the determination of free DP300 in blood withdrawn from rats 2-6 h after they had been intubated with universally tritium-labelled DP300, the data in Table 2 were obtained. The total [^{3}H-]DP300 content of the blood was determined by duplicate combustion of 0.1 ml aliquots in a Packard 305 sample oxidizer and counting the dispensed samples in a Packard 4322 liquid scintillation counter.

Ether extracts were shown [4] by TLC analysis to contain all the extractable free DP300 together with <5% of the conjugated form, which would not be detected by GC analysis. However, the extract of the acidified blood contained much higher levels of DP300, due to hydrolysis of approximately 60% of the conjugate form. Complete extraction of free DP300 was shown to be achieved with 3 × 10 ml diethyl ether, and this forms the basis of the procedure developed for blood analysis.

Extraction of total DP300

In view of the signifi-
cant level of deconjuga-
tion of DP300 that
occurred in the·presence
of cold acid (Table 2),
the effect of both acid
concentration and heating
time were examined using
blood from rats intuba-
ted with [³H-]DP300. The
results in Table 3 show
that the extent of de-
conjugation of bound
DP300 increased with both
acid concentration and
the duration of heating
at 60°. The level of
background interference
that produced GC peaks in
the vicinity of that for
DP300 also increased with
heating time. This
interference was negli-

Table 1. Recovery of DP300 added to blood *(in vitro)*.

| Level of addition, μg/ml | *Mean recovery (%) by each extraction procedure* | | |
	Hexane	Diethyl ether	Acid/ hexane-acetone
100	75	105	99
10	67	95	97

Table 2. Determination of free DP300 after intubation.

Procedure	DP300, mg/l	% of total counts
Scintillation counting	5.9	(100)
Diethyl ether extraction pH 2.2	0.65	11
Acid desorption	3.7	6.3

gible after 0.5 h but would have assumed significance with low level analysis after
heating periods of 1 h or more. It was therefore decided to adopt an 0.5 h heating
period at 60° and, in order to minimize the strength of sulphuric acid handled, to
hydrolyze in 9 M acid.

The acid hydrolysis, performed at 60° for 0.5 h in 9 M sulphuric acid, was
compared with an enzymic hydrolysis using β-glucuronidase/aryl sulphatase (Calbio-
chem). The enzyme solution in pH 4.5 buffer was added to blood and incubated for
16 h at 37°. Preliminary experiments confirmed that, following enzymic hydrolysis,
low recoveries (60%) were obtained after exhaustive extraction with hexane. Accordingly, to reduce protein-binding effects, the hydrolysate was acidified prior to
extraction. This precluded the use of diethyl ether as extractant due to solva-
tion effects in the strong acid which resulted in poor separation; therefore the
hexane/acetone system was used. Complete recovery of [³H-]DP300 was obtained by
either enzymatic hydrolysis (98%) or acid hydrolysis (104%), on the basis of the
counts for oxidized blood samples.

Gas chromatography

Various stationary phases were investigated for GC analysis of DP300. The mixed
SE30/QF1 system was preferred, as it gave the best resolution from trace impurities
present in the solvents and from a low level of background co-extractives from
blood. Sensitivity and specificity were better with ECD then with FID. Under the
conditions detailed, DP300 gave a well-shaped peak at a retention time of 5 min, a
detection limit of <10 pg, corresponding to a sample detection limit of 2 μg/l in
blood or urine, and a linear dynamic range of up to 250 pg. Other workers have [2]
preferred to derivatize DP300 prior to analysis. We prepared the acetyl derivative;
but the slightly increased response and shorter retention time did not, in our
opinion, justify the extra process time or the increased risk of losses.

Interferences with GC analysis

During the course of the investigation it was noted that on occasions the GC column
deteriorated throughout the day, that the baseline became temporarily very unstable

Table 3. Effect of acid concentration and time of heating at 60° on recovery of DP300 from blood (after intubation).

Sulphuric acid concentration (M)	Recovery (%) after heating, h						
	0	0.25	0.5	0.75	1	1.5	2
3		23					
6		30					
7.5		50					
9	59	73	92	94	98	102	96
9.8		90					

and that the plunger of the injection syringe became increasingly difficult to move smoothly in the barrel. These effects were shown to be due to variable carry-over of sulphuric acid into extracts from the total DP300 method. Shaking with an equal volume of water removed this excess of acid from most, but not all, of the offending extracts. Neutralization of extracts with dilute alkali was a tedious and risky procedure, as formation of the phenate and its extraction into the aqueous phase readily occurred if the pH was allowed to rise over 7. Satisfactory removal was most readily achieved without loss of DP300 by shaking with an equal volume of citrate/phosphate buffer pH 6. This step is included in the final method.

Throughout the investigation, variable levels of DP300 (5-25 µg/1) were apparently detected in chromatograms of blood samples from animals maintained on a germicide-free diet. The contaminant was also present at a similar level in reagent blanks, irrespective of whether or not the solvents were purified by distillation prior to use. Using MS we confirmed that the contaminant peak was DP300. The source of contamination was identified as the liquid soap dispensed in our washrooms, which contains 2% added DP300. Efforts were made to ensure that technicians involved in DP300 analysis did not use this liquid soap or any other product known to be formulated with the germicide; but this unfortunately did not completely remove the background interference. Consequently the practical sensitivity of the procedure in our experience is limited to 10 µg/1 blood.

GC-MS analysis

GC-MS has been used with single ion monitoring as a highly specific means of confirming DP300 levels in some sample extracts. The second isotope parent ion at 289.95 m/e was chosen for the analysis, as it was more abundant than the first isotope parent ion and associated with a lower level of background interference. The sensitivity of the procedure was, however, much lower than that using ECD, viz. 1 ng DP300 compared with 10 pg. Satisfactory agreement amongst the three methods presented in this paper for determining total DP300 residues in blood is evident from Table 4.

CONCLUSIONS

Enzymic hydrolysis is usually preferred to acid hydrolysis for deconjugation, since the latter lacks specificity and often gives artefacts: e.g. mercapturic acids are formed from 'premercapturic acids', phenols are formed from cyclohexadiene-dihydro-diols and steroids are partially degraded [5]. We have shown that either the acid hydrolysis method, or the enzymic hydrolysis method followed by addition of acid, gives good agreement with results obtained by scintillation counting and by GC-MS. In practice we have preferred the acid hydrolysis procedure as it is

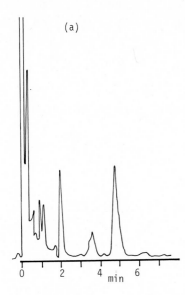

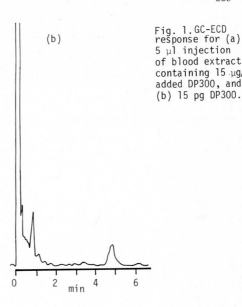

Fig. 1. GC-ECD response for (a) 5 μl injection of blood extract containing 15 μg/l added DP300, and (b) 15 pg DP300.

quicker, allowing a result within 1.5 h, and generally gives a slightly higher recovery. Cleaner chromatograms (Fig. 1) are also obtained since sulphuric acid sulphonates troublesome material, particularly unsaturated compounds [3].

Table 4. Analysis of [³H-]DP300 in blood by three different methods.

Level of addition μg/l	Replicate No.	Scintillation counting	GC-MS	GC-ECD
1000	1	1020	1030	940
	2	1050	1125	1030
	3	1050	970	925
100	1	114	109	93
	2	104	96	92

The methods have been used to measure the proportions of free and conjugated forms in both human and rat blood and urine. In all the samples the proportions of free and conjugate forms were ∿10% and ∿90% respectively. Enzymic hydrolysis of an extract of fish bile releases free DP300, supporting the evidence of Lech [6] that some fish do have the biochemical mechanism necessary for glucuronide synthesis.

Acknowledgements

We wish to acknowledge the work of Mr. C.T. James in synthesizing the labelled material and of Mr. E. Hammond in obtaining the radiochemical data; Dr. J. Schultze of Ciba Geigy gave us information in advance of publication.

References

1. Black, J.G., Howes, D. & Rutherford, T., *Toxicology 3* (1975) 33-47.

2. Schultze, J., Marquardt, F., Lyman, F. & Spitzer, C., *J. Am. Oil. Chem. Soc.* *52* (1975) 215-218.

3. Stretz, P.E. & Stahr, H.M., *J. Assoc. Offic. Anal. Chem. 56* (1973) 1173-1177.

4. Black, J.G. & Howes, D., *in preparation.*

5. Parke, D.V. *The Biochemistry of Foreign Compounds,* Pergamon, Oxford (1968) pp. 8, 41 & 81.

6. Lech, J.J., *Toxicol. Appl. Pharmacol. 24* (1973) 114-124.

Analytical case history

T-10 MICROBIOLOGICAL ASSAY OF CEPHRADINE IN BLOOD AND URINE

Thomas C. Forster
Squibb International Development Laboratories
Moreton, Merseyside L46 1QW, U.K.

Requirement	*Assay of cephradine in blood and urine by a microbiological procedure.*
Chemistry & metabolism	*A semi-synthetic cephalosporin, 7-D(-)-2-amino-2-(1,4-cyclohex-adlein-1-yl)acetoamido-3-methyl-8-oxo-5-thia-1-azabicyclo(4.2.0)oct-2-ene-2-carboxylic acid, hydrate. Cephradine remains unchanged in the body, and no metabolite is formed; 6% protein-bound.*
End-step	*Agar-diffusion microbiological assay (modified from [1]) with part-automation.*
Sample preparation	*Direct dilution of serum and urine in 0.1 M phosphate buffer pH 6.0.*
Comments & alternatives	*Non-specific for cephradine using test strain organism* Sarcina lutea *ATCC 9345. Sensitivity 0.055 µg/ml in serum, 3.0 µg/ml in urine. Recoveries good and reproducible as assessed by spiked control samples. Other methods available: fluorimetric, iodometric.*

Although many chemical and physico-chemical methods are available for the assay of antibiotics, the microbiological assay has been and still is the method of choice for the determination of antibiotics in pharmaceutical preparations, in formulations undergoing long-term stability tests, and in biological fluids and materials. Cephradine is no exception to this, and this presentation highlights the method used in our laboratory for the assay of this antibiotic along with data obtained for blood and urine using this methodology.

Cephradine is a semi-synthetic cephalosporin, being a cyclohexadienyl derivative of 7-amino-cephalosporinanic acid. It is a white crystalline powder, freely soluble in water, sparingly soluble in acetone and ethanol, and virtually insoluble in diethyl ether and chloroform. It has a broad spectrum of bactericidal activity *in vitro*, and has been shown to be highly effective against many Gram-positive and Gram-negative organism infections when administered orally or parenterally. This antibiotic has also been shown to have the advantage of rapid absorption by both routes, to be only 5-6% protein bound and to give optimum excretion rates; 98% is excreted unchanged in the urine within 24 h [2].

ASSAY APPROACH

Cephradine may be assayed in a variety of ways, e.g. iodometric, fluorometric, hydroxylamine, and microbiological. As mentioned earlier, however, the microbiological assay is the preferred method and conforms with registration and legal requirements for data derived from bioavailability studies. It is, therefore, the method used in our laboratories.

There are in turn diverse microbiological assays, but they are normally divided into two categories — agar diffusion, and turbidimetric. Because of the system within our laboratories we rely almost entirely on agar diffusion, and gear methodology towards it. When using agar diffusion methods for cephradine several organisms may be used, e.g. *Sarcina lutea, Staph. aureus, B. subtilis* and *B. pumilus*. In the routine assay of pharmaceutical preparations containing cephradine, *B. pumilus* is the organism of choice, its advantages being good zone definition, reasonable sensitivity and the utilization of a spore suspension

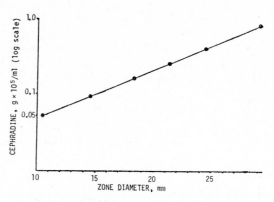

Fig. 1. Cephradine dose-response curve using *Sarcina lutea* ATCC 9341.

[3]. However, in the assay of cephradine in biological materials *Sarcina lutea* ATCC 9341 is employed because it gives greater sensitivity than the other organisms. This organism demonstrates a linear response between 0.025 and 0.8 µg/ml, with sensitivities of 0.05 µg/ml in serum and 3.0 µg/ml in urine when allowing for minimum dilution (Fig. 1).

In assaying serum for cephradine, as for many other antibiotics, the final standard curve and samples were at one time prepared in pooled normal serum. However, because of its low protein-binding capacity this procedure can be omitted without substantial differences in the results. In addition, as cephradine has been found to remain intact in blood and urine, total activity is recorded and no special requirements are necessary in the interpretation of the final activity demonstrated.

Assay methods

The methods utilized in our laboratory are the petri dish/cylinder method or large plate/well method, using 12 × 12 assay plates in an 8 × 8 latin square design. The preparation and spotting of samples is shown schematically in Fig. 2.

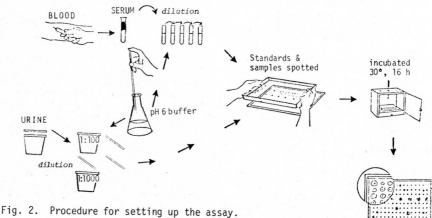

Fig. 2. Procedure for setting up the assay.

When bioavailability studies are being performed to determine blood and urine levels of antibiotics, samples are frequently received in an unbroken coded form and are, therefore, blind to the analyst. In assaying 'blind samples' we have found it advantageous to carry out exploratory 'siting' assays (sample volumes permitting) using six levels of standard in the range 0.05 to 0.8 µg/ml of cephradine, with serum samples diluted 1:2 and 1:10 (sometimes greater) in 0.1 M phosphate buffer pH 6.0 and urine samples diluted 1 : 100 and 1 : 1000 (and greater) in the same buffer. Once a good estimate of the cephradine level in the sample has been obtained by this siting assay, a more precise and accurate result can then be obtained using an 8 × 8 design, with 2 + 2 standards (one high and one low level of standard, in a 4 : 1 ratio) and samples diluted more appropriately to parallel the two standard concentrations. With this design, 2 samples are spotted over the 8 × 8 latin square design, resulting in 8 responses for each level of standard and sample. Further advantages of this design are that it lends itself to the standard procedures of our laboratories in respect of dilution, punching (if wells are used), filling designs, and automatic reading and calculations using Biocoder (made by R.N. Saxby, Ltd., Liverpool) and Autobiocoder systems which will not be elaborated on here. Details of the performance characteristics of the method are shown in Table 1.

Table 1. Performance characteristics of the assay.

CEPHRADINE IN SERUM	CEPHRADINE IN URINE
ACCURACY	ACCURACY
Theory 10 µg/ml	Theory 357 µg/ml
Recoveries	*Recoveries*
10.6	336
10.6	360
10.4	330
10.4	366
9.5	360
9.5	350
9.5	348
9.5	350
9.5	-
9.6	-
10.4	-
11.0	-
9.2	-
9.2	-
9.2	-
9.2	-
Mean 9.8 µg	*Mean* 350 µg
BIAS -2%	BIAS -2%
PRECISION ±0.62 µg/ml S.D.	PRECISION ±1.2 µg/ml S.D.
SPECIFICITY	Not specific for cephradine.
ASSAY TIME	More than 50 samples can be assayed per day per operator.

CONCLUDING COMMENTS

The assay described may be used for the assay of single samples. However, laboratories that are required to process large numbers of samples, running into hundreds, require some form of automation in the reading and calculation part of the procedure to bring about an efficient sample throughput. Similarly, when faced with coded samples where the cephradine concentration is completely unknown and may range from 0 to 50 µg/ml or greater in a blood sample and 0 to 1000 µg/ml or greater in urine, some form of siting assays has to be performed. Examples of the levels that may be obtained with different dosage regimes are shown in Fig. 3, and evidently vary greatly.

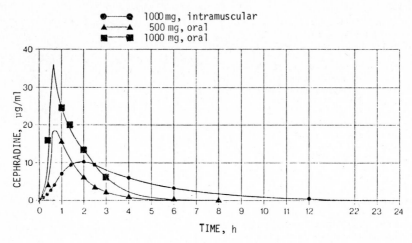

Fig. 3. Concentrations of cephradine found in blood, by microbiological assay, after intramuscular and oral administration to human subjects.

References

1. Isaacson, D.M., *Squibb R & D New Brunswick, Internal Report* (1973).

2. Poutsiaka, J.W. *et al., Proc. 8th Internat. Congr. Chemotherapy, Athens* (1973).

3. Cosgrove, R.F., *Squibb I.D.L., Internal Report* (1974).

Note added in proof (arising from a Discussion query by R.H. Moore): Turbidi-metric methods as now used are frequently more rapid than agar diffusion. There are several automated systems for this procedure (e.g. Autoturb) which are also claimed by many to be more accurate and precise. In our laboratories, however, we choose the agar diffusion method as this technique gives better accuracy, precision and reproducibility in our hands and lends itself more easily to the established routine and automatic procedures in our laboratory, and thus enables a more efficient sample throughput.

Analytical case history

T-11

DETERMINATION OF ETHAMBUTOL IN PLASMA AND URINE
BY CHEMICAL IONIZATION GC-MS USING A DEUTERATED
INTERNAL STANDARD

Andrew D. Blair, Arden W. Forrey, T. Graham Christopher,
Barbara Maxwell and Ralph E. Cutler

*Dept. of Medicine, University of Washington,
Harborview Medical Center, 325-9th Ave., Seattle,
Washington 98104, U.S.A.*

Requirement   *Assay sensitive to ∿10 ng/ml, for plasma and urine.*

Chemistry   *A basic aliphatic compound.*

End-step   *Chemical ionization GC-MS after derivatizing, with a deuterated internal standard.*

Sample
preparation   *Extraction with chloroform.*

Comments &   *Retractable-top probe for the MS is advantageous. Assay superior in
alternatives   sensitivity etc. to 'classical' assays.*

In order to study the pharmacokinetics of ethambutol (a tuberculostatic drug) in patients with renal insufficiency, we have developed a chemical ionization GC-MS analytical procedure which overcomes the problems inherent in the existing colorimetric [1, 2], microbiological, radiochemical [3] and GC methods [4, 5], relating to specificity, sensitivity and reproducibility. The method involves the use of a tetradeuterated ethambutol internal standard.

EXPERIMENTAL

(+)-2,2'-(Ethylene-d_4-diimino)-di-1-butanol (ethambutol-d_4) was synthesized by refluxing 1.00 g L-2-amino-1-butanol (11.27 mmol) with 0.54 g ethylene dibromide-d_4 (2.8 mmol) at 100-105° for 18 h. The reaction mixture was dissolved in 10 ml of water and 10 ml of 20% sodium hydroxide, and extracted three times with 20 ml of chloroform, which was removed by rotary evaporation. The resulting oil crystallized on standing. The material was recrystallized twice from benzene to yield 0.24 g of white crystals (41.8% yield). The material was identified as ethambutol-d_4 by MS and NMR analysis. It was necessary to use the optically active amino-alcohol corresponding to that used in the synthesis of ethambutol to ensure that the extraction ratio from plasma and urine would be identical for ethambutol and the internal standard.

Extraction procedures

One millilitre of a 5 μg/ml solution of ethambutol-d_4 in methanol was pipetted into a series of 15 x 1.5 cm screw-capped (teflon-lined) vials, and one drop of 1 M HCl was added to each. The methanol was evaporated under a stream of nitrogen at ambient temperature. The vials, after addition of 1 ml of plasma or urine, 1 ml of 4 M KOH and 5 ml of chloroform, were shaken on a wrist action shaker for 10 min. The vials were centrifuged at 1900 rev/min for 10 min and the aqueous layer was aspirated. The chloroform was transferred to a 10 ml conical centrifuge tube, three drops of 1 M HCl was added, and the chloroform evaporated to dryness under a stream of nitrogen at ambient temperature. The HCl is necessary in both evaporation steps to prevent evaporation of the ethambutol free base.

Trimethylsilylimidazole (100 µl; Pierce Chemical Co.) and anhydrous pyridine (100 µl) were added to the dried residue and swirled on a vortex mixer just prior to introduction into the GC-MS apparatus.

Mass spectrometry

Originally, the method was attempted using an AEI-MS9 with electron bombardment and the material was introduced into the MS chamber by the direct insertion probe. Under electron impact, ethambutol does not exhibit a parent ion at m/e 204, but loses CH_2OH to give an apparent molecular ion at m/e 173, with the ethambutol-d_4 giving an ion at m/e 177. Whilst the 177/173 ratio could be measured in standard samples, when ethambutol was extracted from plasma a large contaminating component from the plasma at m/e 177 made it impracticable to pursue the method further.

Prior to derivatizing with trimethylsilylimidazole, an attempt was made to quantify ethambutol using methane chemical ionization on a Finnigan Model 3200E GC-MS apparatus with the direct insertion probe, since under chemical ionization conditions ethambutol exhibits a large $[M + 1]^+$ ion at m/e 205. Again, the problem of contaminants from plasma carried over in the extraction step enhanced the $[M + 1]^+$ ion of ethambutol-d_4 at m/e 209.

After derivatizing with trimethylsilylimidazole, 1-2 µl of the reaction mixture was injected onto either an OV-17 or an OV-225 GC column in a Finnigan Model 3200E GC-MS apparatus, interfaced with a Finnigan Model 6100 data system. The ethambutol and ethambutol-d_4 were eluted with methane gas at a flow rate to maintain a source pressure of 1 torr and column temperature maintained at 140°. Mass fragmentography was monitored at m/e 349 and 353, the $[M + 1]^+$ ions for the di-TMS derivative of ethambutol and ethambutol-d_4 respectively, and at m/e 333 and 337, corresponding to the M-CH_3 ions for ethambutol and ethambutol-d_4. The data were also captured using the Finnigan PROMIM, and concentration ratios were determined by measuring the peak heights of each of the four previously mentioned ions.

RESULTS AND DISCUSSION

A secondary problem to using the direct insertion probe was the extreme volatility of ethambutol at MS source temperatures of 150°, since the melting point of the free base is 77°. In the MS-9, a retractable probe tip was used and usable data could be obtained; but with the Finnigan, which did not have a retractable tip, much of the sample was already volatilized by the time the pressure was low enough to turn the ion source on.

Using the GC method, elution of ethambutol from the column was complete in 3 min, allowing up to 20 samples per h to be analyzed. This is a great improvement over the use of the direct insertion probe, which invariably took 15 min to complete each sample and, moreover, contaminated the machine much more extensively than the GC method. The standard curve expressed as a regression of concentration (µg/ml) on 100 x mass ratio (MR) is:

C = -0.546 + 0.092x (100·MR), where C = µg/ml (in original sample),

with a standard error of 0.440 (Fig. 1). The nominal sensitivity on a 0-20 µg/ml range is 50 ng/ml, and the ultimate sensitivity for a 1 ml sample is 10 ng/ml. The specificity of the GC-MS method for the analysis of ethambutol is clearly an improvement over existing methods, since ethambutol is doubly separated from other interfering compounds, i.e. by chromatographic elution and by mass-to-charge ratio. Since the deuterated internal standard is added prior to sample workup and the internal standard most closely mimics the physical properties of ethambutol, problems such as extraction efficiency and accurate pipetting, and GC injection techniques are of little consequence. This has been very evident in the studies performed to date,

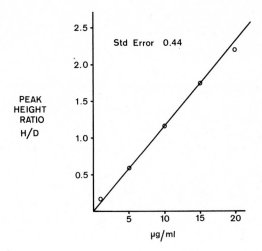

Fig. 1. Standard GC-MS
curve for ethambutol.
*The concentrations refer
to the original sample.*

in that the extraction efficiency between two samples containing the same amount of
ethambutol may vary by as much as 200%. The sensitivity of the assay (10 ng/ml) is
at least equal to the GC methods reported to date, and far superior to the colorimetric and microbiological methods which range from 0.1 to 1 µg/ml. Since a double
separation technique is being utilized, the method reported here will undoubtedly
prove out to be more reliable at very low concentrations, due to the exclusion of
interfering compounds by elution time and *m/e*.

PHARMACOKINETICS

We were initially studying the pharmacokinetics of ethambutol, using the [^{14}C-]-
labelled compound. In the normal individual, other groups had reported getting
essentially quantitative recovery of ethambutol in the urine, and our preliminary
results bore this out. We recognized, however, that if we used [^{14}C-]ethambutol in
patients with severe renal insufficiency and anephric patients, metabolism of ethambutol would undoubtedly obscure the actual ethambutol serum and urine concentrations.
While we were developing the GC-MS ethambutol assay we did, however, study the
pharmacokinetics of ethambutol in these patients with the [^{14}C-]compound. The
results were highly indicative of metabolite build-up in the anephric patients. The
counts in plasma fell after intravenous injection of ethambutol, to a plateau level
within 4 h, and remained constant for approximately 8 h, at which time the counts
tended to rise until the patient's dialysis period began. During dialysis, the
counts in plasma fell to approximately half the pre-dialysis concentration over a
6 h dialysis period, but then, after dialysis, climbed to the original plateau level.

When the GC-MS method became available, the metabolite build-up was confirmed
by showing that the ethambutol concentration fell to zero. The pharmacokinetics of
ethambutol in anephric patients can be fitted by a two-compartment and, in some
cases a three-compartment open model which has a zero asymptote when the samples
are analyzed by the chemical ionization GC-MS method, as compared to measurement
using [^{14}C-]ethambutol which gives a two-compartment closed model with a positive
non-zero asymptote. When blood samples collected 12 h post-injection were made
alkaline and extracted with chloroform, 95% of the [^{14}C-]material remained

unextracted, indicating the possible presence of a dicarboxylic acid which has previously been reported for ethambutol metabolites in urine. We are, at the present time, synthesizing the tetradeuterated dicarboxylic acid of ethambutol in the hope that we will be able to quantitate ethambutol and its reported major metabolites simultaneously.

References

1. Burger, J.M., Pisano, F.D. & Nash R.A., *J. Pharm. Sci. 58* (1969) 110-111.

2. Gundert-Remy, U., Klett, M. & Weber, E., *Eur. J. Clin. Pharmacol. 6* (1973) 133-136.

3. Kelly, R.G. & Hoyt, K.D., *Gas Chromatographic Method of Analysis for Ethambutol in Biological Fluids (Preliminary Report),* Lederle Laboratories, Pearl River, New York.

4. Richard, B.M., Manno, J.E. & Manno B.R., *J. Chromatog. 89* (1974) $8\frac{1}{4}$-82.

5. Peets, E.A. & Buyske, D.A., *Clin. Pharmacol. 13* (1964) 1403-1419.

Analytical case history

T-12   RADIOENZYMATIC ASSAY TECHNIQUES FOR AMINOGLYCOSIDES

Arden W. Forrey, Andrew D. Blair, Michelle A. O'Neill and Ralph E. Cutler
Dept. of Medicine, University of Washington,
Harborview Medical Center, 325-9th Ave., Seattle,
Washington 98104, U.S.A.

Requirement   *Assay of plasma and urine for therapeutic levels (of the order of 10 mg/l) of antibiotics of the streptomycin, spectinomycin, kanamycin and gentamycin families.*

Chemistry   *Aminoglycosides with groups into which substituents can be introduced enzymically.*

End-step   *Radioactivity measurement.*

Sample preparation   *Incubation with labelled donor and an appropriate enzyme, then separation of product from labelled reactant on ion-exchange paper.*

Comments & alternatives   *With urine the use of kanamycin acetyltransferase is complicated by the presence of inhibitor(s). The radioenzymatic approach is quick and economical, and is more accurate than microbiological assay. The radioactivity data should be processed by computer.*

The radioenzymatic approach now to be considered is particularly helpful in therapeutics because aminoglycosides have a low therapeutic index with $T_{\frac{1}{2}}$ elimination values of 2-72 h in renal failure. Regulation of dosage, though predictable from renal function indices such as serum creatinine or endogenous creatinine clearance, should be carefully controlled by periodic measurement of serum drug concentration. Since the drug permeates into the extracellular fluid space, its concentration at desired sites of action will be reflected by this measurement, as clinicians should come to appreciate.

ENZYMES AVAILABLE

Ligating enzymes were first identified in the laboratories of Davies [1] and Umezawa [2] as the mechanism of transmissible drug resistance to aminoglycoside antibiotics. Partial or complete inactivation of the various antibiotic species occurs by transfer of an adenyl, phosphate or acetyl group to a specific position on the antibiotic molecule. Davies and his colleagues at the University of Wisconsin first utilized these enzymes to measure concentration of antibiotics, and Smith and his colleagues at Harvard [3] pioneered their clinical use for monitoring drug concentrations in serum. Many other workers have now adapted the technique for clinical and clinical-research purposes. Nevertheless, their use is not yet widespread in clinical chemistry.

Streptomycin is adenylated on the 3''-OH of the L-glucosamine ring by streptomycin adenyl transferase (SAT) and phosphorylated at the same position by streptomycin phosphotransferase (SPT), which is relatively specific (Fig. 1). Spectinomycin is adenylated by SAT on the threo-OH(9) of the substituted inositol ring (Fig. 2), but is not phosphorylated by SPT. On the other hand, enzymes such as the kanamycin acetyltransferase (KAT) are non-specific. For the kanamycin and gentamicin families (Table 1), the enzymatic reactivity is shown in Fig. 3. Enzymes identified to date, besides KAT, are gentamicin adenyl transferase (GAT), kanamycin phosphotransferases I and II (KPT), lividomycin phosphotransferase (LPT), gentamicin acetyltransferases I and II (GAcT). The KAT enzyme acetylates the 6'-amino group of the purpurosamine

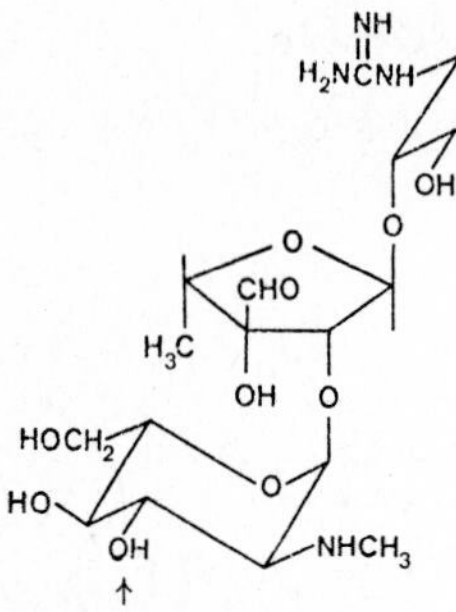

Fig. 1. Streptomycin: site of adenylation by SAT and of phorphorylation by SPT (arrow, ↑)

Fig. 2. Spectinomycin: site of adenylation by SAT (arrow, ↓)

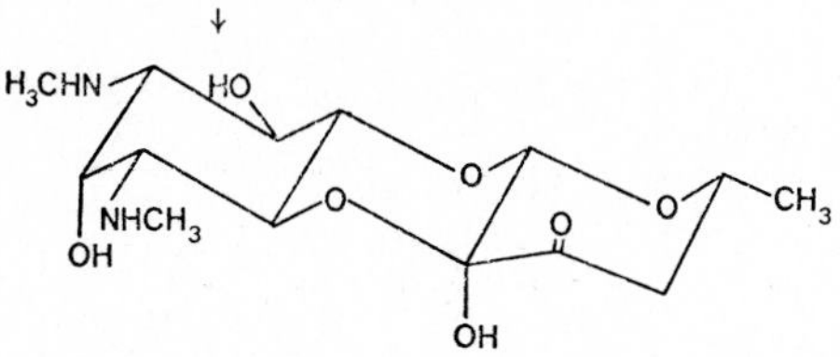

Table 1.   Substituent groups (cf. Fig. 3) in gentamicin and kanamycin antibiotics.

	Species	R_1	R_2	R_3	R_4	R_5	R_6	R_7	R_8	R_9	R_{10}
Gentamicin	A	H	OH	OH	OH	NH_2	CH_3	H	OH	H	H
	C_{1a}	H	NH_2	H	H	NH_2	CH_3	OH	CH_3	H	H
	C_2	CH_3	NH_2	H	H	NH_2	CH_3	OH	CH_3	H	H
	C_1	CH_3	$NHCH_3$	H	H	NH_2	CH_3	OH	CH_3	H	H
Kanamycin	A	H	NH_2	OH	OH	OH	H	H	OH	CH_2OH	H
	B	H	NH_2	OH	OH	NH_2	H	H	OH	CH_2OH	H
	C	H	OH	OH	OH	NH_2	H	H	OH	CH_2OH	H
Tobramycin		H	NH_2	OH	H	NH_2	H	H	OH	CH_2OH	H
Amikacin		H	NH_2	OH	OH	OH	H	H	OH	CH_2OH	$-\underset{\underset{O}{\|\|}}{C}-\underset{\underset{OH}{\|}}{CH}-CH_2-\underset{\underset{NH_2}{\|}}{CH_2}$
Sisomycin		4',5'-dehydrogentamicin C_{1a}									
Verdamycin		4',5'-dehydrogentamicin C_2									

ring, (I), whereas the GAT enzyme adenylates the 3-OH group of the deoxystreptamine ring (II). The KPT enzyme, which also appears in the W667/JR66 sonicates used for preparation of GAT, phosphorylates the 3'-OH (in ring I). The GAcT I and II enzymes acetylate the 2' and 3 amino groups (rings I and II), respectively, of antibiotics related to gentamicin and kanamycin.

Smith's group [3] employed the GAT enzyme for the measurement of gentamicin concentrations. GAT is also effective on tobramycin and kanamycin; but the 3'-OH in gentamicin A and in kanamycin is phosphorylated by ATP if KPT is also present, causing substrate competition and erratic results which can, however, be prevented by purification of the GAT enzyme.

Most reported systems entail the use of either GAT or KAT enzymes in relatively impure sonicates. GAT and KPT, which cause mutual inhibition, occur together in the strains used for enzyme preparation, but can be separated by simple DEAE-cellulose chromatography, although affinity chromatography on sepharose gel may also be used.   Separation is suitably performed with a 30 x 2.5 cm column of DEAE 52 with a gradient formed from pH 7.4 buffer (Tris, 100 mM; $MgCl_2$, 5 mM; dithiothreotol, 1 mM) and the same buffer with NaCl present (0.3 M), at a flow rate of 60 ml/h.   In a

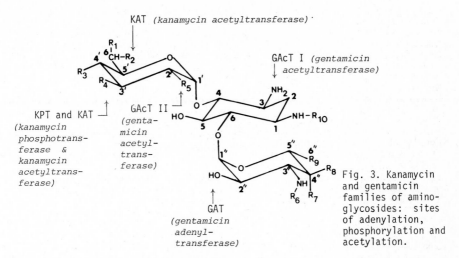

Fig. 3. Kanamycin and gentamicin families of aminoglycosides: sites of adenylation, phosphorylation and acetylation.

column run where the fractions were assayed for KPT in a system containing kanamycin (50 mg/1) and [γ-^{32}P-]ATP, and for GAT in a system containing gentamicin (50 mg/1) and [^{14}C-]ATP, KPT was eluted as a shallow peak mainly at 100-150 min, and GAT more sharply at 250-300 min.

ASSAY PROCEDURE

Reaction conditions entail use of substrates at concentrations above their K_m (shown for GAT in Table 2), generally at 0.1 to 0.4 mM for adenylation and 4×10^{-5} M for acetylation (100-2000 nCi/assay) as shown in Table 3. Reported K_m values for antibiotics may be somewhat inaccurate due to possible KPT contamination of the Sephadex-purified preparation of Smith and Smith [3]. Table 2 also shows K_m values for ATP.

Table 2. Kinetic properties of GAT.
The µg values for V_{max} *refer to protein.*

Reactant		Value
Holmes & Sanford, ref. [4]		
K_m	ATP	4.3×10^{-5} M
	Gentamicin	$<2 \times 10^{-9}$ M
V_{max}	Gentamicin	6.5 p-mol/min/µg
Smith & Smith, ref.[3]		
K_m	ATP	6.1×10^{-5} M
	Gentamicin	1.5×10^{-6} M
	Kanamycin	2.25×10^{6} M
V_{max}	Gentamicin	4.05 p-mol/min/µg
	Kanamycin	0.57 p-mol/min/µg

Table 3. Reaction conditions for radioenzymatic assays.

Reaction vol, µl	nCi /assay	Ligand final concn., M	Vol. spotted on paper, µl	Ref.
For GAT:				
200	400	4×10^{-4}	75	6
110	95	2.5×10^{-4}	75	3
55	80	3.7×10^{-4}	10	7
120	120	1×10^{-4}	50	4
125	75	1.4×10^{-4}	75	8
100	200	4×10^{-4}	75	*this paper*
For KAT:				
45	91	2×10^{-4}	20	9
45	5500	6×10^{-5}	20	5
60	100	6×10^{-5}	40	10
80	82.5	3.4×10^{-5}	70	8

Reactions are carried out in 5-10 mM Tris at pH's from 5.7 to 8.6, in reaction volumes from 45 µl to 550 µl (Table 3). Incubation times range from 30 to 60 min; the GAT enzyme was shown to produce a linear amount of product to 30 min. Aliquots of 20-100 µl (Table 3) are then placed on phosphocellulose paper (P-81; 2 cm circles). The specific binding of the product to the phosphocellulose paper is due to the cationic nature of the product after reaction. Several reported washing techniques employ either Tris buffer or distilled water washes to reduce background counts. We use a brief 2 min, 70°, distilled water wash, followed by a 20 min water wash at room temperature with shaking; the papers are then dried on a glass-topped hotplate. Papers are counted in 15 ml of a toluene-based scintillant; POPOP/PPO and Butyl PBD/PBBO systems can be used, depending upon the liquid scintillation counter available. The dry papers are counted directly when using C^{14} labels, with re-use of the scintillant. Hewitt [5], when using ^{3}H-labelled acetyl CoA, elutes the counts from the papers with 0.3 M NaOH before adding scintillant, but has to use a solublizer in order to count the sample in a toluene scintillant; the latter cannot now be re-used, negating the saving in isotope cost. This latter procedure could serve to advantage to measure low levels of antibiotic, but these levels are generally below those of therapeutic interest.

The anionic nature of the labelled reactants minimizes non-specific binding on the paper. Recently, Hewitt [12] has employed adenosine-soaked phosphocellulose paper to further suppress this non-specific binding. Other more effective exchangers could possibly become available in the future, which, coupled with effective washing techniques, would lower backgrounds even further.

We use 18 standards and the range 0-20 or 0-30 mg/l (depending upon the aminoglycoside), and obtain relative standard deviations of 2-3% or less. Inhibitors of the KAT reaction are present in serum and urine when compared to aqueous samples; this effect is not present with GAT, and standards prepared in all three media are almost superimposable. Only with assay of urine samples does this situation become a problem because of the varying dilution of urine solutes depending on the water load of the subject. Plasma levels of the inhibitor(s) remain constant, hence standards prepared in plasma are adequate. Nevertheless, the nature of the inhibitory substance(s), now demonstrated by several groups, is not yet known.

DATA PROCESSING

Fast processing of the counting data to give sample concentrations and estimated sample precision must be carried out by computer methods. After capture of the data on punched paper tape or on magnetic tape casettes, calculation is carried out either by desk-top programmable calculators or by data communication terminals to time-sharing computer systems. In either case, an unweighted least squares fit of the standards to a straight line (equal variance for each point is appropriate) is used. The system used in our laboratory, with a casette data capture device, is shown in Fig. 4 and a completed report shown in Fig. 5.

For clinical purposes, a selection of the appropriate number of standards based on the requisite precision, drug, number of sample replicates, and laboratory cost factors can be made based on the statistics from this data processing. Quality control of assay developed from time plots and running averages of selected statistics such as intercept, slope and standard error, can ensure that the assay conditions remain predictable. Sample replicates control unpredictable aberrant values and help reduce the error in the predicted sample concentration.

COST AND OTHER ASPECTS

The cost and speed of the assay benefit by the use of small volumes and by the transfer of a large proportion of the reaction mixture to the papers. Costs ranging from 50 ¢ to $3 (U.S.) have been quoted. For GAT, KAT or KPT, we reckon that 100 assays

DATA ACQUISITION & REDUCTION for RADIOENZYMATIC ASSAYS

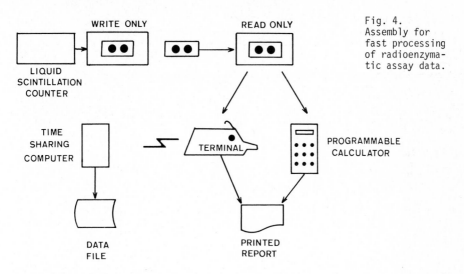

WRITE ONLY

READ ONLY

LIQUID
SCINTILLATION
COUNTER

TIME
SHARING
COMPUTER

TERMINAL

PROGRAMMABLE
CALCULATOR

DATA
FILE

PRINTED
REPORT

Fig. 4.
Assembly for
fast processing
of radioenzyma-
tic assay data.

Fig. 5. Report of
processed data from a
radioenzymatic assay.

```
GENT-TESTH CASSETTE INPUT
T IS 2.583 FOR 95PC CONF.LIMITS
COMP.OPTION IS 3 FOR 17 STANDARDS AND   1UNKNOWNS
    ABS ORPCT    CONC.     ABS.    CALCD.   DIFF.
 1  2774.0000   0.000   2774.0000   0.022 -0.022
 2  2708.0000   0.000   2708.0000  -0.437  0.437
 3  3053.0000   2.000   3053.0000   1.963  0.037
 4  2940.0000   2.000   2940.0000   1.177  0.823
 5  3387.0000   4.000   3387.0000   4.286 -0.286
 6  3479.0000   4.000   3479.0000   4.926 -0.926
 7  3600.0000   6.000   3600.0000   5.768  0.232
 8  3491.0000   6.000   3491.0000   5.009  0.991
 9  4012.0000   8.000   4012.0000   8.633 -0.633
10  3988.0000   8.000   3988.0000   8.466 -0.466
11  4474.0000  10.000   4474.0000  11.847 -1.847
12  5072.0000  15.000   5072.0000  16.006 -1.006
13  4804.0000  15.000   4804.0000  14.142  0.858
14  5550.0000  20.000   5550.0000  19.331  0.669
15  5476.0000  20.000   5476.0000  18.816  1.184
16  7087.0000  30.000   7087.0000  30.022 -0.022
17  7087.0000  30.000   7087.0000  30.022 -0.022
AVE X IS    4293.06 AVE Y IS  10.588
SLOPE IS    0.00696 INTERCEPT IS -19.272
STD ERR OF SLOPE IS   0.0001514 STD ERR OF INT. IS  2.807
STD ERR IS  0.836
```

NO SPEC.NO	ABS OR PCT	DIL		95PC CONF. LIMITS ARE	REL. STD. DEVIATION	FINAL CONC.
1	2794.000	1	0.1614	2.297	1422.8990	0.161
2	4952.000	1	15.1715	2.236	14.7359	15.172
3	4447.000	1	11.6590	2.222	19.0547	11.659
4	4371.000	1	11.1304	2.221	19.9542	11.130
5	4374.000	1	11.1512	2.221	19.9171	11.151
6	4421.000	1	11.4781	2.221	19.3527	11.478
7	2969.000	1	1.3786	2.280	165.4037	1.379
8	3118.000	1	2.4150	2.268	93.9042	2.415
9	3144.000	1	2.5959	2.266	87.2837	2.596
10	3251.000	1	3.3401	2.258	67.5978	3.340

per technician-day (8 h)
are manageable, giving
a labour cost of 44¢ per
tube. Preparation of
sufficient enzyme to
perform 1200 assays
occupies 12 h (or, for
KAT, 16 h), giving a
cost of 5¢ per tube.
Taking account of other
materials, including the
isotope (6.4¢ for GAT,
17¢ for KAT), the cost
per tube becomes:

GAT: 44¢ + 18¢ = 62¢;

KAT: 44¢ + 23¢ = 67¢.

(The 18¢ and 23¢ items
represent total costs
for materials. Data
processing costs are
not taken into account.)

Table 4. Comparison of assay methods — radioenzymatic (Enz.), radioimmuno (RIA) and microbiological (Mic.). The column headings α and β denote intercept and slope respectively for the expression $y = \alpha + \beta \cdot x$.

Comparison	Correlation coefficient	α	β	Remarks	Ref.
Radioenzymatic assay with GAT					
Enz. *vs.* Mic.	0.96	-1.7 (a) -0.03(L)	1.48 (a)* 1.07 (L)*		13
RIA *vs.* Enz.	0.90	0.35	0.99	Compared with Mic. indirectly	11
Radioenzymatic assay with KAT					
Mic. *vs.* Enz.	0.93	3.16	0.86	[^{3}H-]acetate	5
Mic. *vs.* Enz.	0.96	0.03	1.07	[^{14}C-]acetate	8

  * *Uniformly and logarithmically weighted regressions*

Comparisons of radioenzymatic assays with other assay techniques such as radioimmunoassay and microbiological assays are listed in Table 4. Microbiological and radioenzymatic assays correlate closely, although the former tend to give higher concentrations. Reeves [8] and others have shown, however, that in routine clinical laboratories, in contrast with research laboratories, radioenzymatic assays give much better accuracy than microbiological assays, and therefore warrant adoption.

The main clinical use of such assays is for monitoring therapy. Their clinical adoption hinges on convincing practitioners (particularly in infectious diseases services) of their speed, accuracy and economy and of their great usefulness in treating patient infections, especially in cases complicated by renal pathophysiology.

References

1. Davies, J.E. & Rownd, R., *Science 176* (1972) 758-768.

2. Umezawa, H. in *Progress in Antimicrobial and Anticancer Chemotherapy (Proc. 6th Internat. Congr. Chemotherapy) 2,* Univ. of Tokyo (1970) pp. 566-571.

3. Smith, A.L. & Smith, D.H., *J. Infec. Dis. 129* (1974) 391-401.

4. Holmes, R.K. & Sanford, J.P., *J. Infec. Dis. 129* (1974) 519-527.

5. Stevens, P., Young, L.S. & Hewitt, W.L., *Antimicrob. Agents Chemother. 7* (1975) 374-376.

6. Smith, D.H., Van Otto, D. & Smith, A.L., *New Engl. J. Med. 286* (1972) 583.

7. Beneveniste, R. & Davies, J., *Biochem. J. 10* (1971) 1787-1796.

8. Broughall, J.M. & Reeves, D.S., *J. Clin. Path. 28* (1975) 140-145.

9. Haas, M. & Davies, J., *Antimicrob. Agents Chemother. 4* (1973) 497-499.

10. Plantier, J., Forrey, A.W., O'Neill, M.A., Blair, A.D., Christopher, T.G. & Cutler, R.E., *J. Infec. Dis., Supplement* (1976) *in press.*

11. Lewis, J.E., Nelson, J.C. & Elder, H.A., *Nature 239* (1972) 214-216.

12. Dahlgren, J.G., Anderson, E.T. & Hewitt, W.L., *Antimicrob. Agents Chemother. 8* (1975) 58-62.

13. Smith, A.L., Waitz, J.A., Smith, D.H., Oden, E.M. & Emerson, B.B., *Antimicrob. Agents Chemother. 6* (1974) 316-319.

T-NC NOTES AND COMMENTS RELATING TO ANALYTICAL CASE HISTORIES

Assay of endogenous compounds

Editorial comment: From the assay viewpoint, endogenous and exogenous trace substances present similar problems, except for the difficulty of getting valid blanks for the former. There is an especially useful source [1] of documented information on normal levels. Also recommended is a general book on hormone assay [2]. For prostaglandins, as touched on earlier (p. 9), a recent review article may be helpful [3].

1. Diem, K. & Lentner, C. (eds.), *Scientific Tables,* 7th edn., Geigy, Basel (1970).

2. Loraine, J.A. & Bell, E.T. ,   *Hormone Assays and their Clinical Application,* 3rd edn., Livingstone, Edinburgh (1971).

3. Russell, P.T., Eberle, A.J. & Cheng, H.C., *Clin. Chem.* 21 (1975) 653-666.

ASSAY OF URINARY METADRENALINES (A.A.A. Aziz *et al.,* Art. T-2)

Answer to remarks by J.R. Salmon.— P.T. Kissinger's HPLC assay of urinary catecholamines with an electrochemical detector, after a concentrating step with alumina, seems impressive although tricky. We hear that he is able to separate authentic metadrenalines on a pellicular cation-exchanger, but is still seeking a satisfactory way of preparing the sample for the HPLC analysis. *Comment by* W.N. Jenner.— HPLC would be unlikely to separate the desired 3-o-methyl compounds from the 4-o-methyl compounds, which are present at ∿10% of the levels of the former. *Reply by* E. Reid.— We have no information on the latter isomers; but the contamination we described is vastly greater than 10% and so cannot be thus explained.

Comments by G. Schill.— Adrenaline and similar compounds can be extracted quantitatively into chloroform as ion-pair adducts with bis(2-ethylhexyl)phosphoric acid. The pH optimum is 8.3. The same system has also been used in reversed phase chromatography of a number of aminophenols and similar compounds (adrenaline, noradrenaline, symphrin, etc.), and good separations have been obtained. All studies [1] were made on pure compounds (*not* urine) with UV measurement.

1. Modin, R. & Johansson, M., *Acta Pharm. Suecica 8* (1971) 561-572.

Assay of drugs acting on the nervous system

ASSAY OF METHAQUALONE (S.S. Brown, Art. T-3)

The author acknowledges the following useful comments from A.J. Clatworthy.—

Interferences in GC are minimal with a suitable column, such as 3% SE-30 on Gas Chrom. Z, run at 200°. With a nitrogen detector as little as 10 ng/ml of blood can be measured. A neutral blood fraction in ethanol, if from 5 ml of blood, allows UV determinations even at therapeutic levels with little interference. MS determination usually requires derivatives in the case of hydroxylated metabolites, the main metabolite in blood being the 2'-OH compound (non-phenolic) as shown by GC-MS.

    In pharmacokinetic studies, the other drug most likely to be encountered (perhaps influencing methaqualone) is another hypnotic, diphenylhydramine. The spuriously high assay results for 'methaqualone' obtained with a non-specific assay such as UV after extraction with solvents such as chloroform and ether, in comparison with GC, is due to co-extraction of the 2'-OH metabolite. It is not found in blood after a single dose, but appears to build up over a period of continual dosage probably partly due to the long half-life of methaqualone; it is the main unconjugated urinary metabolite in man (whereas any urinary methaqualone is likely to be conjugated). The use of a non-polar solvent such as hexane, followed

[Continued on lower part of next p.

Brief analytical case history

GC-MS AS APPLIED TO THE ESTIMATION OF PHENACETIN, PARACETAMOL AND ACETANILIDE IN PLASMA AND URINE

J.D. Baty and P. Robinson
Department of Medicine
University of Liverpool
P.O. Box 147, Liverpool L69 3BX, U.K.

Assay requirement	*Assay methods for studying the oxidation of acetanilide to paracetamol and the de-ethylation of phenacetin to paracetamol.*
Chemistry & metabolism	*All 3 compounds can be derivatized for GC by silanization with N,O-bis-trimethylsilylacetamide (BSA). Paracetamol gives rise to conjugates.*
End-step	*GC-MS (mass fragmentography), with a voltage switching technique to monitor one ion characteristic of the compound and the corresponding ion from the deuterium analogue (e.g. for phenacetin the ions at 251 and 254 are monitored).*
Sample preparation	*To prepare deuterium analogues as internal standards for addition to the sample, react the appropriate amine with deuteroacetic anhydride; the -NH.COCD$_3$ group is stable to hydrogen exchange below pH 8. After enzymatic hydrolysis of the paracetamol conjugates and addition of internal standard, the plasma or urine is buffered to pH 5 with 3 M NAH$_2$PO$_4$ and extracted with ethyl acetate. The residue obtained by drying down with a stream of nitrogen is derivatized.*
Comments	*The amount of a compound in a particular sample is calculated from calibration curves relating differing weight ratios of the H and D compounds to their respective signals from the GC-MS. The assay method is more fully described elsewhere [1].*

1. Baty, J.D., Robinson, P.R. & Wharton, J., *Biomed. Mass Spectrom.* (1976) *in press.*

Reply to H. de Bree, *who asked:* Do you monitor two ions simultaneously or use a jumping mode ? — A voltage switching technique is used to sample each ion alternately.

ASSAY OF METHAQUALONE, *continued from previous p.*

by back-extraction into dilute acid (the pH is critical), does allow an accurate determination of the blood level of methaqualone.

    Comment from S.S. Brown.— Because methaqualone is such a powerful 'inducer', it is quite feasible that its own metabolic pattern may change with time. It would be very interesting to have qualitative and quantitative data on this point. I have always been puzzled at the lack of published information [the above work from the Metropolitan Police Laboratory is unpublished - *Ed.*] on the circulating metabolites (and possibly their conjugates) in blood, and on the status of the *N*-oxide [1].

    Questions (and answers by S.S. Brown) relating to the absorption studies in Art. T-3.— Could the apparent inter-subject differences in absorption rate be due to differences in the volume of distribution ? (D.B. Campbell). *Ans.:* This might have some bearing, but it is doubtful if there would have been all that much variation in the volumes of the different subjects in the trial.
Would the group A-H show the same sequence in the 0.5 h plasma levels if you had given the same formulation twice ? *(question by* F. Battig, *relating to the inter-pretation that individuals differ in the response to different formulations.)* *Ans.:* If it were possible to repeat the two parts of the study, I suspect that

subjects A and H would again rank top and bottom respectively, as 'fast' and 'slow' absorbers. I doubt whether the physiological variables in such experiments could be controlled rigidly enough to obtain a consistent ranking for all of the subjects.

Comment by V.P. Butler.— Dr. John Lindenbaum (of Columbia Univ., New York) has administered the same batch of digoxin tablets to individual subjects on 2 or, in some instances, 3 separate occasions; with this drug the subjects (all tested in the fasting state on each occasion) varied unpredictably in the time required to attain peak levels of digoxin in serum.

Supplementary refs. from S.S. Brown: [2] deals with the excretion of the 2-hydroxy derivative, studied with GC (N detector), and [1] relates to [1] in Art. T-3:

1. Reynolds, C.N., Wilson, K. & Burnett, D., *Xenobiotica* 6 (1976) 113-124.

2. Burnett, D., Reynolds, C.N., Wilson, K. & Francis, J.R., *Xenobiotica* 6 (1976) 125-134.

References contributed by the Editor.— For GC assay of serum methaqualone, a simple extraction with chloroform at pH 10.5 has been claimed [3] to work as well as earlier, more lengthy procedures. Urinary methaqualone and certain unconjugated metabolites, the pattern of which was examined by GC, could be satisfactorily estimated with a commercial RIA kit [4].

3. Evenson, M.A. & Lensmeyer, G.L., *Clin. Chem.* 20 (1974) 249-254.

4. Berman, A.R., McGrath, J.P., Permisohn, R.C. & Cella, J.A., *Clin. Chem.* 21 (1975) 1878-1881.

Brief analytical case history

ASSAY OF TETRAHYDROCANNABINOL (THC) AND SOME OF ITS METABOLITES BY RIA

L.J. King
Biochemistry Dept., Univ. of Surrey, Guildford GU2 5XH, U.K.

Requirement   *A specific assay for THC in blood or urine.*

Chemistry &   *THC, the main psycho-active constituent of the plant* Cannabis sativa, metabolism   *has very poor water-solubility and very high lipid-solubility, and has a very high affinity for plasma lipoproteins. It forms several metabolites in vivo.*

End-step   *RIA, with dextran-coated charcoal to finally separate antibody-bound THC from unbound THC. To raise the sheep antiserum, used at a final dilution of ∿1:2,000, the THC was conjugated to bovine serum albumin by use of succinic anhydride; the inclusion of a trace amount of [³H]THC indicated that ∿20 THC residues were bound to each BSA molecule.*

Sample   *To obviate high non-specific binding due to the solubility properties,* preparation   *0.1% Triton-X-405 is included in the buffer and the protein content in the assay is kept to a minimum. Plasma samples are extracted with 2 vol. of ethanol, releasing the THC from lipoprotein; 20 μl of this extract can be used in the assay without any ethanol effect on the antibody binding. Up to 50 μl of urine can be assayed direct without extraction.*

Comments   *The assay [1] can detect 50 pg of THC, and also responds to several THC metabolites although several other cannabinoid derivatives do not interfere. Various other drugs of addiction did not cross-react.*

1. Teale, J.D., Forman, E.J., King, L.J., Piall, E.M. & Marks, V., *J. Pharm. Pharmac.* 27 (1975) 465-472.

Brief analytical case history

ASSAY OF THIORIDAZINE AND METABOLITES IN PLASMA

E.C. Dinovo and L.A. Gottschalk
Dept. of Psychiatry & Human Behavior,
University of California, Irvine, Calif. 92664, U.S.A.

Assay
requirement
Specific determination of unchanged drug at levels well below 1 µg/ml.

Chemistry &
metabolism
A phenothiazine, which gives rise to an S-sulphoxide (mesoridazine) and at least 2 other major metabolites in human plasma.

End-step
GC with carefully optimized FID (dual) and with chlorpromazine as internal standard.

Sample
preparation
Plasma (4 ml) extracted at alkaline pH with n-heptane:toluene, back-extracted with aqueous HCl, and re-extracted into a small vol. of the solvent mixture containing chlorpromazine.

Comments &
alternatives
Thioridazine is measurable at 0.3 µg/ml or, by concentrating the final extract, at 0.04 µg/ml. Metabolites are also extracted, but are measurable separately with the GC method (which is based on that of Curry & Mould [1]) although not with a spectrofluorimetric method [2] which, in consequence, over-estimates the thioridazine.

For the GC method, as described elsewhere [3], a Hewlett-Packard 5831A gas chromatograph with 3% OV-17 columns and with programming of oven temperature from 280° to 295° was used. The major modifications from the method of Curry & Mould [1] are the inclusion of a concentration step to allow a larger portion of the heptane: toluene extract to be injected into the GC, thereby increasing the sensitivity of the assay, and the addition of an internal standard, chlorpromazine, in the final heptane:toluene extraction to accurately follow the volume changes. Three standards at 1, 5 and 10 µg/ml were always run concurrently with the unknown specimens.

Pharmacokinetic information was obtained from a study of hospitalized psychiatric patients on a thioridazine or mesoridazine regimen. For single doses, thioridazine conversion into mesoridazine and thence into the sulphone is the predominant metabolic pathway.

1. Curry, S.H. & Mould, G.P., *J. Pharm. Pharmacol. 21* (1969) 674-677.

2. Pacha, W.L., *Experientia 25* (1969) 103-104.

3. Dinovo, E.C., Gottschalk, L.A., Nandi, B.R. & Geddes, P.G., *J. Pharm. Sci. 65* (1976) *in press.*

EDITOR'S NOTE: Dr. Dinovo's account was not actually presented at the Techniques Forum.

ASSAY OF PHENOTHIAZINES — *FURTHER NOTES & COMMENTS*

The following questions and answers relate to Art. T-4 (S.H. Curry).—

Answer to W.D.C. Wilson: Ether is unsuitable as an extraction solvent because of flammability, its volatility, and its constituent peroxides which oxidize phenothiazines. Even so, it is still necessary to use it for 7-hydroxychloropromazine.
Answer to E.L. Crampton: It is difficult to quantify the actual extent to which

sulphoxide formation actually occurs during ether extractions. *Answer to* D.B. Campbell: Chloropromazine and its metabolites in urine are surprisingly stable under normal conditions of temperature, but do go off in extremes of light and heat; storage in the dark is essential. *Further answer to* W.D.C. Wilson: For reduction of *N*-oxides such as CPZ-NO, metabisulphite is effective; other reagents such as $TiCl_3$ also work, but additionally reduce sulphoxides.

Question by O.R.W. Lewellen: You consider that in the clinical situation a crude assay of urine for total chloropromazine metabolites forms a good guide as to whether the patient is taking his or her tablets; in view of the well-documented excretion of CP2 metabolites over a long period of time *after* cessation of dosing, is this test really satisfactory? -*Ans.*: The rate of metabolite excretion during dosing is 10 or more times that in the long wash-out period after stopping dosing. qualitative tests are useless, but quantitative work is very valuable. *Question by* A.J. Clatworthy: Is there a correlation between plasma CP2 levels on a therapeutic regime and the anti-schizophrenic action ? *Ans.*: As is evident from the Article, this is very complex.

The following questions and answers relate to Art. T-5 (D.A. Cowan)

Question by S.H. Curry.— Have you observed conversion of chlorpromazine-*N*-oxide into demonomethylchlorpromazine under the influence of SO_2 or metabisulphite ? This reaction has occurred in my own studies. *Ans.*— There is a report [1] of the non-stoichiometric conversion of chlorpromazine-*N*-oxide into the secondary amine and formaldehyde under the influence of SO_2. However, we find that the *N*-oxide when complexed with methyl orange is converted by SO_2 into the parent chlorpromazine.

1. Fok, A.K. & Ziegler, DM., *Biochem. Biophys. Res. Commun.* 41 (1974) 534-540.

Question by G. Schill.— You made a group separation of the metabolic products by ion-pair extraction with methyl orange. Have you tried ion-pair chromatography ? It might give you the possibility of directly isolating the metabolites and quantitating from the chromatogram if a UV detector is used. *Ans.*— We are investigating the use of HPLC for separating metabolic products, and it would indeed be interesting to attempt their isolation by ion-pairing. *Ans. to* O.R.W. Lewellen.— The quantitative studies were done *in vitro*. The proportion of the total metabolic pattern represented by the *N*-oxides has indeed been studied in animals with the aid of $[^{14}C]CP2$ and $[^{35}S]CP2$.

Question by R. Whelpton.— Is your 'pink' spot' extracted into organic solvents ? When we have extracted urine from patients receiving large doses of several phenothiazines, on occasion deep red residues have been seen. This 'pink' material is extractable into heptane. *Ans.*— We have found that the pink spot is indeed extracteed into organic solvents such as ether and, to a lesser extent, heptane. It would appear that you are extracting compounds similar to the hydroperoxides which we have found.

Question by J.J. de Ridder.— The temperature effect on the mass spectrum is most pronounced in the low-mass region. What is, however, the effect in the molecular weight region ? Does the ratio $M^+/(M-16)^+$ change with a temperature increase ? If so, there is a possibility that when this ratio decreases, you are measuring not the *N*-oxide any more, but merely the parent compound. *Ans.*— We did see an increase in the intensity of the M-16 ion peak compared with that of the molecular ion with increasing probe temperature in the solid inlet mass spectra of the *N*-oxides. This supports the hypothesis that the *N*-oxides lose oxygen thermally prior to ionization at elevated temperatures.

ASSAY OF BENZODIAZEPINES (cf. Art. T-6)

Remarks by A.J. Clatworthy *(Metropolitan Police Forensic Science Laboratory)*.— In the U.K. the benzodiazepines are now the most presented and possibly abused group of drugs, having recently overtaken the barbiturate group in the number of prescriptions issued. Fortunately the benzodiazepines are considerably less toxic than the barbiturates, and I still await a substantiated death due directly to a benzodiazepine alone (most are in conjunction with alcohol or death due to inhalation of vomit). In our work in the forensic laboratory we routinely screen for the presence of any of this group, by conversion into the benzophenone in all blood and urine samples where asked. We find indications of this group in at least 25% of our cases; the problem is merely one of interpreting the results in terms of which one has been ingested (they are inter-metabolized) and of what the blood level means.

Of the group, chlordiazepoxide is probably the most toxic, but is not particularly useful in all cases where it is presented; the main bulk of those prescribed are diazepam and nitrazepam, which appear to differ very little in their actions and are relatively less toxic. The problem is likely to escalate in the very near future with the routine prescribing of flurazepam/flunitrazepam and possibly clonazepam, which are very much more potent; we have already started to receive cases of overdosage and abuse of flurazepam in the short time that it has been marketed.

Supplementary comments by D.B. Faber, who supported the above remarks about relative toxicities.— There are few interactions between benzodiazepines and other drugs as used in multi-drug therapy, where there is a need for rapid and specific analysis of the various drugs and their metabolites, just as in toxicology.

Assay of 'somatic' drugs *(Nortriptyline, below, is really in the foregoing class)*

Nortriptyline and digitoxin assay (D.B. Faber - *p. 39 and on opposite p.*)

Question by A. Clatworthy: what methods are used for the estimation, for example, of nortriptyline *in situ* on a thin-layer plate ? D.B. Faber *replied thus.* - In the account (Art. E-4 in this Vol) of the analytical procedure for the fluorodensitometric assay, methods for fluorimetric activation in general are indicated. In the case of nortriptyline the spots are rendered visible by immersing the TLC plate in dilute perchloric acid and subsequently heating it in a drying oven. More detail is given in our paper ([9] *in the contribution opposite).*

Comment by V.P. Butler: Values for the total levels of active glycoside and active metabolites (digitoxigenin and its mono- and bis-digitoxosides) *might* be more useful clinically than a measurement of serum digitoxin alone.

ASSAY OF NIFLUMIC ACID (T. Cowen & J.R. Salmon, Art. T-7)

Reply to question by J.V. Jackson.— As the samples were from a controlled clinical trial, the question does not arise of possible interference in the niflumic acid estimation by other drugs extractable by acid-ether (e.g. metenamic acid, aspirin). *Comment by* V.P. Butler.— Whilst there may indeed be differences between the fasting and post-prandial states in the configurations of the serum level *versus* time curves after absorption of a drug, this does not *necessarily* reflect decreased *total* absorption of the drug. This can be better evaluated by measuring total urinary excretion of the drug or by performing longer-term 'steady-state' studies. *Follow-up comment, by* A.W. Forrey.— When a decreased rate of absorption is encountered, a better idea of total drug absorption can be obtained by measuring 'AUC' (area under absorption curve) for longer periods of time.

Assay of anti-microbial and other agents *(For points arising from Art. T-11,*
see p. 54)

ASSAY OF IRGASAN (D.R. Hoar & D.J. Sissons, Art. T-9)

Reply to question by D.B. Campbell.— The glucuronide is not active as a germicide. It was assayed so as to satisfy the various safety committees.

ASSAY OF CEPHRADINE (T.C. Foster, Art. T-10)

Question by V.P. Butler.— Can microbiological assay be used in a clinical situation if the patient is receiving another antibiotic ? *Ans.*— Yes, if the organism used for the assay is resistant to the second antibiotic.

Brief analytical case history

DETERMINATION OF DIGITOXIN IN HUMAN SERUM

D.B. Faber[1], A. de Kok[1] & U.A.Th. Brinkman[2]
[1]*Laboratory of Toxicology and Biopharmacy,*
 Academic Hospital of the Free University, de Boelelaan 1117, and
[2]*Department of Analytical Chemistry, Free University,*
Amsterdam, The Netherlands.

Requirement *A specific assay for therapy control purposes and toxicology, sensitive enough for the range 10-60 ng/ml of serum.*

Chemistry & metabolism *Dixitoxin is an heart-glycoside with a steroid skeleton. Fluorescence can be generated by HCl vapour under the influence of artificial light. Metabolism gives rise mainly to digitoxigenin bisdigitoxoside, digitoxigenin monodigitoxoside and digitoxigenin, as well as digoxin and metabolites to a lesser extent.*

End-step *Fluorodensitometry, following one-dimensional TLC on Kieselgel 60.*

Sample preparation *Solvent extraction of the serum sample (2 ml) with chloroform; dry down at 40° in dry air stream, and dissolve residue in chloroform for TLC.*

Assay results & comments *Sensitivity of 1-2 ng digitoxin by applying spots with a small diameter. Linearity observed between 2 and 20 ng. Overall recovery 99.1% with $S.D. = 11.2\%$. The time needed for one analysis is about $4\frac{1}{2}$ h, the real time of analysis being $\sim 2\frac{1}{2}$ h; in serial studies 20-24 determinations could be done daily.*

Whereas most method descriptions do not mention whether digitoxin metabolites are co-determined, the present assay separates the digitoxin completely from the other compounds in serum, and thus enables the total fate of digitoxin in relation to the clinical effect to be studied more specifically than by radioimmunoassay (RIA).

Since digitoxin is prescribed in cardiac failure and has a notably small therapeutic index, a method has to be available which is very sensitive, accurate, really specific, rapid, low-cost and can be performed in any clinical laboratory. This, and the therapeutic use of digoxin, pose a challenging analytical problem. Various procedures published for digoxin during the past ten years are mostly very time-consuming or not specific enough [1-4]. Smith [5] developed an RIA method which is very sensitive, accurate, simple, and requires only one hour; but there are some disadvantages related to digitoxin metabolism [6] and to the fact that patients on maintenance dosages of digoxin give false positive values corresponding to levels of digitoxin of ~ 1-2 ng/serum. Another disadvantage is that laboratories which lack radioisotopic equipment cannot perform this procedure. Therefore, to eliminate these disadvantages, we decided to develop a new method [7], now outlined. It is based upon a fluorodensitometric approach as already applied to cyclobenzaprine [8] and to amitriptyline and nortriptyline [9]. Although the recoveries and other features as outlined above were acceptable, there were differences between the values obtained by fluorodensitometry and those by RIA. This might be due to co-determination in the RIA method of digitoxin metabolites or other structurally related substances. (In 11 patients, the ratio TLC value/RIA value ranged from 0.09 to 0.95; mean 0.47.)

Improvements may come from investigating not only the extraction procedure and the use of programmed multiple development (PMD) [10, 11] and of high-performance TLC-material [12], but also a better detection calculation system. The result could be a fluorodensitometric method having advantages at least comparable to those of RIA. Since the fluorogenic reaction of digoxin and methyldigoxin surpasses even that of digitoxin, it seems possible that digoxin (lower therapeutic level 1-2 ng/ml) could likewise be assayed by fluorodensitometry.

Operational notes. —   The solvent system was chloroform-methanol-acetone-water (64:6:28:2); the development ($\sim$20 min) was done in a non-saturated tank. After generation of fluorescence by HCl and light, and heating the plate for a few minutes to remove the acid, the fluorescence can be measured quantitatively with the Vitatron TLD-100 densitometer at 536 nm (excitation 365 nm). When kept in the dark the fluorescence is stable for weeks. The unknown concentration of the sample is determined by interpolation between two standards. A scan is illustrated in Fig. 1.

The efficacy of the solvent in separating digitoxin from metabolites and interfering substances (Table 1) was not matched by that of other solvent systems that were tried [cf. 6]. Specificity for digitoxin comes in part from the use of chloroform as the extractant [13]. By generating the fluorescence with HCl vapour (at saturating level, for at least 1 h in the dark followed by 12 min under a quartz halogen lamp), the plate gets homogeneous exposure, and sensitivity is better than with other reagents. The fluorescence intensity is improved by covering the plate with a non-volatile film of a fluid such as liquid paraffin.

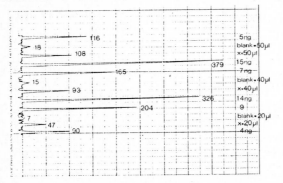

Fig. 1. Densitogram to show the determination of an unknown sample of digitoxin, x. The integrated value for each spot is given at the top of the curve.

Table 1. hRf values for digitoxin and main metabolites and digoxin, with the TLC system described. (hRf = *distance travelled, mm.*)

Substance	hRf
Digitoxin	35
Digitoxigenin-bisdigitoxoside	39
Digitoxigenin-monobisdigitoxoside	44
Digitoxigenin	56
Digitonin	origin
Digoxin	24

1. Lukas, D.S. & Peterson, R.E., *J. Clin. Invest. 45* (1966) 782-795.

2. Lowenstein, J.M. & Corrill, E.M., *J. Lab. Clin. Med. 67* (1966) 1048-1052.

3. Burnett, G.H. & Conklin, R.L., *J. Lab. Clin. Med. 71* (1968) 1040-1044.

4. Oliver, G.C. Jr., Parker, B.M., Brasfield, D.L. & Parker, C.W., *J. Clin. Invest. 47* (1968) 1035-1042.

5. Smith, T.W., *J. Pharmacol. Exp. Ther. 175* (1970) 352-360.

6. Züllich, G., Braun, W. & Lisboa, B.P., *J. Chromatog. 103* (1975) 396-401.

7. Faber, D.B. & de Kok, A., *to be published.*

8. Faber, D.B., *J. Chromatog. 74* (1972) 85-98.

9. Faber, D.B., Mulder, C. & Man in't Veld, W.A., *J. Chromatog. 100* (1974) 55-61.

10. Perry, J.A., Jupille, T.H. & Glunz, L.J., *Anal. Chem. 47* (1975) 65A-74A.

11. Perry, J.A., Jupille, T.H. & Curtice, A., *Separation Science 10* (1975) 571-591.

12. Ripphahn, J. & Halpaap, H., *J. Chromatog. 112* (1975) 81-96.

13. Vöhringer, H.E. & Rietbroek, N., *Clin. Pharmacol. Therap. 16* (1974) 796-806.

INDEX of Subjects

The emphasis in the Index is on methodological developments (cf. title of the book Series). Accordingly, there has not been systematic indexing of all applications of a technique such as GC, or of all text mentions of particular drugs or other compounds. Yet many of the latter are indeed indexed (seldom by rigorous chemical names), either individually or under class names such as Phenothiazines.

Page entries such as 25- signify that ensuing pages are also relevant, i.e. the - denotes a major entry.

CORRECTIONS TO VOLUME 4

p. xi: *To* R.H. Hinton *entry, add* Art. 19

p. 199: *In top line,* 2m/g *should read* 2 ml/g

pp. 286 & 287: *Transpose the Figures (but not their Legends)*

p. 306: *Insert Table heading:* Table 1. Zonal fractionation data summary.